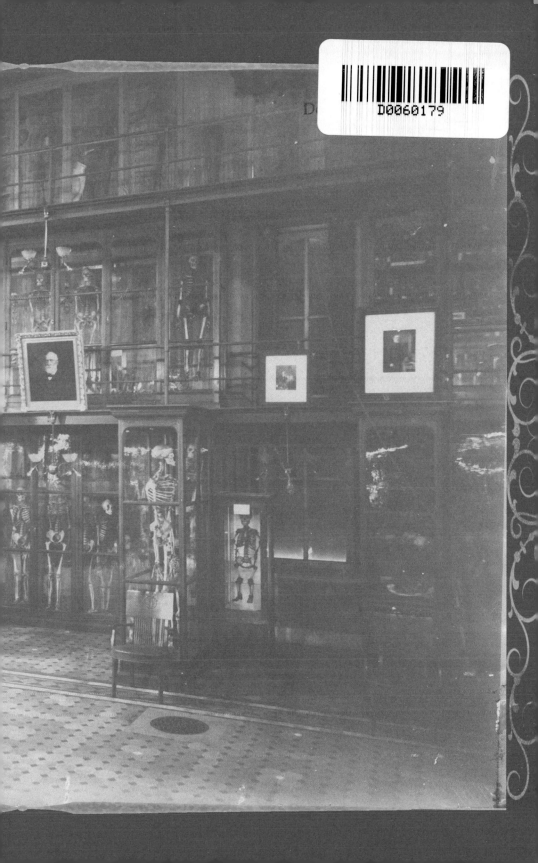

DR. MÜTTER'S
MARVELS

DR. MÜTTER'S MARVELS

A TRUE TALE *of* INTRIGUE *and* INNOVATION *at the* DAWN *of* MODERN MEDICINE

By

CRISTIN O'KEEFE APTOWICZ

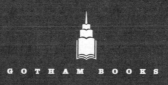

GOTHAM BOOKS

GOTHAM BOOKS

Published by the Penguin Group
Penguin Group (USA) LLC
375 Hudson Street
New York, New York 10014

USA | Canada | UK | Ireland | Australia | New Zealand | India | South Africa | China
penguin.com
A Penguin Random House Company

LIBRARY OF CONGRESS CATALOGING-IN-PUBLICATION DATA
Aptowicz, Cristin O'Keefe, author.
Dr. Mütter's marvels : a true tale of intrigue and innovation at the dawn of modern medicine /
by Cristin O'Keefe Aptowicz.
p. ; cm.
Includes bibliographical references and index.
ISBN 978-1-59240-870-2 (hardcover)
I. Title.
[DNLM: 1. Mütter, Thomas D. (Thomas Dent), 1811-1859. 2. Mütter Museum. 3. General Surgery—Pennsylvania—Biography. 4. Physicians—Pennsylvania—Biography. 5. General Surgery—history—Pennsylvania. 6. History, 19th Century—Pennsylvania. 7. Museums—history—Pennsylvania. 8. Pathology—history—Pennsylvania. WZ 100]
RD27.35.D74
617.092—dc23
[B]
2014014747

Printed in the United States of America

5   7   9   10   8   6   4

Set in Adobe Caslon
Designed by Sabrina Bowers

This project is supported in part by an award from the National Endowment for the Arts. Art Works.

CONTENTS

—PART THREE—

DR. MÜTTER'S
MARVELS

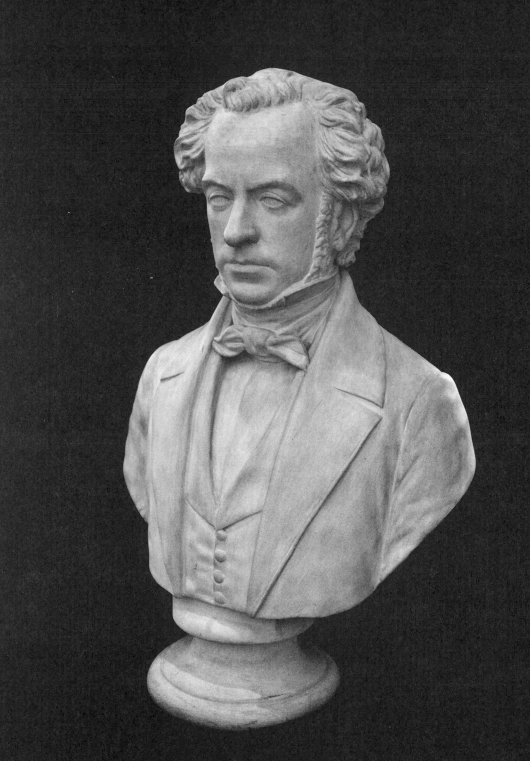

Thomas Dent Mütter

PROLOGUE

———————————

Thomas Dent Mütter *is dead and the world will forget him.*

That is what Richard J. Levis thought, feared really, the day he heard the news. Mütter's death should not have come as a surprise. In his last years, he was a man who struggled to keep the demons of his ill health at bay. And though he worked hard to make sure his ambitious surgeries, his quick wit, and his charmingly ostentatious style of dress were always center stage, even Mütter couldn't hide how broken his body had become by the endless torture of pain and disease, the same foes he battled his entire career. Perhaps that was why it was still a shock when he finally succumbed to them. Mütter always seemed to be someone who could beguile death to stay away just a little while longer.

Levis had been Mütter's student at Philadelphia's Jefferson Medical College. It seemed bitterly ironic that 1859, the year Levis would be named lead surgeon at Philadelphia General Hospital, would also be the year the greatest surgeon he'd ever studied under would die at the age of forty-eight.

Levis remembered walking into the Jefferson Medical College surgical clinic—which Mütter himself had fought to have built—and how Mütter stood at the lectern, giving an ardent joyful greeting to every student as they entered the room. His surgical lectures were universally acknowledged to be unrivaled. Unlike other professors in his time, he always addressed his students in a plainspoken manner, endeavoring to be clearly understood even as his lectures and surgeries became more complex and ornate.

And my God, his surgeries! thought Levis. His ingenuity, his early excellence, the attention he paid to the poor and humble. Would future generations remember how Mütter's office was thronged with patients from every part of the Union, rich and poor, old and young, attracted by his fame and

1

the promise of his genius, waiting patiently for hours just to consult with him? How the patients in the crowded receiving room at the college's clinic would gather around him with a confidence and infatuation when he entered, as if to say, "If I may but touch his garment, I shall be whole."

And how Mütter made these people whole again.

The broken. The diseased. The cursed. People who were considered monsters, even by medical definition. Mütter welcomed them all. An expert and efficient surgeon, he systematically rehearsed every procedure in his mind before beginning it; each assistant was accurately assigned special duties; and each instrument and requisite appliance was cleaned and laid out before the operating table.

In every view of him, he was a great doctor, even at a time when the definition of what that meant was ever changing, when the path was filled with the poisonous bramble of his critics, obstinate men in power who thought they knew best.

Despite the constant physical struggles that made Mütter's too-short life blaze so brightly, those who loved him did not see him as a man tormented by the failings of his own body. Mütter was a man who embraced life: He hosted lavish parties; spent late nights with students—current and former—drinking cold beer and eating fresh oysters, laughing loudly; took numerous trips across the Atlantic, where he was greeted warmly by the most eminent medical men of London and Paris; and spared no labor or expense in securing the most valuable material to illustrate his lectures, and thus acquired one of the best private surgical cabinets of his time. A collection of human curiosities so strange and shocking that finding it a permanent home would prove to be one of Mütter's last great trials.

It seemed impossible to Richard Levis that a man like this could ever be forgotten. Yet he knew it happened every day.

Levis brought a fresh inkpot and pen to his desk. He was not a poet, just a surgeon doggedly working in the second-largest city of a country on the brink of war, but he still considered it his duty to craft a worthy remembrance.

"The subject of this memoir needs no eulogium from us, before the medical profession," read the piece later published in *The Medical and Surgical Reporter*, "and our humble hands would attempt to wreathe no new laurels for his brow. . . . The short life of Doctor Mütter, illustrated the most remarkable mental abilities, and the gentlest qualities of heart. For years, we have viewed him at what seemed the zenith of professional eminence, and yet he continued struggling under the oppression of the severest bodily infirmities, to elevate the science to which he was devoted and to relieve the miseries of others.

"His life, until his retirement, was one of incessant labor. His lectures and immense practice occupied the day, and midnight found him still toiling. The allurements of pleasure and the couch of indolence could not attract him from his great pursuit, and he continued to be active until unable to hold up longer against his fate, he sought retirement and repose, a calm well suited to the close of a useful life. . . .

"What an epitome of this life it is to know that so much mental activity has ceased here, forever; that the eye which so lately gleamed with enthusiasm is closed; the cheek which glowed with ardor is pale; the voice which rang so loud and clear with eloquence, is hushed in the endless silence of the tomb."

Then Levis added one final small plea, that his voice not be the only one to recall this bright and brilliant star. Looking into the future, the brokenhearted former student humbly asked that "other and abler pens write for him, to coming ages" so that his idol could achieve the immortality Levis thought he deserved, and to make Mütter "a deathless name . . . forever blended with the history of American Surgery."

PART ONE

THE MEDICAL MAN MUST
OBTAIN A THOROUGH MEDICAL EDUCATION

To secure true eminence, not popularity, not notoriety,

not the distinction that friendly or family

> *influence or wealth may for a time confer,*

the medical man must,

as the first and most important requisite,

obtain a thorough medical education.

But I would caution you against attempting eminence

in any other department of science:

"One science only will one genius fit,

So vast is art, so narrow human wit."

Thomas Dent Mütter

CHAPTER ONE

MONSTERS

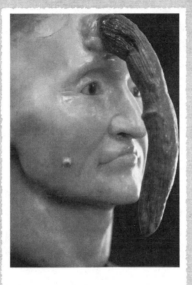

Even in the middle of the ocean, Mütter could not get her out of his mind. He excused himself early from dinner, stopped well-meaning conversationalists mid-sentence, and rushed down to his sleeping quarters just to hold her face in his hands.

To an American like him, she appeared unquestionably French: high cheekbones, full upturned lips, glittering deep-set eyes. For an older woman, she was impressively well preserved, her temples kissed with only the slightest crush of wrinkles. When she was young, Mütter imagined, she must have been very beautiful, though perhaps girlishly sensitive about the long thin hook of her nose, or the pale mole resting on her lower left cheek. But that would have been decades ago.

Now well past her childbearing years, the woman answered only to "Madame Dimanche"—the Widow Sunday—and all anyone saw when they looked at her was the thick brown horn that sprouted from her pale forehead, continuing down the entire length of her face and stopping bluntly just below her pointy, perfect French chin.

THE YOUNG DR. THOMAS DENT MUTTER HAD ARRIVED IN PARIS less than a year earlier, in the fall of 1831. Even for Mutter, who had always relied heavily on his ability to charm a situation to his favor, it had not been an easy trip to arrange.

He was just twenty years old when he graduated from the University of Pennsylvania's storied medical college. To an outsider, he may not have seemed that different from the other students in his class: fresh-faced, eager, hardworking. But he knew he was different—in some ways that were deliberate and in other ways that were utterly out of his control.

Perhaps the most obvious of these was Mutter's appearance. He was, as anyone could plainly see, extraordinarily handsome. Having studied his parents' portraits as a child—one of the few things of theirs he still possessed—he knew that he inherited his good looks. He had his father's strong nose, impishly arched eyebrows, and rare bright blue eyes. He favored his mother's bright complexion, her round lips, and sweet, open oval face. His chin, like hers, jutted out playfully.

Mutter made sure to keep his thick brown hair cut to a fashionable length, brushed back and swept off his cleanly shaven, charismatic face. His clothing was always clean, current, and fastidiously tailored. From a young age, he understood how important looks were, how vital appearance was to acceptance, especially among certain circles of society. He worked hard to create an aura of ease around him. No one needed to know how much he had struggled, or how much he struggled still. No, rather he made it a habit to stand straight, to make his smile easy and his laugh warm. He was, as a contemporary once described him, the absolute pink of neatness.

The truth was that, financially, he had always been forced to walk a tightrope. Both his parents had died when he was very young. The money they left him was modest, and thanks to complicated legal issues, his access to it was severely limited. Over the years, he grew practiced in the art of finessing opportunities so that he could live something approximate to the life he desired. At boarding school, he was known to charge his clothing bills to the institution and then earn scholarships to pay off the resulting debts. When he wanted to travel, he secured just enough money to get him to his destination and then relied on his wits to get him back home.

And now that Mutter had achieved his longtime goal of graduating from one of the country's best medical schools, he focused on his next goal: *Paris.*

Paris was the epicenter of medical achievement: the medical mecca. Hundreds of American doctors swarmed to the city every year, knowing that in order to be great, to be truly great, you must study medicine in Paris. And that had always been Mutter's plan: to be great. More than that: to be *the greatest.*

GETTING TO PARIS, HOWEVER, WAS NOT AN EASY ENDEAVOR. HE knew—as all gentlemen of limited means did—that sailing as a surgeon's mate with a U.S. naval ship in exchange for free passage to Europe was an option open to him, but competition was always considerable and fierce. Mutter spent months submitting letters and applications to the secretary of the Navy, trying to use charm, logic, and bravado to secure a position. He even implored his guardian, Colonel Robert W. Carter, to ask prominent men close to President Jackson to write letters on his behalf, explaining, "[I] am afraid that I shall not be able to obtain an order unless I can get my friends to make some exertions for the furtherance of my plan." Despite all the effort he expended, no position ever materialized.

Mutter could only watch as the wealthier members of his graduating class departed for Europe with financial ease. Others returned to their hometowns with their new degrees, bought houses with their fathers' money, and started their practices using their families' connections. Mutter remained in Philadelphia, and his hopes remained fixed on Paris.

Mutter felt his luck about to change when he read about the *Kensington* in a local Philadelphia paper. For months, the Cramp shipyard had been building a massive warship. The rumor was that it was being built for the Mexican Navy, and that upon seeing its immense size—and cost—they opted to back out of purchasing it. However, the most recent update was that the giant ship had sold after all, to the Imperial Russian Navy.

Mutter saw an opportunity. He went to the Cramp shipyard and asked if the American crew in charge of sailing the *Kensington* to Russia was in need of a surgeon's mate. That he was just twenty and only a few months out of medical school was a minor detail. He hoped that being present, able, and willing would be enough. Luckily for Mutter, it was. A few weeks later, he boarded the ship (later to be renamed the *Prince of Warsaw* by Tsar Nicholas himself), and left America for the first time.

THE OCEAN WAS LIKE NOTHING MUTTER HAD EVER EXPERIENCED: vast and wild and so incredibly loud. He had hoped the enormity of the newly built warship—with its four towering masts and immense spiderweb of rigging—as well as its extensively trained crew would offer him comfort during the weeks at sea, but the experience was more taxing than any book or anecdote portended.

He did not anticipate that whether he was holed up in the bowels of the ship or clinging to the aft railing, his body would be trapped in a relentless cycle of emptying itself. That his stomach would never become accustomed to the rolling blue-black swells of the sea. Nor did he realize how intimate he would become with the ship's beastly stowaways—bedbugs and fleas, weevils and rats. He would wake to bugs crawling in his hair and mouth, and fall asleep to sounds of the rats chewing through his clothes, attempting to suss out even the smallest morsel of food. And then there were the storms, the nights when he felt certain the vessel would break in two as mountainous waves crashed over it, the ship itself painfully groaning with each hit. The ocean seemed nothing but a frothing black maw, hungry to devour him.

When the sea was calm and the sky bright and blue, he forced himself to stand on the ship's deck and look toward what he hoped was Europe. He tried to enjoy these moments, but he didn't know true relief until the crew pointed out birds appearing in the sky, a sign that they were approaching land, after more than a month at sea.

WHEN MUTTER FINALLY ARRIVED IN PARIS, IT IMMEDIATELY reminded him of the ocean; it too was vast and wild and incredibly loud. Unlike at sea, however, in Paris he felt perfectly at home.

Its streets were packed, people and buildings in every direction. His world was suddenly and delightfully filled with new sounds, new scents, new music. There were colorfully dressed women sweeping the streets, and strapping men carrying enormous bundles on their heads. There were strange-looking carriages that seemed like relics of a barbarous age, which were in turn being pulled by enormous and brash horses. Even the food being eaten at street-side cafes seemed strange and exotic to Mutter. The city avenue was a vast museum of wonderful new sights to gawk at, and it seemed that the French wanted it that way. They loved to look, and to be looked at. It was true what Mutter had heard: Those French who could spare the time would flamboyantly promenade every day. And on Sundays, absolutely everyone did.

Once Mutter had secured modest student housing, he set out to promenade himself. He'd been sure to pack his finest clothes for the journey: suits cut close to his slim frame (his natural thinness being perhaps one of the only benefits he'd gained from the illnesses that had plagued him since childhood) and made from the most expensive fabrics he could afford in the brightest colors in stock. Years earlier, a schoolmaster once wrote to Colonel Carter, Mutter's guardian, that his pupil's "principal error is rather too

much fondness for a style of dress not altogether proper for a boy his age."
Clearly, that schoolmaster had never been to Paris.

Mutter enjoyed the moment, peacocking on Parisian streets for the first
time, a master of his fate. The lines between Mutter's starting points and
his destination were not often straight, but he took pride and comfort in
knowing that he always got there. And the next morning, he would begin
the next phase of his mission, his true goal in Paris: to learn everything he
could about modern medicine until his money, or his luck, ran out.

IN 1831, OVER A HALF MILLION PEOPLE CALLED PARIS THEIR HOME,
and by royal decree, each French citizen was entitled to free medical treatment from any of the dozens of hospitals within the city limits. The hospitals were typically open to any visiting doctors, provided one could show
them a medical degree and, when necessary, place the right amount of
coins into the right hands.

Studying medicine in Paris became so popular that guidebooks were
written just for the visiting American doctors. Nowhere else in the world,
one wrote, could "experience be acquired by the attentive student as in the
French capital . . . where exists such a vast and inexhaustible field for observation . . ."

And it was true. Where else but Paris would there be not one but *two*
hospitals devoted entirely to the treatment of syphilis? Afflicted women
were sent to the Hôpital Lourcine, a hospital filled with the most frightful
instances of venereal ravages. The men were sent to the Hôpital du Midi,
which required that all patients be publicly whipped as punishment for
contracting the disease, both before and after treatment.

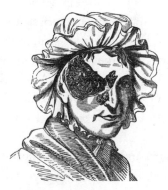

Woman with Ulcer of the Face

Hôpital des Enfants-Malades was a hospital for ill children, and was nearly always filled to capacity. It had a grim mortality rate—one in every four children who came for treatment died there—but the doctors on staff assured visiting scholars that this was because most of the patients came from the lowest classes of society and thus were frequently brought to the hospital already in a hopeless or dying condition.

Doctors specializing in obstetrics could visit Hôpital de la Maternité. It served laboring women only, and averaged eleven births a day. Some days, however, the numbers rose to twenty-five or thirty women, each wailing in her own bed, as the doctors and midwives (called *sages-femmes*) rushed among them. New mothers were allowed to stay nine days after giving birth, and the hospital even supplied them with clothing and a small allowance, provided they were willing to take the child with them. Not all of the women were.

So the Hôpital des Enfants-Trouvés for abandoned children was founded. Newborns arrived daily from Hôpital de la Maternité from women unable or unwilling to keep their children, as well as those infants whose mothers died while giving birth, as one in every fifty women who entered Hôpital de la Maternité did.

The Hôpital des Enfants-Trouvés also allowed Parisian citizens to come directly to the hospital and hand over a child of any age. The hospital encouraged families to register and mark the children they were leaving so they might reclaim them at a later date, but the families who chose to do so were few. In fact, the vast majority of the children there had arrived via *le tour*.

Le tour d'abandon ("the desertion tower") was merely a box attached to the hospital, constructed with two sliding doors and a small, loud bell. An infant was unceremoniously placed in the box, the door firmly closed behind it, and the bell was rung. Upon hearing the bell, the nurses on duty would go to *le tour* to remove the infant, replace the box to its original position, and wait. Every night, a dozen or so infants were received in precisely this way.

For a while, it had been in vogue for wealthy, childless individuals to adopt children from the Hôpital des Enfants-Trouvés to bring up as their own, but the practice had long since fallen out of fashion. At the time of Mutter's visit, more than sixteen thousand children were considered wards of the Hôpital des Enfants-Trouvés, and of those, only twelve thousand would live to adulthood.

There were hospitals for lunatic women and for idiot men, hospitals for the incurable, for the blind, for the deaf and dumb, and even for ailing elderly married couples who wished to die together—they could stay in the same large room provided that the furniture they used to furnish their room became the property of the hospice upon their deaths.

And perhaps most astonishing to the visiting American doctors, Paris had the École Pratique d'Anatomie, which provided any doctor, for six dollars, access to his own cadaver for dissection. In America, cadaver dissection was largely illegal. Many doctors resorted to grave robbing to have the opportunity to examine the human body fully. In Paris, twenty doctors at a time would whittle a human body down to its bones—provided they could stand the smell and the ultimate method of disposal of the dissected corpses: At day's end, the decimated remains were fed to a pack of snarling dogs kept tied up in the back.

However, more than any single hospital, what most attracted Mutter to Paris were the surgeons: brilliant and daring men who were to him living gods, redefining medicine and at the zenith of their renown.

MUTTER HAD ALWAYS LOVED SURGICAL LECTURES AND MADE sure he secured seats as close to the front as possible. In Philadelphia, there were two great medical colleges—the University of Pennsylvania and Jefferson Medical College—and it was customary for the rival schools to hold surgical demonstrations so that prospective students could choose between them, a glorified public relations exercise. Mutter loved the daringness of the surgeries attempted during this time. The lectures were often packed, as eager established and prospective doctors thrilled at the city's best surgeons attempting to outdo one another with their skill and showmanship. However, the combination of ambitious surgeries and unprepared young men sometimes proved disastrous. On one occasion, a Jefferson Medical College professor attempted a daring removal of a patient's upper jaw, using marvelous speed to incise the face and rip out the bones with a huge forceps. But the surgery was perhaps too much for a public display. Doctors who were present would later recall the spectacle of it, how the partially conscious patient spat out blood, bones, and teeth, while unnerved students in the audience vomited and fainted in their seats.

But regardless of how brutal or simple the case, all surgical lectures were a challenge to watch. The anxious patient would be publicly examined and forced to listen to his surgery loudly outlined to an audience of strangers. Next, the patient would nervously drink some wine with the hope that it would dull the nerves and lessen the pain. (In Paris, the need for medicinal wine was so great, the hospital system maintained its very own wine vaults, spending more than 600,000 francs a year on an extensive collection of red and white wine housed exclusively for its patients.)

The patient was then instructed to lie on the surgical table, where he would be held down by the surgeon's assistants and told to stay as still as possible. Everyone—the patient, the doctor, even the students in their seats—knew how impossible this command would be to follow.

The first incision usually brought the patient's first scream—the first scream of many. Soon came the blood, the struggle, the shock. The patient would beg the surgeon to stop, plead and shout, and yell to the students to come save him, his voice cracking, tears streaming down his face. The surgeon was expected to ignore it all, to move forward swiftly and surely, and to hope that his assistants were strong men with equal resolve. Every student had heard stories of patients who were able to struggle free, who leapt off the table and attacked their doctors—often with the surgeon's own instruments!—before running out of the room, leaving a trail of their own blood behind them.

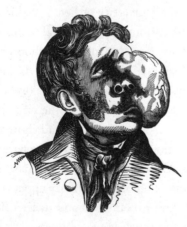

Man with Tumor of the Jaw

To Mutter, ignoring the patient was one of the most difficult parts of surgery. He struggled to develop the ability to temporarily see past the patient's pain—their wide and desperate eyes—and focus solely on his goals as the surgeon.

It had always been explained to him that the most important quality of a good surgeon is confidence, born of both education and experience. You needed to know you were right and that your actions were right, regardless of what was happening around you. Mutter understood this, but in the moment, it was often still a difficult instruction to follow.

Of course, in spite of the skill and care of the surgeon, the patients often died. Sometimes they died in the middle of surgery, the trauma to their bodies becoming too much. Sometimes they would die after, because their wounds were unable to stop bleeding, or the unwashed tools of their own surgeon had given them a fevered infection that consumed their flesh from the inside out. Under the best circumstances, the patient not only lived but lived a better life.

And it was this opportunity to improve a life that caused Mutter to be deeply attracted to studying surgery. Having spent so much time as a patient when he was a child—being bled by lancet or by leech, fed tinctures and bitter weeds, left to sweat it out alone in his bed or soaked in a special bath—he was perhaps too familiar with other, nonsurgical branches of medicine, where recovery was often a guessing game. Sometimes, the relief would be almost immediate once treatment had begun, but more often, the results were undefined, his chest rattling for weeks, his body left to grow gray and thin.

Surgery, however, was not a guessing game; it was an art. People came in need of relief, and the surgeons used every ounce of their skill and knowledge to provide it.

THERE WAS ONE MORE REASON MUTTER REVERED SURGERY ABOVE all other medical pursuits. Surgeons, unlike other professionals of the medical field, were successes of their own creation. While other doctors found their patients—and their positions in society—based on the family they were lucky enough to be born into, surgeons earned their place through hard work, study, and skill. In fact, it seemed to Mutter that the best surgeons came from the lower or middle classes. It was a "natural consequence of this state of things," one doctor from the era wrote, seeing that "very few persons entitled by birth or other advantageous circumstances . . . would condescend to study, much less engage in the practice of medicine," thus "poor and ambitious young men from the provinces were induced to repair to Paris and enter upon the study of the only profession through which they could expect to obtain distinction and worldly prosperity."

It was well known that several of the best-respected surgeons and physicians in France had risen from the lowest castes of life and many from the uttermost depths of poverty. Even the acclaimed chief surgeon of Hôtel Dieu, Guillaume Dupuytren, who was often referred to as the Emperor of Surgery, had been born poor and had struggled. Furthermore, he was not ashamed of it, but rather credited his background with his success, telling his students that "had not Monsieur Dupuytren been compelled from poverty to trim his student's lamp with oil from the dissecting-room, he never would have succeeded in becoming Monsieur le Baron Dupuytren."

MUTTER KNEW THAT SURGERY WAS HIS CALLING, AND RACED through the streets of Paris to study the work of its greatest practitioners. He was aggressive in his pursuits, pushing through crowds to secure the best seats at the surgical lectures, or firmly staying as close as possible to the lecturing doctors as they made their rounds in hospital, no matter how much the other students pushed. Meals of spiced mutton and fresh bread went half-finished as he plotted the next week's schedule. Bowls of café au lait were abandoned so he could make an early start every morning, eager to begin his day.

He had come to Paris assuming it would be the doctors themselves who would have the greatest influence on him, these men who were legends in their own time. Chief among them was Guillaume Dupuytren, who ruled over the Hôtel-Dieu, the city's largest hospital, and single-handedly changed how surgery was done. An immensely brilliant operator, exhibiting marvelous dexterity, proceeding with almost inconceivable speed, his boorish arrogance became as famous as his accomplishments in the surgical room. Jacques Lisfranc de St. Martin was head of the Hôpital de la Pitié, the city's second-largest hospital. He was Dupuytren's greatest friend turned into his most bitter rival, and spent most of his life trying to escape Dupuytren's shadow. Lisfranc was known to refer to Dupuytren as "the bandit of the river bank," while Dupuytren frequently called Lisfranc "that man with the face of an ape and the heart of a crouching dog." There was Philibert Joseph Roux—who so dazzled his classes with his graceful and brilliant work that it was said "his operations were the poetry of surgery," but who had also earned Dupuytren's scorn years earlier by winning the hand of the woman they both loved. And Alfred-Armand-Louis-Marie Velpeau, whose textbook on obstetrics was so influential, it had been translated into English by one of America's most respected obstetricians: Philadelphia's own Charles D. Meigs.

Mutter was deeply impressed with the audacity of each of these surgeons' talents and their seemingly inexhaustible work ethic. However, it was not any single man who ended up changing the course of Mutter's life but, rather, a new field of surgery freshly emerging in Paris, which even the French referred to as *la chirurgie radicale*.

Who sought out this radical surgery?

Woman with Severe Burns of the Face

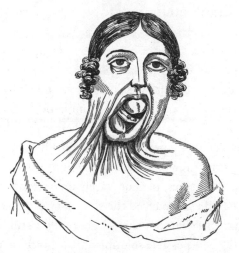

Monsters. This is how the patients would have been categorized in America. Mutter was used to seeing them replicated in wax for classroom display, or hidden in back rooms away from the public eye. He had seen them in jars, fetuses expelled from their mothers, irreparably damaged. MONSTER, the label would read.

Some of these monsters were born that way: a cleft palate so severe the face looked to have been split in two with an ax. Hardly able to eat or drink, spit collected in pools on the child's clothing as his tongue lolled around the open hole of his mouth, awkward and exposed.

Others were born "normal," but their bodies would slowly turn them into monsters, as tumors laid siege to their torsos or limbs, swelling their legs like soaked wood, their eyes strained and nearly popping.

Other times, the monsters were man-made: men whose noses were cut off in battle, or as punishment, or for revenge, the centers of their faces evolving into a large weeping sore; women whose dresses caught fire, becoming houses of flames from which their owners couldn't escape, the skin on their faces turned into melted wax, their mouths permanently frozen in screams.

Monsters. This is what they were called, and this was how they were treated. For such tortured people, death was often seen as a blessing.

In Paris, however, the surgeons had a solution. They called it *les opérations plastiques*.

Was it quackery? Mutter wondered when he first heard about it. Was it a trick? Would these unfortunates be presented like a sideshow? Were the doctors in the audience there to learn or to gape? What could surgeons possibly do to help such hopeless cases?

At the very first lecture, Mutter began to understand the difference between regular surgery and *les opérations plastiques*.

The patient, often greeted with gasps of horror and pity, stood stock-still and unafraid as the surgeon made his examination. These regrettables didn't show the unease normal patients did; their eyes didn't wander back to the door from which they entered and through which they could also escape. Gradually, Mutter grew to understand why.

In regular surgical lectures, patients rarely understood the trouble they were in. When the knife first pierced the skin, they could come to the sudden realization that a life without this surgery might still be a happy one. Thus, escape was the best possible solution and a choice they wanted to exercise right away.

Patients of *les opérations plastiques*, however, were often too aware of their lot in life: that of a monster. It was inescapable. They hid their faces when walking down the street. They took cover in back rooms, excused themselves when there were knocks at the door. They saw how children howled at the sight of them. They understood the half a life they were condemned to live and the envy they couldn't help but feel toward others—whole people who didn't realize how lucky they were to wear the label HUMAN.

It was not uncommon for these patients to enter the surgical room fully prepared to die. Death was a risk they happily took for the chance to bring some level of peace and normality to their mangled faces or agonized bodies. The surgeries weren't physically necessary to save their lives; rather, they were done so the patient might have the gift of living a better, normal life. That is what *les opérations plastiques* promised.

Plastique was a French adjective that translated to "easily shaped or molded." That was the hope with this surgery: to reconstruct or repair parts of the body by primarily using materials from the patient's own body, such as tissue, skin, or bone.

The surgeries, of course, were not always successful—if a patient's problem had been so easy to fix, it would have been corrected by lesser doctors years ago. But other times—and these were the times the audience waited for, the ones that made Mutter's hair stand on edge—the end result was nothing short of miraculous.

With a careful hand, a steady knife, and a piece of bone, a surgeon could reconstruct a man's nose with a twisted portion of his own forehead. A burned woman's eye could close for the first time in ten years, thanks to a surgeon's knife cutting the binding scar tissue and replacing it with skin from her own cheek. Cleft palates were fused back together—trickier than it might seem, for the sensitivities when working on the roof of the mouth meant the patient was in constant threat of vomiting, which would tear open delicate sutures and ensure infection.

Mutter seized every opportunity to witness these plastic operations firsthand. He used his charms to become an *interne* at the hospital to which Dupuytren was attached so he could watch the great master at work. But he didn't limit his focus to Dupuytren, and soon became so familiar with each surgeon—their style and flourishes, their weaknesses and strengths—that he began to view them as his friends, even though they never shared a single word. He took copious notes, drew detailed diagrams, and bought every relevant book he could find and afford. It became his happy obsession.

Mutter hadn't been in Paris even a year when he realized his time was running out. His limited funds were being swiftly exhausted, and he still needed to fund his trip back home. His newly made friends in the Parisian medical society tried to dissuade him. They adored the dashing young doctor with the "quick, active, appropriative mind . . . readily imbued with the spirit of his distinguished [Parisian] teachers." They implored him to stay, pointing out how much work a charming American doctor could get in a bustling city full of English-speaking tourists.

Mutter loved his time in Paris, but his desire to return to Philadelphia was even stronger. He was twenty-one years old and felt healthier than he ever had in his entire life. He felt like a new man. He had even given himself a new name. He was no longer Thom D. Mutter from Virginia.

He had reinvented himself as Thomas Dent Mütter—with a perfectly European umlaut over the *u*.

With the last of his money, he purchased a wax model from a shop that specialized in reproductions for doctors. It was the face of Madame Dimanche, the French washerwoman who grew a large, brown horn from the center of her forehead. At first, the old woman hadn't known what to make of the strange brown nub that appeared like an ashy smudge in the center of her head, but she knew to hide it from view, starting a decade-long habit of avoiding eye contact. But the nub grew relentlessly, larger and larger, until it was as thick and dark as a tree branch.

When she finally allowed it to be examined, she followed a chain of doctors that ended with a surgeon who told her he could remove it if she would trust him. She did. And so it happened the surgeon—practiced in this new art of *les opérations plastiques*—who promised her relief was able to actually deliver it. How happy she was to walk down the streets, her head unhidden. How thrilling it was to feel the wind kiss her bare face.

Mütter purchased a replica of Madame Dimanche's presurgery face, her long, thick horn still intact. And on the long journey back to America, he took it out often, the sea bucking the boat beneath him. He took out her face and stared into it. In it, he saw his future.

CHAPTER TWO

The City of Brotherly Love

AN

ACCOUNT

OF THE

Bilious remitting Yellow Fever,

AS

IT APPEARED

IN THE

CITY OF PHILADELPHIA,

IN THE YEAR 1793.

By *Benjamin Ruſh*, M.D.

PROFESSOR OF THE INSTITUTES, AND OF CLINICAL MEDICINE,
IN THE UNIVERSITY OF PENNSYLVANIA.

PHILADELPHIA,
PRINTED BY THOMAS DOBSON,
AT THE STONE-HOUSE, N° 41, SOUTH SECOND-STREET.
MDCCXCIV.

THE PHYSICIAN SHOULD BE
AN AMBITIOUS MAN

To say to a young man "be not ambitious,"
*   is to say to him live the life of a drone.*
If ambition were a sin, is it probable that a wise Creator
*   would have endowed nine-tenths of his people with it?*
The love of praise is so congenial to our nature,
*   and so powerful a spur to every undertaking,*
*   that the moral world would be a chaos*
*   without its animating influences.*
It is like the sun; it gives life and heat to all around.

Thomas Dent Mütter

PHILADELPHIA IN THE EARLY 1800S WAS AN EASY PLACE TO DIE.

The simplest thing could end your life: a broken bone from a fall, a leg gouged by a loose nail, a hand burned by a pot of boiling soup. In a time before antibiotics, infections could ravage a body in days. You could die from allergies. You could die from asthma. You could die from a single rotten tooth.

The food you ate and the water you drank could kill you just as easily as the guns that were bought and sold without regulation. Of course, there was cancer and diabetes, gout and heart disease. There was murder and suicide and accidental drownings, as well as executions by city and state.

Infectious diseases ran rampant through populous cities like Philadelphia, wreaking havoc on everything they touched.

There was smallpox, spread simply by human interaction. It caused the body to burst into blisters, lesions, and scabs, affecting adults and children equally and brutally. If you were lucky enough to survive it, the scars left behind—including sterility—could haunt you the rest of your life.

There was yellow fever, which no one knew was spread by mosquitoes and which earned its name by turning its victims yellow, before forcing them to bleed from the eyes and mouth and erupt with the black vomit of partially digested blood.

In 1793, yellow fever struck a rain-soaked Philadelphia so hard that the entire government shut down. Once symptoms were seen, the infected person was all but abandoned by friends and family. To protect their own patients, the Pennsylvania Hospital and Almshouse refused to receive yellow fever victims, forcing ailing citizens to eventually die alone in the streets. It became such a problem that local authorities annexed a circus ground on the outskirts of the city as a "depository [for] victims of the plague who had nowhere to go and nobody to care for them." The city's most prominent physician, Dr. Benjamin Rush, advised that all his patients leave the city at once, and anyone forced to remain should immediately engage in "heroic bleeding and purging." Rush's advice only caused more death. By the end of the disease's reign, more than one-tenth of the city's entire population was dead.

There was cholera, spread through contaminated drinking water, which painfully dehydrated its victims, the affected bodies retching liter upon liter of a fluid that looked like rice water and smelled like fish.

In 1832, cholera spread across the East Coast, finally hitting Philadelphia in July. It became such an overwhelming problem that Philadelphia publishing house Carey, Lea & Blanchard (at the time, the country's leading publisher of medical books) began publishing *The Cholera Gazette*, a weekly publication designed to inform the public of the progress and hopeful treatment of this terrible disease. It became wildly popular as the death toll from the disease caused Philadelphia to log in sixty to seventy deaths a day. It took nearly four months for the city to rid itself of the disease, and as testimony to the "heroic role of the medical profession in battling the infection," the city council would eventually reward the physicians in charge of the hospitals during this time with silver pitchers of recognition.

There was also malaria and croup, diphtheria and dysentery, measles and whooping cough, consumption and scarlet fever. Even something as simple as the flu could kill hundreds in a city over one winter.

The swiftness and brutality of disease and death in the nineteenth century was something with which Mütter was already intimately familiar. It was a lesson he'd been forced to learn at an early age.

Lucinda Mutter was nineteen years old and in love when she became pregnant with Thomas in the summer of 1810. She and her husband, John Mutter, had happily married on Christmas Eve three and a half years earlier, when she was fifteen and he was twenty-five.

The two could not have been more different.

Lucinda had been born into the established Gillies family, which was connected, via marriage and blood, to some of the most prestigious families in the South: the military elite Armisteads (five Armistead brothers would fight in the War of 1812, and the British bombardment of George Armistead's fort would later serve as the inspiration for "The Star-Spangled

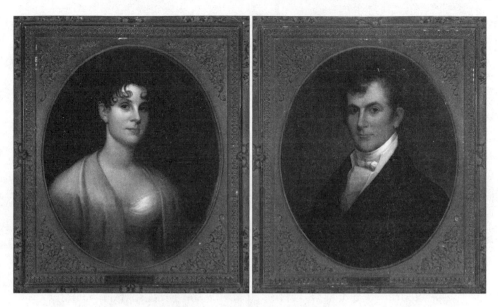

Lucinda and John Mutter

Banner," the future U.S. national anthem); the prominent political family of the Lees (whose family would include not only governors, business leaders, and two signers of the Declaration of Independence, but also General Robert E. Lee, the future leader of the Confederate Army); and the influential Carters (whose patriarch, Robert Carter, was so powerful that he earned the moniker King Carter and, when he died in his late sixties, left behind fifteen children, three thousand acres of farmland, and more than one thousand slaves).

At age fifteen, Lucinda was a young bride even for an ambitious era in which women were frequently married in their late teens. However, she was bright and proudly educated. Early in their marriage, when she and her husband decided to have their portraits painted, she insisted that she be painted with an open book in her hand. John Mutter, on the other hand, was a scrapper. He was a first-generation Scottish immigrant whose father endeared himself to his new countrymen by fighting alongside them in the Revolutionary War. John, like his father, was a hard worker. He was also smart, ambitious, and extremely handsome, and was known to be a good neighbor and a good citizen. By the time he and Lucinda were ready to start their family, John ran a healthy business as a factor and commission agent. To have success in that field, you needed to be both resourceful and multitalented, for these men not only aided farmers in selling their crops but also helped them purchase farming supplies, gave advice concerning the condition of the market or the advisability of selling or withholding a crop, and sometimes even orchestrated the sale or purchase of slaves for a client. Mutter had built his reputation on his charm and his work ethic.

Lucinda gave birth to their first child on March 9, 1811, in the bedroom of their newly purchased home at 5th and Franklin Streets in Richmond, Virginia. The baby was born healthy and pink, and Lucinda named him Thomas, after her husband's late father.

It was a happy time for the young family, but a troubled time for the nation. When President James Madison declared war on Britain in June, the ensuing two bloody years of unpopular battles forced the fledgling American economy to its knees. Businesses in both the North and South suffered, but luckily for his young family, John Mutter's success continued. His businesses flourished and, as was expected during this time, so did his family.

Lucinda was soon pregnant again, and a second son was born in May 1813. She named him James, after her own late father, a beloved doctor who had died almost a decade earlier.

For a year, they were a family of four: John and Tom and James and Lucinda, living in a sunny house in Richmond, Virginia, flush with money and all in good health. But in 1814, the family's uninterrupted string of good luck began to run out.

First, baby James got sick and declined rapidly. Just thirteen days after they celebrated his first birthday, James died. He barely beat a grim statistic, which noted that one in every five children born during this period died before their first birthday. John and Lucinda buried his thin, illness-ravaged body in the cemetery of St. John's Church in Richmond, Virginia.

The family grieved all in black during a long hot Virginia summer. When autumn finally came, John thought a trip might brighten his sorrow-struck wife's spirits and improve her unstable health, but this proved to be a mistake. Lucinda only grew more ill and weak as the journey progressed, and her body finally gave out in a Maryland inn. When she died, she was only twenty-two. Her stunned husband buried her small body in Baltimore's St. Paul's Church before traveling home.

Within a five-month span, John Mutter had buried his beautiful wife and youngest son. He was now thirty-three, a widower, and a single father to Thomas, who was only three.

The year after Lucinda died, John bought a large house in Henrico

County, Virginia—a gesture meant to confirm that he intended to marry again, and that his family would continue to grow. He called it Woodberry, and he tried his best to make it a home for his young son, whom he loved deeply and spoiled often. But the next few years proved to be a relentless boot on John's neck: His business and health begin to fail at an alarming rate; he was forced to sell all the furniture he had bought for his and Lucinda's first home at 5th and Franklin Streets in Richmond, Virginia, and then finally to sell that home itself. He was tired all the time and couldn't shake a rattling cough that took up residence in his chest. Sometimes he would return home from a long day of work with a handkerchief full of his own blood.

If you fell ill in the northern half of the United States, it was popular advice to go south to restore your health: the heat, the fresh air, the clean water and sulphur springs.

But if you already lived in the humid South—and especially if you ran in moneyed circles—you were told to go to Europe.

And so, in 1818, John Mutter left his young son behind and sailed to Europe with the hope that their doctors, the climate, and their medicine could bring him back to his former self. John assured everyone that he would make a full recovery, and even brought with him both a secretary for his correspondence and a private physician who would ensure his well-being every leg of the journey. But perhaps even he knew the truth: Before he left America, he penned a detailed will.

John Mutter said good-bye to young Thomas, now seven, on an autumn day in Virginia, placing him in the care of Tom's grandmother, Frances Gillies, his late wife's widowed mother. The boy sobbed at his father's waistcoat once the carriage had been loaded. With his usual charm and a reassuring smile, John promised his son that he would return to him as quickly as he could, before climbing into the carriage and being driven away.

Thomas would never see his father again.

Four months into this journey, on a winter's passage of the Alps, John Mutter died.

It would, of course, take weeks for the news to make its way to America. In Thomas's mind, his father was still very much alive when the first alarming symptoms of his grandmother's illness began to show.

Frances had been a martyr for many years to gout, a cruel and painful disease that caused various joints on her body—her fingers, her toes, her elbows, her knees—to swell painfully. The affected parts would turn bright red and become hot to the touch. She could scarcely stand for Thomas to be in the room with her when it got really bad, as air whipped up by his energetic body felt like a thousand needles piercing her skin.

But his grandmother's health now seemed worse. As her body grew weaker, the pain grew more oppressive. A doctor's widow, Frances tried to self-treat her ailment with food, drink, and rest, but nothing was working. Doctors were eventually called, and young Thomas could do nothing but watch as his grandmother endured the same treatments he'd watched both his parents suffer through: Her arms were sliced with small razors to "bleed out" her bad blood; heated glass cups were applied to skin to force out more "bad humors"; and unknown purgatives were given to her in liquid and solid form, causing her to vomit and her bowels to loosen and empty violently.

It was a truth that everyone in that era knew: Oftentimes the treatment was even worse than suffering with the disease itself.

Frances Gillies lived just long enough to hear the news of the passing of her son-in-law, and to share it with her devastated grandson. Then she passed away too.

Thomas Dent Mutter was just seven years old, and every person who had ever loved him was dead.

THOMAS DENT MÜTTER'S STORY IS NOT SO SURPRISING IF YOU consider that a man did not need a medical degree to practice medicine in early nineteenth-century Philadelphia. In fact, he didn't even need a license—a practice that Philadelphia would not embrace until the final decade of the nineteenth century.

Although the tide was changing, the clear truth was that anyone who wanted to put out a shingle and call himself a doctor could do just that.

Even those doctors who followed due process—apprenticed under local doctors, went to medical colleges and studied hard, practiced often and kept as up-to-date as possible with the latest innovations—still struggled with the medical limitations of the day.

Medicine was performed literally in the dark. Electricity was newfangled and unpopular. Almost every act a doctor performed—invasive examinations, elaborate surgeries, complicated births—had to be done by sun or lamplight.

Basics of modern medicine, such as the infectiousness of diseases, were still under heavy dispute. Causes of even common diseases were confusing to doctors. Benjamin Rush thought yellow fever came from bad coffee. Tetanus was widely thought to be a reflex irritation. Appendicitis was called peritonitis, and its victims were simply left to die.

The role that doctors—and their unwashed hands and tools—played in the spread of disease was not understood. "The grim spectre of sepsis" was ever present. It was absolutely expected that wounds would eventually fester with pus, so much so that classifications of pus were developed: A "yellow ooze" was seen as a good "laudable pus" while an "ichorous pus" (a thin pus teeming with shredded tissue) was viewed as "the stinking herald of cadaverous putrefaction."

Medicine was not standardized, so accidental poisoning was common. Even "professionally" made drugs were often bulky and nauseating. Bleeding the ill was still a widespread practice, and frighteningly large doses of purgatives were given by even the most conservative men. To treat a fever with a cold bath would have been "regarded as murder."

There was no anesthesia—neither general nor local. Alcohol was commonly used when it came to enduring painful treatments, although highly addictive laudanum (a tincture of ninety percent alcohol and ten percent opium) and pure opium were sometimes available too. If you came to a doctor with a compound fracture, you had only a fifty percent chance of survival. Surgery on brains and lungs was attempted only in accident cases. Bleeding during operations was often outrageously profuse, but, as comfortingly described by one doctor, "not unusually fatal."

Physicians working in this time period were largely unaware that innovations were on the horizon that would make "a pauper in the almshouse more comfortable and cared for better after an operation than a king," as one late-nineteenth-century Philadelphia doctor described the state of medicine in the first half of his century.

And it was a strictly enforced male-dominated field. In the early 1800s, there was not a single female physician in Philadelphia. More than that, women's role in medicine in any form was often disparaged. In a speech given at the Philadelphia County Medical Society, female nurses were described as "very generally ignorant, often dirty and sometimes drunk." *The Boston Medical and Surgical Journal* ran a letter to the editor decrying an ad for a woman practicing medicine, stating, "Science itself is not only disgraced by being made the instrument of a petty income to an ignorant, presuming, flippant-tongued female, but she thus brings contempt upon the sex, of whom better things are expected."

"Individual discoveries are glorious and worthy, but we must give due need of praise to the hard working, obscure practitioners, who regardless of fame and wealth apply them," a late-nineteenth-century doctor noted in a speech about mid-century medicine. "Our fathers did wonders with the resources they could command. The lesson of their lives is largely one of dignity, self-sacrifice, devotion to science and regard for the bonds of professional conduct and duty and carelessness as to wealth or fame. Men come and men go, but science lives and advances."

And it was into this world that Thomas Dent Mütter, an orphaned boy now grown up and fresh from his experiences in Paris, returned.

CHAPTER THREE

TO RENDER EVIL
MORE ENDURABLE

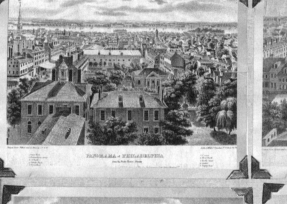

Philadelphia in the 1830s

THE WILLING MANSION SEEMED LIKE A PERFECT PLACE FOR Thomas Dent Mütter to open his first office for the practice of surgery. Built by former Philadelphia mayor Charles Willing, the mansion was a lovely brick building, three stories high with eleven large windows facing bustling Third Street just below Walnut. It was a stately and impressive place to start what he was sure would be a distinguished career.

Mütter knew that to become distinguished would require not only earning a favorable reputation with the public as a reliably successful surgeon, but also attaining distinction within a wide circle of his professional colleagues. He was sure he would do both and build an impressive practice by showcasing the fantastic techniques he'd learned in Paris.

"Adopting, with all the enthusiasm of his nature, the new precepts which he had been taught for the relief of these affections, he settled down among us," a colleague would later write of Mütter's first year in Philadelphia, "with such a trusting belief in his own resources, such a just confidence in the brightness of his future, that it seemed almost as if he felt that he would be able to renew the marvelous times of old, when supernatural powers came to mingle themselves with men in order to render their evils more endurable."

But even months after opening his office, Mütter sometimes spent long mornings and afternoons alone. Patients were not forthcoming, even though he tried his best "to be agreeable, to be useful, and to be noticed." In fact, Mütter had developed a reputation of "cut[ting] quite a swathe" as he rode around Philadelphia in a low carriage behind a big gray horse, driven by a servant in livery.

"Youthful looking, neat and elegant in his attire," he was described by a fellow doctor, "animated, cheerful, and distinguished in his bearing, whether observed in the social circle, or encountered, as, with his tall gray horse and handsome low carriage, he traversed our fashionable thoroughfares."

Mütter's colorful silk suits were a shocking contrast to the staid black, gray, and brown Quaker-inspired fashions found on Philadelphia's streets. But as always, he didn't mind the stares. He wanted to be memorable during his relentless attempts to curry favor with the city's best-known medical men by attending gatherings where they ate and drank and by trying to join the private societies they founded.

But unfortunately for the struggling physician, many of the doctors he tried so hard to impress thought this "immaculately dressed young man riding about Philadelphia" was "something of an intrusion." They complained that his conversation was often too full of his French masters, and how he boasted, openly and often, of their superiority, explaining how when it came to surgery, "one Frenchman [is] equal to a dozen Americans." The oft-repeated stories of the daring surgical exploits of his French idols "were not received with pleasure in every quarter." He was often accused of exaggerating, or *drawing a long bow,* as it was referred to in nineteenth-century slang.

"Mütter's early disappointment professionally was ironically due in part to the fact that he succeeded rather too well, both in his desire to be helpful as well as to be noticed," a Virginia historian would later note. It seemed an odd stumble for someone whose welfare and happiness since the age of seven seemed wholly dependent on endearing himself to near strangers.

WITH THE PASSING OF HIS MATERNAL GRANDMOTHER, SEVEN-YEAR-old Thomas Dent Mutter entered a very vulnerable type of orphanhood. His life and future were now entirely dependent on the emotional charity of people who were all but strangers to the boy.

Patrick Gibson—John Mutter's business partner and the trustee of John's will—had trouble at first trying to secure Thomas a new home. He was a spoiled boy, having been heavily doted upon by his father and grandmother, and in a time before the medical world fully understood how diseases were transmitted, there were concerns about risks a family might be taking by inviting into their home a little boy whose entire immediate family had been felled by illness.

But Gibson was able to downplay young Thomas's lack of discipline and disquieting family illnesses by shining a spotlight on his better qualities— specifically his keen intelligence and an unfailingly amiable disposition. To Thomas's good fortune, Gibson convinced a very wealthy and prominent man to take the boy on as his ward.

Robert Wormeley Carter, known as Colonel Carter for most of his life, was born into one of the best-known families in the South, and was also a distant cousin through marriage to Thomas's mother, Lucinda.

Once the agreement was struck, Thomas was taken directly to Sabine Hall, the Carter family's sprawling estate. Built in the early 1700s on four thousand acres of rich Virginia soil, right on the lush banks of the Rappahannock River, Sabine Hall had been passed down through several generations of Carters. Colonel Carter was now its owner, and there he lived with his wife, his children, and several hundred slaves.

When young Thomas arrived at Sabine Hall, he brought along everything he could from his old life: two trunks of clothing, a small toy hobby horse, and a working single-barreled gun. He also brought a Shetland pony, with bridle and saddle, and a satchel filled with his dead mother's jewelry: two gold lockets, two gold rings, a pearl necklace, and a pearl pin. He brought paintings of his parents and a small red book that contained only one thing: a drawing of his mother in ink. He brought with him a bright mind, a willful stubbornness, and a moderately effective charm.

And he also brought along a deep and troubling cough.

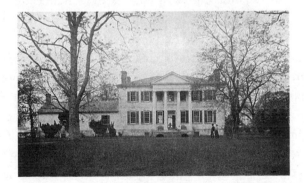

Sabine Hall

To a little boy who had known only the bustling energy and modest homes of Richmond, Virginia, Sabine Hall was an intimidating place to try to call home.

Robert "King" Carter—the family's legendary eighteenth-century patriarch—had spared no expense in building the house for his son, Landon. The enormous brick and stone building featured four large white cypress columns that rose all the way to the second floor and were surrounded by six meticulously curated gardens extending over five opulent terraces, from the top of the hill down to the plantation's fields. Entering the house, visitors were greeted by an enormous front parlor flanked by a hand-carved staircase. The house was decorated with numerous oil paintings of the Carter family: King Carter, Landon Carter, portraits of each of Landon's three wives, and, of course, now, Colonel Carter himself.

Colonel Carter was just twenty years old when he took in seven-year-old Thomas, and while Carter was born into a comfortable life, he was not afraid of change. During Thomas's stay at Sabine Hall, he made many dramatic alterations to the building and its environment. He constructed a giant portico on the front of the house, a broad classical pediment was added to the roof on the river facade, and a sixty-foot veranda that stretched the entire length of the house was built facing the river, taking more than seventy days of relentless carpentry to finish. Carter then requested that the entire redbrick exterior be painted white, and even demanded that the roof and chimneys be lowered.

In an odd coincidence—which might explain Mütter's later attraction to the city—it was said that Carter's main catalyst for making these changes was a visit he made to Philadelphia. He was deeply impressed with the "gay and splendid city" and was especially taken with its architecture, later writing in his journal that he found its streets "as beautiful as any in the world." And indeed the new Sabine Hall did resemble some of Philadelphia's best-known architecture. Philadelphia's First Bank of the United States had a similar oversize portico and light-colored facade, and the city's new Masonic Temple (designed by William Strickland), which Carter would later call "one of the most elegant buildings in America," had a gate lodge of a style very similar to the Gothic one he had built for Sabine Hall.

However, the attention to detail and visionary execution that Carter had lavished on the reinvention of Sabine Hall did not extend to the small boy he had just accepted as his ward. From the beginning, Carter made it clear to Patrick Gibson that he would provide a roof over Thomas's head, food on his plate, and a bed for him to sleep in, but it would fall to others to guide the boy in his life.

"I felt for our friend Mr. Mutter the most sincere friendship, and would most willingly do anything I could to promote the welfare and to place a foundation for the respectability and happiness of his son," Carter wrote to Gibson shortly after receiving Thomas at Sabine Hall. "I should however wish clearly to understand the situation of the amount of the fund that Thomas must depend upon for his future subsistence and wishing at the same time to have as little to do with the fund of the Estate as possible."

And perhaps feeling a bit of remorse at taking on such a large responsibility—and the criticism that might come with it—the twenty-year-old Carter noted, "I certainly feel much delicacy and reluctance by assuming a character which requires me so much judgment, care and attention, and which procures for you in return little less than actual loss, or unremitted condemnation."

Money proved to be a constant source of frustration and concern for both Thomas and his guardian. Carter brought the boy in with the promise that his costs would be covered by his late father's estate, but it wasn't long before Carter himself would be forced to sell both Woodberry—the only home Thomas knew after the death of his mother—and its contents to pay off debts that no one knew John Mutter had.

Hopeful that the rest of the estate's money would be free eventually (though he could have no idea that it would take years for the court system to release the funds to him), Carter kept strict records of the money he spent on the boy and began keeping him under a strict budget. It was during this examination of the budget that Thomas's fondness for expensive garments was first documented.

"The charge Mr. Bradley makes for the child's clothes, $23 apiece for his last two suits, is so very extravagant that they should if possible be made elsewhere," a stunned Carter noted, "but not having his measure I must for the present submit."

But if there was one area that Carter refused to cut corners on, it was the boy's education. Charles Goddard, the man who had tutored Thomas when his father was still alive, was brought to Sabine Hall and continued to serve in that role for another four years. The established rapport between tutor and pupil was a huge comfort to Thomas, and had the added benefit of relieving the Carter household of some of the disciplinary duties associated with the puckish, outspoken boy.

However, when Thomas turned twelve, Carter decided it was time to look at boarding schools. He eventually selected for Thomas the Llangollen School in Spotsylvania County, a grammar school that prepared boys to attend college. There, for a bargain price of $140 a year, Thomas learned English, French, and Latin, studied geography and mathematics, and boarded with his own teacher, John Lewis, who wrote Carter often about his growing ward's progress.

Thomas proved to a bright and willing student, and Lewis's letters always showcased the latest subject in which Thomas was excelling. However, Lewis's letters to Carter also revealed that the growing boy continued to struggle with his health problems.

"Early in the spring he had a slight attack of intermittent fever which soon yielded to the ordinary medicines . . . ," Lewis wrote Carter before adding, "his general health I think is greatly improved from last month. He is stronger and more active and is considerably grown."

The following year, Lewis wrote, "His general health has been better than it was the last year," though he was forced to add that the boy was still "occasionally attacked by bilious colic," a painful condition marked by severe cramping, vomiting, and jaundice.

In his own letters to Carter, young Thomas rarely mentioned his health or his scholastics. Rather, his letters were marked with frequent pleas for new clothing.

"I wrote to Aunt to send me two pairs of shoes as I have not any at present," he wrote Carter in 1824. "Please write Aunt to get my winter clothes and some shoes and socks as I am in want of them."

Six months later, he wrote, "As the warm weather is coming very fast I should like to get my summer clothes in time as I have but one very old suit. . . . I shall want some shoes about that time also. I do not wish to have any more made here as they cost as much as at Fredericksburg and are spoilt in the making."

A few months later, in his first letter to Carter since returning to school, Thomas told his guardian, "I am in great want of shirts as I have but two in the world and they are very old and tattered. I got some summer clothes from Mr. Lewis, but they are not sufficient for me nor nice enough to wear in town."

Thomas's desire to appear stylish only grew when, in 1826, he finally left Llangollen School to attend college at Virginia's Hampden-Sydney College. There, he ran up extravagant clothing bills and simply charged them to the school, with the hopes of earning scholarships and additional funds to pay off the debts. It was a ploy that didn't always work. At the end of his first year there, a frustrated merchant sent Colonel Carter the overdue bill directly, demanding payment for the more than one hundred dollars' worth of clothing and accessories Thomas had purchased on credit during the school year (and for which Thomas had only been able to pay back half).

The bill shows that Thomas—who was just sixteen years old—had made such eclectic purchases as a fashionable leghorn hat, several patterned vests, jackets and pants, yards of ribbons made from silk and velvet, several pairs of silk stockings, dog biscuits, a buck knife, and even several dozen cigars. In fact, Thomas's clothing choices were so flamboyant in style that the college's theater department was known to have borrowed from his wardrobe to outfit the actors in their plays.

When Colonel Carter received the bill, he was understandably furious, and threatened to withdraw his support if Thomas didn't fix his disobedient ways. Thomas promised he would.

At Hampden-Sydney, Thomas continued to blossom scholastically. He was written up for being distinguished in scholarship, industry, and behavior, though he did find himself in trouble more than once for skipping chapel without an excuse. He grew so popular, well liked, and respected that he was elected by his class to write and give a speech representing the college; the experience proved to be a shaping one for the developing young man.

Having felt largely invisible for much of his adolescence, Thomas thrilled at being center stage. His skills at charming tutors, professors, and caretakers to get his way translated well to engaging an audience, and he was praised for his natural gifts as a captivating presenter and for his voice, which was seen as being remarkable for both its range and amplitude.

Thomas also began traveling more around the South, visiting the areas where his parents grew up and meeting with distant family members. He did this without Colonel Carter's permission or approval, usually by borrowing enough money to make it to his desired destination, and then using his charms to secure the funds to get back home. Every so often, Colonel Carter would hear a tale of his ward's wanderlust ways from friends or acquaintances who had bumped into the boy during his travels. Again, Colonel Carter would threaten to remove his support of the boy, and again the boy would vow to do better.

But there was something within Thomas that compelled him to want to

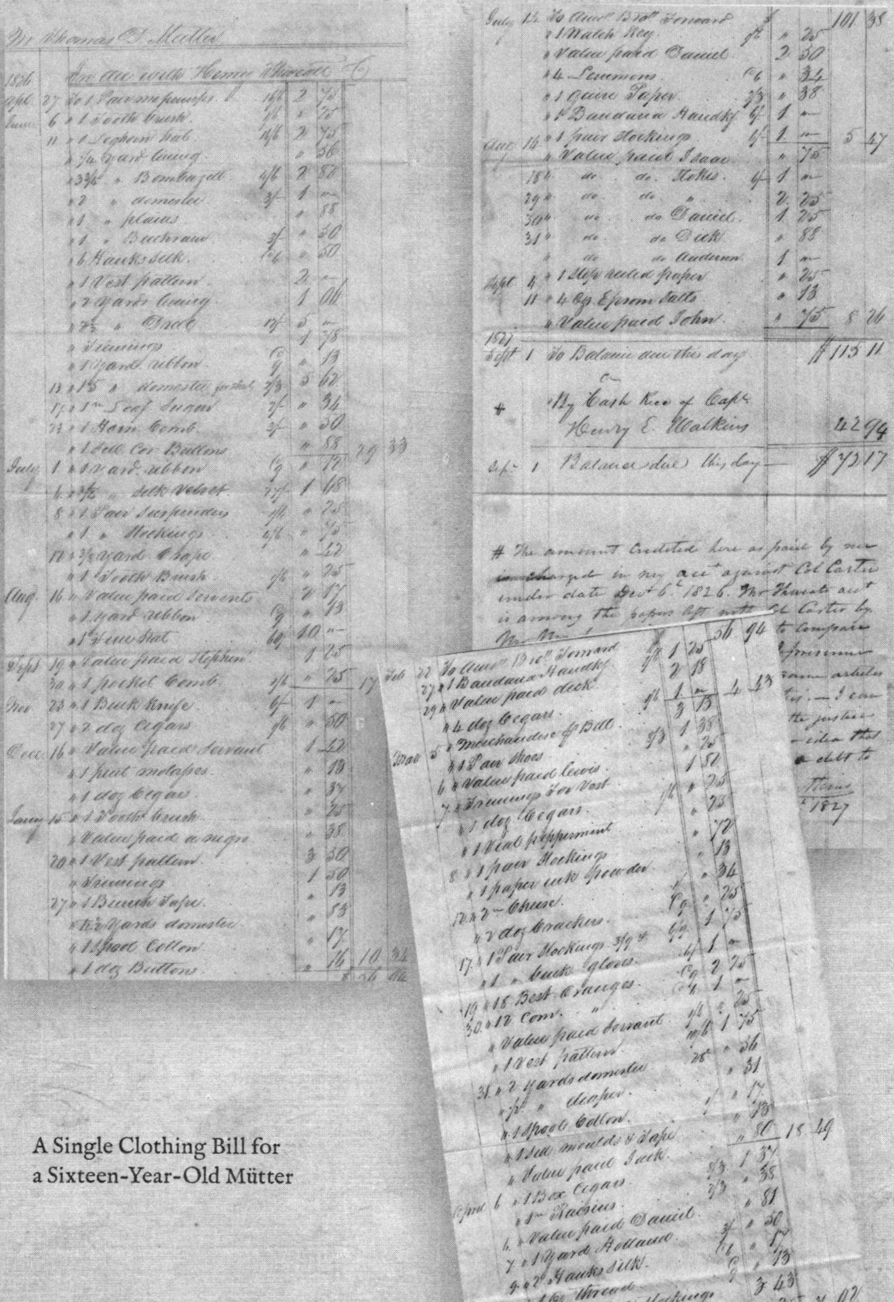

A Single Clothing Bill for
a Sixteen-Year-Old Mütter

see the world outside of Virginia. He even convinced the initially reticent Colonel Carter to support his decision to spend a semester at Yale, a college of growing reputation located in the northern city of New Haven, Connecticut. But this adventure proved to be disastrous as Thomas's weakened health came into immediate odds with the frigid northern winter. He was eventually sent home when none of the Connecticut doctors could stop him from coughing up blood—but not before he ran up outstanding bills with a tailor and a shoemaker, which Colonel Carter would again be contacted to pay.

Thomas risked Colonel Carter's ire one last time when, instead of returning to college after leaving Yale, he decided to spend time in Fredericksburg and Alexandria, places where his family once lived, again without Colonel Carter's permission. But it turned out to be a wise choice.

Thomas's family still had connections in that area. He was able to meet with knowledgeable and helpful doctors who agreed to help the troubled seventeen-year-old, the grandson of their long-dead friend, Dr. James Gillies. The news from these consultations was not reassuring—Thomas would be too ill to return to college anytime soon, they advised, and this unsettling condition would likely plague him for the rest of his life.

Thomas took the news with fortitude and equanimity, impressed with and grateful for the doctors who analyzed his situation with speed, and gave him advice with honesty and clarity.

It proved to be a watershed moment for Thomas. He suddenly realized what he wanted to do with his life: to study medicine and become a compassionate, trustworthy, and humanistic doctor like these men were.

Though he knew that Colonel Carter was upset with him and his erratic behavior, he felt compelled to write him immediately with the news:

> My dear Sir
>
> Owing to your short stay in the District, I was unable to have any conversation with you concerning my future course of studies. My present ill health will I am afraid prevent my returning to College, at all events for some time. I have therefore with the advice of several of my friends determined to study Medicine, which course I hope will meet with your approbation. I propose studying with Dr. Semmes of Alexandria. I feel I had best study here as my expenses would be much less than in any other place. You will perhaps say that study is study in whatever way one may pursue it, but you must recollect that there is a

very great difference between a college life, which requires you to be
up both late and early, and the life of a student of medicine. I should
like therefore to commence as soon as I am a little better for my time
is very precious and I wish to be able to commence practice by the
time I am twenty-one. And I do assure you if you will give your
consent to this plan and assist me with your counsel and friendship
you shall have no cause to repent; and although you have been led to
think rather too harshly of me, yet, I hope it is all forgotten and that
you will be to me, as I have every reason to suppose you were before,
my sincere friend.

THOMAS D. MUTTER

COLONEL CARTER GAVE HIS SUPPORT, AND NEARLY A DECADE
later—after graduating from the best and oldest medical school in the country, and after much studying under the most impressive doctors in the United
States and Europe—Thomas Dent Mütter became a doctor. One who was
now floundering in his always empty office in Philadelphia.

Colonel Carter supported his dream of being a doctor, just as seventeen-
year-old Thomas had hoped. It was a dream to which Mütter had been so
enthusiastically and devotedly focused that every financial request he made
of Colonel Carter was met with generous response, as the guardian grew
more and more impressed with the actions of his young ward.

But now that Mütter's extensive schooling was over and he had officially
"come of age," Colonel Carter felt it was time for his generosity to be with-
drawn and for Thomas to stand on his own. With that news, Mütter knew
the safety net that Carter's resources and name provided was vanishing.
And Mütter's own already strained funds were swiftly being depleted by
the incredible upkeep of his office and lifestyle.

Mütter felt he could do nothing but sit frustrated in his empty office and
watch as other doctors in the city used the currency of their well-known
and well-connected family names to secure their first patients. From the
beginning, Mütter knew his success would have to depend on his own efforts alone, but even he was not prepared for how difficult it would truly be.
How was it possible that he was able to endear himself to respectable figures in France, where haughtiness and disdain were almost an art form, and
yet it was such a struggle here?

When 1834 arrived in typical frigid Philadelphia fashion, Mütter found himself in feeble health. Worried his condition would deteriorate in Philadelphia's cruel winter, he decided the best course of action would be to temporarily close his practice and make an extended visit to one of Virginia's famed health spas. There he could do some thinking about what he should do about his situation.

Mütter chose a spa in Monroe County (in what would later become West Virginia) and was drawn in by the promise of warm weather and familiar foods. But he was also more than a little curious about the spa's claims for the healing qualities of their saltwater springs. While most doctors agreed that the warm humid air of the South encouraged the body to heal itself quicker—especially when it came to ailments of the lungs—than the dry and bitterly cold air of the wintry North, many spas took it one step further and claimed that dipping in their saltwater or sulphur springs could cure a person of disease. Mütter was eager to investigate.

In a fateful twist, Mütter was also able to make some extra money in the weeks he spent at the spa, by using his charm to develop a sizable practice among the spa's clientele. While his own besieged body slowly healed, Mütter was able to slightly rebuild his beleaguered finances and collect material for what he hoped would be an insightful article on "watering spas" and whether they deserved the considerable confidence certain segments of the medical profession (and larger segments of the greater population) had in their healing properties.

HOWEVER, WHEN MÜTTER RETURNED TO PHILADELPHIA, HE realized he had more pressing issues than writing the article. He had spent a year trying to establish himself as a reputable doctor in the City of Brotherly Love, with very little to show for it. Mütter saw only one solution: He would shutter his practice, leave Philadelphia for good, and return to Paris, where he felt he would have excellent prospects of success.

While he had been studying there, he had noticed there was not a single English or American physician actively working, despite the constant influx of American and English-speaking visitors. And Mütter thought that, because he had formed such associations and acquired such favorable influences during his residence in Paris, and was proficient in both French and German, he could likely anticipate receiving the patronage of the English, American, and German tourist as he developed his reputation with the

French. Considering all of this, Mütter began to feel foolish for even considering staying in Philadelphia.

A doctor whom Mütter had first met at the University of Pennsylvania, Samuel Jackson, asked him to wait. Jackson was an assistant to one of the medical college's best-known professors and had met Mütter when he was a bright, eager but puckish student (the subject of Mütter's doctoral thesis was "Chronic Inflammation of the Testis"). Even then, Jackson believed that Mütter had extraordinary potential.

Jackson asked that Mütter give Philadelphia one more year.

"If at the end of that time the prospect should then seem no brighter," he offered, "return for a permanent residence in Paris."

However, this additional year would be different. Instead of attempting to establish himself by starting his own practice, Mütter would agree to work as an assistant to the popular, and increasingly sickly, Dr. Thomas Harris. Harris was a teaching surgeon at the summer school of medicine, the Medical Institute, and Jackson sensed that Mütter might have a chance of establishing his reputation in Philadelphia if he aligned himself in this way—not just as a surgeon, but as a teacher too.

It wasn't clear if that was the path Mütter wanted to take, but he decided to accept the challenge Jackson offered.

And with this decision, Mütter's fate became forever entwined with the chaotic, turbulent, and cutting-edge history of Philadelphia's medical schools.

CHAPTER FOUR

THE MEDICAL ATHENS
OF AMERICA

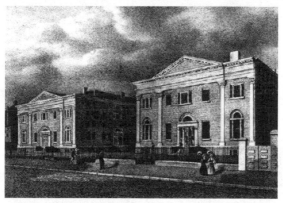

The Medical School of the University of Pennsylvania

THE PHYSICIAN SHOULD
POSSESS SELF-RESPECT

In no profession, probably, does a man more need
the possession of this truly honorable attribute.
The very nature of his avocation, which places him
at the beck and call of every one,
tends to diminish his self-respect; and
the desire to please all drags him still lower.
Bear always in mind who you are and what your
office is, and determine never to add another
to the disgraceful herd.

Thomas Dent Mütter

IT COULD RIGHTFULLY BE SAID THAT MEDICAL EDUCATION IN America was born in Philadelphia.

The University of Pennsylvania School of Medicine became the first and only medical school in the thirteen American colonies in the fall of 1765, making the school more than a decade older than the country in which it was founded.

Prior to its existence, all serious American aspirants toward the medical profession were compelled to go to Europe to complete their education.

But the medical school at Benjamin Franklin's own University of Pennsylvania made it possible for American students to study "anatomical lectures" and "the theory and practice of physik."

To earn a medical degree in these early years, a student had to: attend at least one course of lectures in anatomy, materia medica (now known as pharmacology), chemistry, and the theory and practice of *physik* (the art of healing, or medicine); attend at least one course of clinical lectures; study for one year under the doctors working at the Pennsylvania Hospital; be examined privately by medical trustees and professors; and, finally, be examined publicly.

It should go without saying that in addition to being at least twenty-four years of age, the student would also need to be both white and male. Being white and male, of course, were the two main prerequisites for successfully undertaking most any profession at this time.

But even from the beginning, the Philadelphia school earned a reputation for attracting the brilliant and the strange. Dr. John Morgan, who founded the medical school at the University of Pennsylvania in 1765, was regarded as "something extra among the people," and was seen as possessing "some of the eccentricities of genius." He was known in the city for being the first male public figure who ventured to carry a silk umbrella in Philadelphia (then "a scouted effeminacy"), but he was also credited with being the first doctor to send his patients to an apothecary—a person whose profession was the preparation and selling of medicine—instead of feeling responsible for creating and distributing the various herbs, tinctures, and salves himself.

In his first public address about his vision for the school, Morgan said, "Perhaps this Medical Institution (the first of its kind in America), though small in its beginning, may receive a constant accession of strength and annually exert new vigor. It may collect a number of young men of more than ordinary abilities, and so improve their knowledge as to spread its reputation to distant parts, and, by duly-qualified alumni, may give birth to other institutions of a similar nature."

This statement proved prophetic. For sixty years, the University of Pennsylvania was the defining medical institution for Philadelphia. By 1825, Philadelphia's population had exploded to over 138,000 people; more than 1,000 of these citizens were medical students. Not all of these students attended the University of Pennsylvania, where the total medical school population of closer to 500 packed into the undersize classrooms and lecture halls, to the students' growing discomfort. Every physician had private students who apprenticed under him, and this tradition continued even after other schools opened. But what the students learned through these apprenticeships was not standardized. Students who came to Philadelphia because of its reputation as America's medical center could not be guaranteed a slot in a medical school, nor could they be assured that the doctor under whom they studied was teaching them information that was up-to-date, or even correct.

Additionally, many in the community began to be more critical of how the University of Pennsylvania was being run. There was criticism of its cramped classrooms and overstuffed student rolls; accusations of favoritism in filling its department chairs and teaching positions; criticism of the faculty's recent duplicitous practice of operating private schools that would then feed into the university's medical school, ensuring that they could collect double the fees for teaching their classes; and most damning, an air of infallibility when it came to their opinions, which was not at all in keeping with scientific progress.

It became obvious to some in the community that "for Philadelphia to retain her position as the medical Athens of America," another major medical school in the city was needed.

Philadelphia at that time could have supported several colleges with the medical talent within its city limits. Several physicians in the city were popular enough to necessitate the building of personal lecture rooms connected to their offices. But the University of Pennsylvania—not wanting any competition to their obvious monopoly—was always quick to downplay such claims. And as the call for more medical schools grew louder, the University of Pennsylvania would use its political power to thwart any attempt to start a new school and, furthermore, would ostracize any doctor who didn't share its belief that Penn should be the only medical school in Philadelphia.

Several efforts to establish a second medical school were made in the 1810s and early 1820s, but all efforts to obtain a charter from the state legislature were unsuccessful.

This would all change in 1824, when the irascible Dr. George McClellan's ongoing quarrels with the University of Pennsylvania's Medical Department resulted in his leaving to found his own school: Jefferson Medical College.

George McClellan had received his medical degree from the University of Pennsylvania in 1819 and yearned to be one of the "duly-qualified alumni [who] may give birth to other institutions of a similar nature," of whom the medical school's founder John Morgan had spoken fifty years earlier.

McClellan was a brilliant physician, a true natural who saved a man's life before he even entered the medical school by fully amputating a leg that was almost completely severed, "swiftly stopping the hemorrhage" and instinctively leaving enough skin to make flaps for the stump. As a teacher, he was popular, a persuasive and forceful speaker with "a resounding voice that bespoke authority." His ability to attract all kinds of people to his lectures—students, practitioners, and laymen—led him to be one of those Philadelphia doctors who needed their own lecture hall.

But he was also extremely erratic and temperamental.

"Some of his best friends indeed would say that [McClellan] was impolitic, and unwise, and, at times, even inconsiderate and imprudent," a peer would later write.

He thought of himself as an excellent judge of character and wasn't shy in expressing those opinions. A bombastic figure, he was even known to heckle other surgeons while they were performing surgical lectures. His

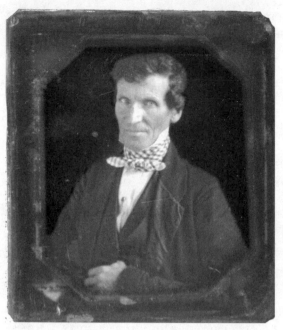

George McClellan

friends attempted to explain his galling behavior as simply the "*sans cere-monie* and *en avant* spirit" of his "sleepless genius."

"In public, he was inconsiderate and irregular," his friend explained, be-cause "alone, he was the grave, profound Philosopher."

When McClellan's repeated attempts to obtain a charter for a second school failed, the sly McClellan channeled his rage toward simply circum-venting the issue. Instead of wasting time and energy fighting the city for the permission to found a brand-new school, he instead coordinated with Jefferson College in Canonsburg, Pennsylvania, to simply establish a med-ical department of that college in Philadelphia.

Canonsburg's Jefferson College was founded a half century earlier and had earned a prominent place as a literary institution. It proudly laid claim to "a respectable contingent of educated intellect to our country . . . spread all over this land, engaged in the various departments of trade and manu-factures, in agriculture, statesmanship, in the professions of law, medicine, and theology, and in establishing and conducting other seminaries of learning."

McClellan knew that while the University of Pennsylvania might find it easy to squash the ambitions of one man, it would be tougher to deny such a respectable and established institution—which prided itself "in extending the benign influences of sound learning and an elevating morality"—from the same opportunity.

And it worked.

Much to the chagrin of the University of Pennsylvania—which had remained unrivaled in the city for well more than a half century—Jefferson Medical College became the city's second such institution in 1824.

But getting the school started was a tricky endeavor. While Jefferson had been able to secure a talented faculty, they did not have an endowment or any buildings in which to teach. McClellan rented the Tivoli Theater on the south side of Prune Street and remodeled it as best he could to fit a college setting. He also had the school's top three professors—including himself—give public demonstrations and lectures every day and night until the school opened, to help advertise the merits of the new school to the medical students arriving in the city every week.

It proved a successful gambit. The first class numbered an impressive 107, with 20 graduating at the end. The faculty and founders were highly satisfied with its first session, which they had considered to be only "an experiment."

But even in its first year, Jefferson Medical College broke new ground in teaching medicine. McClellan insisted that his own audacious idea be instituted from year one: that all students must take an active part in the care of patients. He considered it to be a deeply important factor in the training of medical students that they be taught by having them observe and work with their own professors as they treated patients. It was an idea that had never been tried before, and this revolutionary concept would prove to be McClellan's most important contribution to medical education, reshaping the way medicine would be taught throughout the world.

FOUNDING THE NEW SCHOOL, HOWEVER, ALSO MADE PHILADELPHIA a battleground, for now there were two rival medical institutions, filled with brilliant, eccentric, and outspoken professors, clashing in private and in public, to earn the moniker of the best medical school in the country.

And young Thomas Dent Mütter was just about to jump into the fray.

CHAPTER FIVE

A FALCON FLIGHT

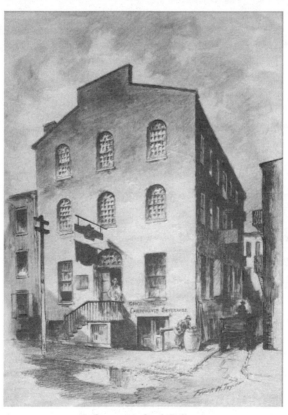

Jefferson Medical College

THE PHYSICIAN MUST ALSO BE A THINKING, OBSERVING, AND REASONING MAN.

Let me advise you to commence at once observing
for yourself.
Don't trust what you are told in lectures, or read
in books, but make the knowledge your own,
by your own labors.
Lectures and books will serve as guides and beacons,
but the goals can only be reached
by travelling the road yourself.

Thomas Dent Mütter

From the absolute beginning, Mütter's students adored him. Dr. Harris, for whom Mütter served as assistant at the Medical Institute, a "summer school of medicine," was sick often. Mütter began to fill in for him regularly, much to the delight of the students, many of whom were not much younger than Mütter himself.

Stylish and fresh, quick with his wit and flashy in his presentation, Mütter was delighted and relieved that all the things that seemed to frustrate and alienate him from the staid medical establishment endeared him to this younger generation of students.

But it wasn't just Mütter's charm or flash that mesmerized his pupils. His lectures grew a reputation for being well devised, amply demonstrated, and outstandingly delivered. His love of the material, his eagerness to have the latest information spread quickly and accurately, and his natural energy and enthusiasm, combined with his clear demonstrations, unusual teaching specimens, and "sprightly oral elucidations," helped fix his students' attention on his lucid and methodical arrangements of his often extremely complicated subjects.

The art of teaching came so readily to him, those around him would say his ability seemed "almost intuitive."

"At his first essay from this perch," a colleague would later write, "he seems to have taken a falcon flight."

"In orators, this early perfection is not often seen," a peer noted, comparing Mütter's great skill as a professor to "great generals, who learn to fight by fighting, and whose only real school is war."

And perhaps that war metaphor was more apt than the speaker knew. As

Mütter was just beginning his career in the late 1830s, Philadelphia was entering one of the most turbulent periods of its medical history.

Two long-simmering crises were coming to a head and would dramatically implode before the decade's end. They would have a profound effect on the course of American medicine and, consequently, on the career of Thomas Dent Mütter.

The first crisis grew out of a challenge to the old private system of medical training, whereby various physicians around the city gave a series of private lectures to as many students as could be convinced to pay. When a pupil felt he had learned what he needed, he would undergo an examination for an MD degree. Needless to say, it was a highly profitable system for the medical community, especially those physicians lucky enough to be paid both by private students and by the university with which they were associated. But it had enormous flaws. There was no guarantee of the quality or accuracy of the lectures. Being a great physician didn't always guarantee that you had the ability to be an effective teacher. Similarly, an impressive word-of-mouth reputation could be earned by a charismatic and outgoing professor, with the students never knowing that the information he was teaching was out-of-date, not entirely correct, or sometimes flat-out wrong. Lecturers worked in isolation, largely viewing one another as competitors, so there were no systems in place to correct the dramatic difference in quality among the various professors.

Even organized schools or lecture halls, like the Medical Institute (where Mütter was getting his first taste of success), were "purely private enterprise[s] whose standards derived entirely from the conscience and abilities of the individuals involved."

Perhaps shaken by the new competition presented by Jefferson Medical College, the University of Pennsylvania began to seriously rethink how their medical training should and would be conducted. Their new objective: to standardize medical teaching by bringing it more consistently under the regulation of the administration.

The impulse came from a good place, but it was nonetheless met with strong resistance by private instructors. The University of Pennsylvania immediately set about crushing anyone who tried to oppose them, often using what their detractors called "rather unwholesome tactics." One example, among many: The university was accused of conspiring to monopolize the supply of cadavers in the city, thus forcing out of business any private anatomists not in the university's favor.

These tactics worked, and by the end of the 1830s it was said, and not without several notes of frustration and bitterness, that no man could look for success as a private teacher in any branch of medicine unless he be directly or indirectly connected with the university.

The second crisis the Philadelphia medical community faced was *itself*. Or rather, that the more contentious members of the community were becoming more flamboyant in their public battles with one another, and the situation was finally reaching a breaking point.

When Dr. George McClellan's problems with the Philadelphia medical establishment led him to found Jefferson Medical College in 1824, it was certainly not the end of his clashes with the University of Pennsylvania or its faculty.

In the ten years following Jefferson's founding, the "period of accommodation" between the university and its new rival was marked by bitter, unrelenting public confrontations, often instigated and led by the two public faces of these medical schools: McClellan for Jefferson and Dr. William Gibson for the University of Pennsylvania. Both men were chairs of surgery at their respective colleges, and both men had legendarily fiery tempers and sharp tongues.

"It is said that one should not speak ill of the dead. Far be it from me to do so," a contemporary would later write of Gibson, "but I cannot ignore the fact, known to most of his professional contemporaries, that Gibson was not an amiable man. His ill temper often betrayed him into unkind expressions, even in the lecture-room."

Indeed, though Gibson had rightfully earned his reputation as an "impressive lecturer" who never failed to command the attention of his classes with "clearness, accuracy and earnestness," it was also a well-known fact that his practice—both as a surgeon and a physician—was extremely small, a situation owed largely to his temper and acerbic nature.

Gibson, like McClellan, often indulged in offensive language against his opponents. When the two encountered each other in public, they were not shy in expressing their mutual disdain.

In one oft-repeated story, while teaching in a packed University of Pennsylvania lecture hall, Gibson openly accused McClellan of falsehood for having asserted that he had repeatedly performed an operation (an "extirpation of the parotid gland" or removal of a large salivary gland in the back of the mouth) that Gibson himself thought "unfeasible." For a long time, there was what was delicately referred to as "a warm controversy" on this subject between the rival schools, with McClellan feeling personally attacked. The medical community at large soon became divided by the issue, though most seemed to side with McClellan.

Finally, Gibson—in a totally unexpected move—invited McClellan to the University of Pennsylvania to bear witness to Gibson's performing the surgery he had previously denied was possible, in front of Gibson's own class. McClellan agreed and, when the day arrived, was delighted to see the classroom packed not only with students from both schools, but also many local physicians "who had come to see the fun."

Gibson, too, thrilled at the size of the eager audience, and skillfully performed the surgery with a trademark flourish. But when the operation was over, Gibson turned toward the audience and announced, "Gentlemen, I have performed what is generally called extirpation of that gland. However, the mass I have removed is only a *tumor* overlying that gland, *not the gland itself.*"

"Gentlemen," McClellan coolly replied while standing up, "my distinguished friend has extirpated the parotid gland, but, unfortunately, doesn't know it."

The remark caused "convulsions of laughter" in the large assembly. The story of the surgery would go on to be written in medical journals across the country, only further intensifying the rivalry between the two great surgeons . . . and their schools.

Mütter's entry into the Philadelphia medical school community in the mid-1830s coincided with a period second to none in America's medical history. Gibson himself would later say that this time would be remembered for "rivalry marked with jealousy and unfairness." Medical lore and literature would record abundant evidence of the personal abuse and criticism that medical men of the day rained upon one another, and of the bitter acrimony that often characterized any public discussion of important questions, especially that of treatment.

Because of this unhelpful and seemingly unending infighting, Philadelphia's reputation as a medical mecca was slipping. It still possessed two great schools, and its doctors were still revered far and wide. Even with all this bitter discourse, every ambitious medical man in the United States looked toward a chair in a Philadelphia college as the crowning point of any serious career. But no one could deny that the city was gaining rivals in places like New York, Baltimore, and Chicago, and the current fractured state of the Philadelphia community did nothing to stop these other cities in their bid for the top.

Perhaps this is why the Philadelphia medical community began to pay attention to Mütter more closely in the wake of his professorial successes. Young, smart, ambitious, and blessed with extraordinary talents, Mütter was gaining a reputation as "one of the best of good fellows" and not just in the lecture hall.

"He possessed spontaneously, as it were, the art both of making and holding friends," a fellow doctor would write of him, "a natural amenity of manner and gentleness of character, a manliness of bearing so intermingled with feminine graces that even children were attracted by it, and a love of approbation that induced him to do what he could to please others."

When Dr. Harris grew too sick to make house calls, he asked Mütter to go on his behalf. Mütter's skill, matched with his comforting and charming demeanor, endeared him to the patients. Soon, other doctors, including and especially the ever-encouraging Dr. Jackson, made a habit of sending Mütter to make house calls in their stead. As a result, within a few months, Mütter began to develop a healthy private practice.

He was also garnering an impressive reputation as a surgeon. His access to the medical school's surgical rooms allowed him to attempt the kinds of ambitious surgeries he had learned about in Paris, many of which defiantly occupied "the difficult domain of reparative and reconstructive surgery."

His first surgical patients found their way to him through the school itself, who promised citizens free surgical treatment, provided they agreed to the surgery's being performed in a public setting.

But it didn't take long for Mütter to also begin receiving surgical patients privately as word of his unusual skills began to spread. The first patients came from the Philadelphia area, but soon, "strangers from various parts of this wide domain . . . sought from his skill the relief which their various sufferings demanded."

"He succeeded with patients for the same reason as with students," it was written of him; "he was both respected and liked." This seemed like a welcome change from the relentless acrimony and open hostility that now marred the reputations of McClellan and Gibson, the city's two top teaching surgeons.

Mütter might have sensed that he was being groomed for something greater when three distinguished Philadelphia doctors—Randolph, Norris, and Anderson, all several years his senior—independently approached him and inquired if they might assist him in one of his next surgeries *radicales*. They each wanted to see firsthand how Mütter took cases so damaged and tragic, and fixed them so seamlessly.

Perhaps the most sensible response would have been to have each doctor come in separately and then select patients whose surgeries would be easiest to perform in front of such an esteemed audience. But that wasn't Mütter's way.

He knew it was risky, but he couldn't help it. He decided to do a very difficult surgery, and asked all of them to be his assistants on it. It took some finessing, but Mütter assured them that each individual would serve a necessary part in the surgery.

Still, it was quite a sight to see: men at the prime of their careers, lining up to assist a twenty-nine-year-old surgeon who was perhaps best known to their wives as the doctor who liked to match the color of his expensive suit to the carriage in which he was riding. But the simple truth was that the doctors were happy to line up by Mütter's side, to witness his surgical prowess, to be close to his quick, sure hands.

Less happy, however, were Mütter's students, who grumbled in their seats on surgery day, upset that their own views of the operation might be blocked.

After a quick contented survey of the scene, Mütter began the process of tuning them all out so that the entirety of focus could be directed to the patient shaking and drooling in the surgical chair.

Nathaniel Dickey was a local Philadelphian whom Mütter had liked from the first time they met: intelligent, funny, and in perfectly good health, aside from the obvious. The twenty-five-year-old's face was dramatically split down the middle. His lips and the top of his mouth were raw and open, and despite Nathaniel's best efforts to prevent it, thick cords of spittle often poured from the opening.

It was Nathaniel who sought out Mütter, asking if anything could be done to help a person like him. With a thick slur but bright eyes, he confessed to Mütter how badly he wanted to have a wife and children, how much he dreamed of walking down the street with this beautiful family he so often envisioned having, and have not a single passing stranger gawk at his deformed face.

Now, weeks later, Nathaniel sat in front of Mütter, his head firmly supported against the chest of a seated Dr. Norris, and his arms held down against his torso by a tight white sheet.

Mütter had already explained the surgery to Nathaniel in detail. In the days leading up to it, Mütter would thrice daily massage Nathaniel's face, attempting to desensitize his vulnerable palate. Even the slightest amount of vomit rising from his throat would threaten the entire operation, ruining the delicate work he was attempting to do, and inviting dangerous infection to nest in his already beleaguered mouth.

The risk of purging was one of the reasons the surgery had to be performed with the patient almost entirely sober. Mütter also needed him to stay still and stiff, to open his mouth wider and wider if need be, and to keep the contents of a nervous stomach in their place.

Nathaniel had to be more than a patient; he had to be a partner in seeing this difficult surgery to its end. Mütter knew this. And so they would meet multiple times a day for facial massages. And as Mütter's hands gently explored Nathaniel's handsome but broken face, he would walk the young man through each moment of the surgery, carefully explaining each danger and tenderly warning of each increasing level of pain. Nathaniel never once wavered in his determination to see it through.

But now on the day of the surgery, Mütter saw Nathaniel's eyes widen and his body become rigid as he moved toward him. Mütter paused for a moment, letting Nathaniel take several deep breaths. Nathaniel's eyes unconsciously wandered to the table where Mütter had laid out his tools: a knife, a hook, a pair of long forceps, needles, waxed thread, scissors, sponges on handles, wine and water, cold water, towels, and—hidden under a handkerchief for emergency use only—leeches, opiates, and a sharp lancet.

After making his opening remarks, being sure to name and thank each of his impressive assistants, Mütter took care to position himself properly. He decided to stand a little to one side of Nathaniel, to obstruct the entrance of light into the mouth as little as possible. He then asked Nathaniel to throw his head back as far as he could and to open his mouth and keep it in this position as long as he was able. He placed a comforting hand on Nathaniel's shoulder, squeezed just once, and then began.

Within moments of the surgery's quick first step—the insertion of a sharp hook into the roof of Nathaniel's mouth used to gently pull the deformed mass of muscle and skin back—the trio of doctors forgot who they were, or that anyone else was in the room. The students groaned and fussed, as the doctors blocked their view, closing their small circle in an attempt to get a closer look at Mütter's whirlwind actions.

The trick to surgeries of this kind, Mütter knew, was twofold: You had to be quick so as to lessen the stress and pain of the patient, but slow enough to make sure you were doing it right. Mütter's hands were a confident blur of motion as he cut and pierced, excised and sutured, flayed and positioned.

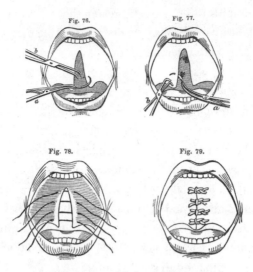

Surgery on Nathaniel Dickey

He checked in with Nathaniel often, offering whatever words of comfort and support he could. And when possible, he tried to involve the doctors who had agreed to assist, but once he realized they were more than content to watch, he focused solely on the job at hand.

If Mütter had chosen to look at them, he would have noticed their faces: mouths pursed, eyebrows gathered in concentration, eyes narrowed in half disbelief. Each one wanted to ask Mütter to stop, to slow down. Mütter's ambidextrousness meant that he could do twice the work in half the time. The doctors grew dizzy and overwhelmed, unsure of which hand to follow, unsure how they would be able to replicate the surgery themselves when it seemed like quick, efficient chaos.

But Mütter paid them no heed. The only thing that could distract him from his work was the face of Nathaniel, which he monitored as a mother would—tracking each wince, each moan, each muffled cry. When Nathaniel's body would quake uncontrollably under Mütter's hand, he would remove all instruments and look into Nathaniel's eyes. With Mütter's hand gently placed in Nathaniel's damp hair, he would feed him a small glass of cold water. Nathaniel gargled it, and spat. The pan turned red as it grew slick with blood.

And when Nathaniel was ready, Mütter returned to his work, his face calm and focused, clear and bright, almost happy.

After just twenty-five minutes, it was done. Nathaniel's face, which just a moment earlier had been an open wound—bleeding, raw, and split—now was tenderly united, the silk thread straining at the incision sites, but holding. Nathaniel, exhausted and drenched in sweat, relaxed into the chair as Mütter walked backward, wiping his hands on a fresh towel.

The doctors were silent, still trying to process what they had just seen. The students sat back in their seats, their journals open and empty on their laps. What notes could they take that could capture what they had just witnessed? It felt as if perhaps they had been given a glimpse of the future, a sign that things were about to change.

But Mütter noticed none of it. Instead, he remained focused on Nathaniel. He stepped again toward the trembling young man, a small sponge in hand. He softly blotted the last remnants of blood from his newly reunited mouth, his hand firm and proud on Nathaniel's shoulder. Where others once saw a monster, Mütter thought, he had revealed the man. And from under the handkerchief on the surgical table, he pulled one more hidden item: a small mirror, clean and shining. With one tender hand cupping the back of his exhausted patient's head, he held the mirror in front of Nathaniel's new and handsome face. Mütter smiled.

And Nathaniel Dickey, disobeying doctor's orders this one time, smiled back.

CHAPTER SIX

CE QUE FEMME VEUT, DIEU LE VEUT AUSSI!

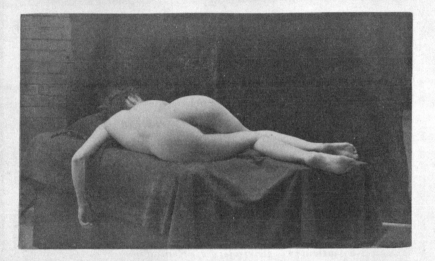

Woman Posed for Gynecological Examination

THE PHYSICIAN
SHOULD ALSO BE A GENTLEMAN

The Dictionary tells us that a gentleman is one raised
　　by birth, office, fortune, or education, above the vulgar.
　　But surely such a definition is far from the truth.
To be a gentleman, something more is necessary
　　than to have had a grandfather.
If fortune was the key to the sanctum of the gentleman,
　　how many a knave, how many a swindler, how many
　　an ignoramus, would find admittance
　　and how many a true gentleman be excluded!
Nor does education alone make the gentleman, without
　　being combined with good-breeding and good morals.
Perhaps I cannot better define the characteristic of
　　gentleman than has been done by a most distinguished
　　writer of our own country—Bishop [G. W.] Doane.
"A gentleman," says he, "is but a gentle man—
　　no more, no less: a diamond polished that was
　　a diamond in the rough; a gentleman is gentle;
　　a gentleman is modest; a gentleman is courteous;
　　a gentleman is generous; a gentleman is slow
　　to take offence, as being one that never gives it;
　　a gentleman is slow to surmise evil, as being
　　one that never thinks it; a gentleman goes armed
　　only by a consciousness of right; a gentleman
　　subjects his appetites; a gentleman refines
　　his tastes; a gentleman subdues his feelings;
　　a gentleman controls his speech; and finally,
　　a gentleman deems every other better than himself."
Of such, doctors should be made.

Thomas Dent Mütter

THE WOMAN GRIMACED, HER SEX OPENED TO THE CLASSROOM full of young men.

"See this unobvious, apparently vile lump of animal texture?" Dr. Charles D. Meigs asked his collection of students, gesturing to the woman's genitals. "Here, in the inner court of the temple of the body? How *can* you study this subject sufficiently?

"Women possess a peculiar trait—it is modesty," he continued, as he walked over and firmly placed another pillow between the woman's legs. "It is one of their most charming attributes.

"But scan her position in civilization, and it is easy to perceive that her intellectual force is *different* from that of her master and lord. I say her master and lord; and it is true to say so," he continued as he casually repositioned the woman for the maximum exposure: moving her buttocks to the edge of the table, pushing her thighs at right angles to her quaking trunk.

"The great administrative faculties are not hers," he continued. "She plans no sublime campaigns, nor leads armies to battle, or fleets to victory. In society, she is still in bonds, manacled by custom and politics. She composes no *Iliad*, no *Aeneid*. Do you think that a woman could have developed, in the tender soil of her intellect, the strong idea of a Hamlet, or a Macbeth? *No.*"

Meigs walked to the table, which displayed the tools of his trade: speculums and scalpels, tinctures and powders, a stack of handkerchiefs, and a large jar of properly starved leeches. He dipped his fingers in a bowl of olive oil and rubbed them slowly together as he looked back at the woman.

"Such is not woman's province, nature, power, nor mission. She reigns in the heart; her seat and throne are by the hearth-stone. The household altar is her place of worship and service," he said, walking toward her. She was staring at the wall in front of her, her hands balled on the thin cotton sheet.

"She has a head too small for intellect," he said, stroking her hair but looking to his audience, "but it is just big enough for love."

DR. MEIGS FELT HE KNEW WHAT HE WAS TALKING ABOUT.

He was the father of ten children, all with the same devoted wife, Mary. She not only survived each of the ten births but nursed all the children herself, and was so faithful to them throughout that, though several had most violent and prolonged attacks of illness during infancy and childhood, only one died. Her fourth son, William Montgomery, passed away at four and a half. The couple's sixth son (and seventh child) would be named William Montgomery as well, in honor of the late child, a custom of the time.

Charles D. Meigs himself was the fifth of nine children and had received his unusual middle name, Delucena, from a Spanish gentleman to whom his maternal grandfather had become strongly attached during the Revolutionary War. Meigs's own father had been the thirteenth and final child of his mother, Jane, who gave birth to him when she was forty-nine years old.

It came as no surprise that the Meigs men felt they knew a little something about women and birth, and Charles D. Meigs, in particular, felt it was his duty to share this knowledge with the world. It was his extraordinary gift to the world.

Meigs was an enormously popular and respected figure in women's health during the mid-nineteenth century. Though he had lost the coveted position of chair of obstetrics at the University of Pennsylvania to Hugh Lenox Hodge (a talented doctor whose failing eyesight forced him out of surgery but for some reason seemed to pose no problem when it came to obstetrics and gynecology!), Meigs was still regarded as one of the leading voices in obstetrics.

Meigs believed that the field of gynecology and obstetrics was handicapped by the prejudices and false modesties practiced by women and encouraged by many religious leaders of the time. How were doctors supposed to treat women effectively when, in many localities, an obstetrician could examine the abdomen of a pregnant woman only through blankets?

Having little patience for women whose bodily shyness proved a barrier to him, Meigs believed and preached passionately that treatment others might view as curt and brutish—but he saw as efficient and gentlemanly—was

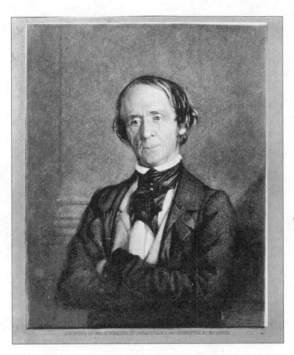

Charles Delucena Meigs

often the quickest route between a foolish patient and the treatment the doctor knew was needed.

In his lectures, he would act out scenes for his students, illustrating brief exchanges he had had with his patients. In one exchange he recounted in his own textbook, a frightened patient told Meigs she'd "rather die" than be subjected to a manual gynecological examination by him. His response was simply to shout at her in French, "*Ce que femme veut, Dieu le veut aussi!*" The translation: "What a woman wants, God wants too!"

If Mütter represented a new, more empathetic vision of how doctors could treat patients, then Meigs was a perfect symbol of the dominant—and dominating—establishment. And these men had no reason to believe that their careers would be so intimately tied to each other. Until, of course, they were.

CHAPTER SEVEN

THE GREAT THAW

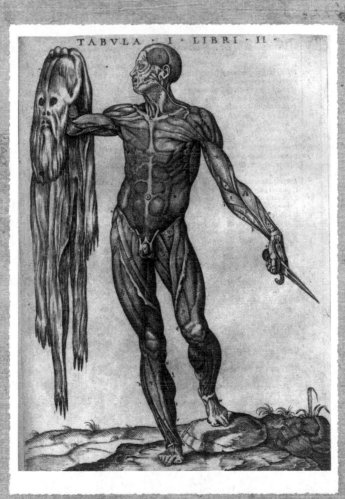

TABVLA · I · LIBRI · II ·

IN PHILADELPHIA, THE YEAR 1841 WAS BORN IN ICE. THE LAST days of 1840 were spent in a torrent of hail, rain, and snow, and when dawn cracked against the cobblestone streets of Philadelphia on January 1, 1841, the city was frozen solid.

"It will, perhaps, long be remembered by the present generation," wrote a historian of the time, "that in the year 1841, there was . . . no spring. Winter commenced on the 15th of November and continued until the 15th of May."

It was during these relentlessly frozen months that the fate of Jefferson Medical College would be decided.

THE PROBLEMS PLAGUING JEFFERSON MEDICAL COLLEGE REACHED a tipping point in the late 1830s. McClellan, the mad genius who founded Jefferson Medical College a decade earlier, would face yet another battle— this time with his own school.

While his students, who warmly called him Mac, still adored him, the board of trustees of Jefferson Medical had grown tired of his antics. Unquestionably a brilliant visionary, McClellan still lacked two important requisites of great surgeons and great professors: judgment and patience. The casual frequency with which he jumped to conclusions, both personally and professionally, coupled with his uncontained temper and unmanageable tongue, led to frequent clashes inside and outside his own college.

The board had other concerns as well. Most recent years of the Jefferson Medical College were plagued with financial problems and it still suffered from continued harassment by the University of Pennsylvania. The board had also created problems for itself by hiring new faculty members who were just as eager to brawl as McClellan, including John Revere (the unruly son of patriot Paul Revere), Granville Sharp Pattison (whose nickname was the Turbulent Scot), and William Barton, whose open hostility toward other members of the faculty was expressed loudly and often through his legendary "Navy vocabulary."

"[Dr. Barton]'s favorite epithet, almost constantly applied when speaking of one of the trustees, was so profane and abusive, that from regard to the highly respectable family of this trustee, I shall not mention it," a shaken faculty member would later write in his memoir.

Jefferson Medical College had hired its faculty precisely because it wanted to be seen as embracing the "spirit of independent thinking," but it did not foresee how this would translate into constant challenges between board and faculty, as well as near-constant clashes among faculty members themselves. When the board decided it had had enough and suggested that a major change must be made, McClellan aggressively resisted. He called the board "a parcel of politicians" and a "blackguard Board of Trustees," before publicly announcing that Jefferson was "rotten and going to the dogs."

But in his rashness, he failed to reckon with the power and stability of the board of trustees.

In 1838, the Jefferson Medical College board decided that the only course to take was to vacate all the chairs and to elect new professors. Current faculty members who still wanted to be a part of Jefferson Medical College were, of course, invited to place their names on the ballot for consideration. McClellan placed his name on the ballot to retain his position as founding chair of surgery, but when the final votes were tallied in July 1839, he didn't make the cut. McClellan's connection with the school he had fought so hard to found had come to an unceremonious end.

Even with the dismissal of McClellan and several other members of the faculty, the college continued to struggle. Two years later, when two faculty members decided to leave and one passed away suddenly, the board decided once again to take drastic measures and vacate all the positions for a second time.

The Jefferson Medical College board knew its institution was at a crossroads. The school, which was born from innovation and blazed a new path in medical education, had been slowly strangled by the same faculty who had once brought it such pride. They knew they needed to hire new faculty, but this time, they tasked one of their best remaining faculty members, Robley Dunglison, to scout out the best candidates.

Dunglison had earned his nickname, the Great Peacemaker, by holding the college together in spite of all the explosive personalities who were happily tearing it apart, and he was tasked with rebuilding the school's lineup yet again. It was not easy. The city was teeming with talented doctors eager to live and work in the prestigious spotlight that a faculty position at Jefferson Medical College afforded, but more than just their skills would need to be considered this time around. Dunglison was asked not only to bring together the most innovative minds in medicine, but also to ensure that the gentlemen hired could form a harmonious family of professors. Nonetheless, the whole city of physicians wanted to be considered, and rumor had it that among those jockeying for a spot were the stalwart Charles D. Meigs and a newcomer by the name of Thomas Dent Mütter.

BY THE END OF AN ICE-COVERED MARCH, DUNGLISON HAD COME up with his list, which he hoped would mark the dawn of a new era at Jefferson Medical College. He offered the list up to the Jefferson Medical College board for their ultimate vote on April 2. On the list were some of the city's best-known doctors.

For some chairs, the decision about who should fill them was easy. Dunglison was able to present the one name he considered the best, and the board unanimously agreed with his choice. But for other chairs, like those for surgery, anatomy, and chemistry, there was serious competition.

It came as little surprise that Charles Meigs would be nominated for the chair of obstetrics. He spoke six languages, had a popular practice in Philadelphia, and was already the author of two wildly acclaimed books on women's medicine. His first, a bestselling translation of *An Elementary Treatise on Midwifery* by the famous French anatomist and surgeon Alfred-Armand-Louis-Marie Velpeau, proved so successful that a second edition was issued just in time for Meigs to publish his first independent work, *The Philadelphia Practice of Midwifery*, which also became a big seller. In print and in practice, Meigs was swiftly becoming his country's leading authority on women's health. As a lecturer, he earned even more raves.

"Meigs possessed all the requisites for success upon the stage—remarkable powers of mimicry, great enthusiasm, and a strong perception of the ludicrous. In the lecture-room, he was the best actor I have ever seen," a contemporary once wrote of him, "and it is deeply to be regretted that there are not more of such teachers in the amphitheatre, especially in the afternoon, when the student, exhausted by the fatigues of the day, finds it difficult to keep awake."

Of course, what student could sleep when being lectured on such topics as the difference in appearance between genitals of virgins and those who had given birth (Meigs described the labia of virgins as being plump, with a "rose tint," while those who had borne children have labia "bluish" and "shriveled or collapsed in appearance, except with fat persons"), as well as the proper treatment of abscesses on the labia (Meigs strongly recommended bleeding the woman from the arms, using small sharp razors, before applying leeches directly onto her genitals).

The board of Jefferson Medical College elected him as chair of obstetrics unanimously.

Joining him would be Dunglison himself, since he had forwarded his name for the chair of Jefferson's Institutes of Medicine and Medical Jurisprudence. This was not an act of hubris. The British-born Dunglison made his name in the 1820s and 1830s, when his seminal medical texts established him as the "father of American physiology," and his long residence in the South had enabled him to act as the personal physician for both Thomas Jefferson and James Madison. The Jefferson chair was created specifically for him, in what would prove to be a successful attempt to lure him north. It would be a position he would hold for over a third of a century, and he would be so dedicated to it that he wouldn't return home to his native England for thirty years. When he finally did, his elderly mother—"still a fine-looking old lady, dressed in the old style, wearing a turban" though now suffering from dementia—could not remember him.

"This, it need not be said, was a great disappointment to Dr. Dunglison," a former student would later recall, "but he showed much equanimity and delighted to talk with her by the hour of by-gone days . . . she would generally conclude [their conversation] by saying to him, 'So you have seen Robley? He was the best boy that ever was . . . ,'" as her afflicted mind was unable to marry the memories of her young son with the old man who sat before her.

Two doctors who, like Mütter, were born and raised in Virginia would be elected to two more of the chairs: John Kearsley Mitchell was elected to chair of the practice of medicine, and Robert Huston was given the chair of materia medica (*materia medica* being the era's catchall term for "the body of collected knowledge about the therapeutic properties of any substance used for healing").

Meigs was likely hoping that, of the six doctors up for consideration for the chair of chemistry, Franklin Bache would ultimately be selected. Bache, the great-grandson of Benjamin Franklin, had taught in tandem with Meigs for more than six years. Their long friendship meant so much to each other that they both named sons after the other.

Meigs named his seventh and youngest son Franklin Bache Meigs, while Bache had given Charles's name to his firstborn—Charles Meigs Bache—who, sadly, passed away shortly after birth. Bache had six children, five of whom were still living when his wife, Aglae, passed away in 1835. Bache, "faithful to her memory," never remarried.

Meigs and Bache made quite a pair. Bache had a full head of hair, thick bushy eyebrows, and a placid, calm sweetness. Meigs was thin, with sallow visage and a large balding head. But they shared a sense of moral righteousness. Both considered themselves austere, honest, and forthright and could not easily lend themselves to any compromise that might lie between right and wrong.

"If I were to describe Franklin Bache, I would speak of him as an entirely upright man—not merely upright in outward dealings, but in thought

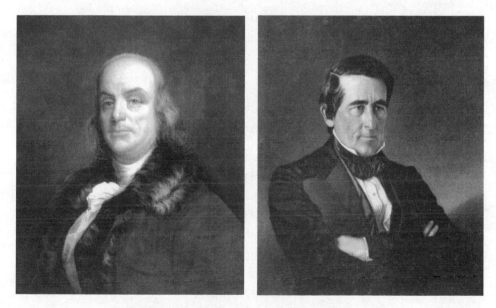

Benjamin Franklin and his great-grandson Franklin Bache

and word and deed," a former student once said of him. "To his mind a matter was either right or wrong, true or false. He could not appreciate, as some do, intermediate shades."

Meigs shared this rigid vision of morality and took it several steps further. If someone in Meigs's family was found guilty of "discrediting" the Meigs name, he simply removed all evidence of them from the family Bible, a tradition he asked his children to keep.

"If all men could be induced to preserve their family records, discarding without mercy every member of their blood-line, whose conduct might stain it," Meigs told his children, "society would derive great security, and virtue a strong support from that course."

"If it should be deemed unfair to ignore discreditable members of a line," he begrudgingly added, "then at least let a mark of disapprobation be set opposite their record."

Unlike Meigs, however, Bache didn't have the best reputation as a teacher. Some argued that his famous family opened doors that would not have been opened for a lesser-known man of similarly limited talents.

"If as a lecturer [Bache] was dull," a colleague would later write of him, "he was earnest and faithful; and the students, if at all intelligent and attentive, could not fail to be instructed by him. But it must be confessed that few of them ever displayed much knowledge of chemistry at their final examination."

But luck was with the old friends, and Franklin Bache—despite stiff competition—was also voted to his position unanimously.

MÜTTER WAS THE YOUNGEST NAME TO BE FORWARDED TO THE Jefferson Medical College board. He was thirty years old, having graduated from medical school only ten years earlier.

Mütter's gifts as a lecturer had been amply demonstrated during the six years he had spent at the Medical Institute, and his reputation—as a surgeon and as a professor—was now firmly established. Still, he faced tough competition with the only other name up for nomination: Joseph Pancoast.

Pancoast was the same surgeon who had beaten McClellan—the founder of Jefferson Medical College—for the coveted chair of surgery. Pancoast was six years older than Mütter and had a reputation as "an extraordinarily versatile man" when it came to medicine. A combination anatomist and surgeon—and prominent in both arenas—he was so skilled across platforms that he was the only doctor to be nominated for more than one chair. In fact, he was nominated for *three*.

Like Mütter, Pancoast was an innovator. He challenged not only how medicine was taught, but how medicine should be practiced. Among his many innovations, Pancoast could claim:

> An early type of cataract surgery (performed while the patient is awake—"a very fine needle, turned near the point into a sort of hook, is introduced three-sixteenths of an inch behind the cornea");

> The invention of the plough and groove, or plastic suture ("in which four raw surfaces, the beveled edges of the flaps, and the margins of the groove cut to receive the flaps, come together");

> A surprisingly "good-looking substitute" for a destroyed eyebrow ("made by raising a flap of the scalp with the soft drooping hairs of the temple, and giving it a long pedicle, to run in a bed cut for it up to the brow");

> And a surgical technique (involving "an abdominal tourniquet with a large roller compress over the lower end of the aorta") that made amputations at or around the hip joint possible, since before Pancoast's innovation, such amputations were "very fatal from the excessive blood loss."

Additionally, Pancoast was known as a man of decided convictions, professional, moral, and political; a kind husband and father; a warm friend; and an upright citizen. Mütter admired Pancoast, and saw in him a potential ally in the work Mütter himself was attempting to do. To Mütter, it seemed as if he and Pancoast shared a common vision: to help free medicine from an inherited body of superstition, both with their patients and within the profession.

As a professor, Pancoast was respected by his peers and his students. And while he earned praise of his work with anatomy, it was Pancoast's surgical prowess that worried Mütter the most.

"He possessed all the attributes of a great operator—quickness of perception, unflinching courage, and rare presence of mind," another surgeon wrote of Pancoast. "It may truly be said of him that his hand never trembled and his eye never winced."

How could Mütter, who was still young both in age and in his career, compete with such a man?

So DESPITE MÜTTER'S GROWING REPUTATION, IT WAS NONETHELESS a surprise that when the votes were cast, it was Mütter, not Pancoast, who was unanimously elected chair for the principles of surgery.

Pancoast was instead elected the chair of anatomy.

And in a surprising move, the college decided to elect a separate chair for the practice of surgery. It was the first time in the institution's history that the study of surgery would be divided in such a way. Pancoast too was up for that position but lost it to Dr. Jacob Randolph, the son-in-law of Philip Syng Physick, whose own work in late-eighteenth-century operating rooms was so profoundly innovative and important that Physick was dubbed the "father of American surgery." But Randolph was utterly unsupportive of splitting the chair of surgery in such a way, and swiftly declined what he saw as a weakened position.

After hearing Randolph's response, the board decided not to split the chairs after all. Instead of having two surgical chairs—one for the "principles" and the other for the "practice" of surgery—they voted to reinstate the one powerful position of chair of surgery. And they voted to give that chair—and the incredible platform it provided—to their youngest and least-tested professor: Thomas Dent Mütter.

Shortly after the election, Philadelphia's frigid weather broke. The thaw was so quick and so great that Philadelphia's Schuylkill River overflowed, flooding into the city almost two full city blocks on each side.

It was equal parts calamity and miracle, for as difficult as the flood was, the city that had felt too long held hostage by the drawn-out winter, finally felt ready for change—no matter the wreckage.

CHAPTER EIGHT

THE NEW JEFFERSON
MEDICAL COLLEGE

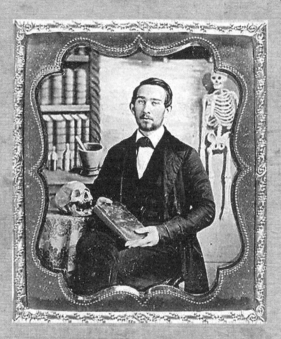

Portrait of a Jefferson Medical College Student

THE PHYSICIAN MUST BE
AN INDUSTRIOUS MAN

Without habits of industry, the finest talents are,
   for the most part, lost.
Each day adds something new
   to the general stock of medical lore,
and it is your bounded duty to diligently
   and carefully investigate
the nature and worth of these additions,
   and endeavor at the same time
to contribute your own might
   towards the elucidation of difficulties,
or the improvement of your art.
Up, then, young men!
You, to whom a future generation has
   to look for the decisions of the questions
   which the feeble light of our day
   prevents us from determining.

Thomas Dent Mütter

THE ADVERTISEMENTS ANNOUNCING THE NEW FACULTY OF Jefferson Medical College began running that summer, and attempted to lure new students in periodicals like *The Boston Medical and Surgical Journal* and *The New York Medical Gazette*:

JEFFERSON MEDICAL COLLEGE.

Session of 1841–42.

The regular Lectures will commence on the last Monday of November.

On and after the first of October, the dissecting room will be open, and the Professor of Anatomy will give his personal attendance thereto. Clinical instruction will likewise be given at the Dispensary of the College.

During the course, ample opportunities will be afforded for clinical instruction; Professors Dunglison, Huston, and Pancoast being medical officers of the Philadelphia Hospital; Professor Meigs of the Pennsylvania Hospital; and Professor Mütter, Surgeon to the Philadelphia Dispensary.

Professor Dunglison will lecture regularly on Clinical Medicine, and Professor Pancoast on Clinical Surgery, at the Philadelphia Hospital, throughout the course.

Added to these facilities, the Museum of the Institution affords essential aid to the student, by its various anatomical, pathological, and obstetrical preparations and drawings, as well as by the diversified specimens of genuine and spurious articles, and plates, drawings, &c. for illustrating the materia medica. These, with the numerous and varied specimens that have been *recently* added from the private collections of the members of the faculty, render the Museum and Cabinets more rich and effective for the purpose of Medical Instruction than they have ever been.

ROBERT M. HUSTON, M.D., *Dean of the Faculty.*

The *New* Jefferson Medical College. That is how the board hoped people would refer to it once the illustrious names of their newly appointed, hand-selected faculty were revealed.

Up until now, the strength of Jefferson had always lain in the personal power of its faculty, and the refined, scholarly Dunglison hoped these men—evenly split between old and new, Northerners and Southerners—would usher in a new era for the vanguard medical institution. And furthermore, that these men would help shape a bolder, more ambitious, more unified vision for what American medicine could be during an important and precarious time in history.

But for now, they had to survive their first year, this brilliant collection of physicians, all with strong personalities, fixed opinions, and the kind of robust, prideful egos that come from making a career of saving people's lives. Now this same group had to compete for resources, attention, and respect from their new peers, their new board, and their new students—and all without bitterly and publicly imploding as other faculties before them had.

FOR THE RETURNING STUDENTS OF JEFFERSON MEDICAL COLLEGE that year, much of their routine seemed the same as it had been in years past . . . at first.

In the morning, the students would enter the Ely Building, the main lecture hall of the college, located on the southwest corner of 10th and Sansom Streets. Recently remodeled to better suit the school's ever-growing population of students, it boasted two "capacious" lecture rooms that could comfortably seat 450 (and seat 550 *uncomfortably*), as well as two additional large halls in the rear of the building.

The first hall would be the territory of Dr. Pancoast, used exclusively for dissecting.

The second hall would be used as an "anatomical museum"—a storage space where professors could keep the physical materials they used in their lectures: models of human faces or body parts made of wood, or wax, or plaster; actual bones, limbs, and organs preserved in jars; and realistic anatomical illustrations, as seen in both paint and pen. It would also be the place where students could view unusual medical specimens and artifacts; for instance, a strange wax model of a French woman with a thick horn growing from her head, donated by the curious new professor of surgery.

Over the years, Mütter had amassed an ambitious collection of unlikely, abnormal, and extraordinary material—intestines pulled from cholera victims; a human heart that had been slowly transforming into bone; cancerous livers, lungs, kidneys, and spines; a cancerous testicle so enlarged by its disease that a special case had to be built to contain it; tumors sliced from noses, throats, eyeballs, and breasts; a finger so brutally ripped from its hand that only a flexor tendon remained attached; a human foot showcasing a horrific compound fracture of the ankle, which had been dried and prepared so that it looked like a wax model . . . but wasn't; the withered heart of a ten-year-old boy whose limbs turned blue because of his body's inability to hold on to oxygen; a wax cast of a hermaphrodite; and much, much more.

"He surrounded himself richly with materials of illustrations," a fellow professor would later write, "to excite, surprise and [inspire] wonder."

Mütter was thrilled to finally have a place to properly store and display his collection. And the students reveled in the chance to examine specimens and artifacts that—up until the moment they fixed their gaze upon them—they had assumed could only be the impossible product of a wild imagination.

For six long hours each day—in frigid cold and relentless heat—students sat upon hard benches in Jefferson's overcrowded lecture rooms, listening to their professors intently while taking notes with journals balanced on their knees, the nibs of their pens dipping often into small pots of ink positioned perilously on the corners of portable writing desks.

Some professors allowed for questions at the end of each lecture, but for the most part, they were largely one-sided affairs. It was the job of the professor to share what he knew, and the job of the student to "task to the utmost [his] powers of memory and analysis."

When evening finally came, the exhausted students would retire to their rented rooms to eat small meals of potatoes, oysters, beer, and bread, and "trim [their] lamps for a toilsome study."

"Many a time, in the midnight rambles of my medical duty, I have looked up from the street to the pale light of the student's room," later recalled John Mitchell, a fellow Jefferson faculty member, "and heaved a sigh at the thought, that one so young and playful should there be thwarting the gentle instincts of his nature."

This was a pattern that would last for months, or even years, as medical students were encouraged to take two yearlong sessions of courses prior to their final examination. At this point, it was the tradition, and the students entering Jefferson Medical College had no reason to think it would change when they first entered Mütter's lecture hall in November of 1841.

MÜTTER STOOD AT THE LECTERN AND WATCHED HIS STUDENTS enter the lecture hall. Novembers were (and are) typically frigid months in Philadelphia, and this one was no exception. The young men stumbled in, looking nearly identical in brown and black coats, their hats pulled down to cover their foreheads and the frozen tips of their exposed ears.

The students hailed from all over the newly formed country: Virginia, New Hampshire, Pennsylvania, Delaware, Ohio, Kentucky, New York, Tennessee, Mississippi, Connecticut, Maryland, Georgia, Maine, Alabama, and South Carolina. There were even men from Canada and Ireland who had traveled all the way to Philadelphia to learn medicine in this institution and from these men.

Mütter greeted each one loudly as they walked in, catching many by surprise. Surely, they thought, this gregarious young man at the lectern must be playing a prank of some sort. After all, it was customary for the professor to wait until the room was full before making his entrance, lest their learned, lauded, and in-demand instructor waste even one second of his precious time.

So who was this strange gentleman—small in stature and delicately framed, with a clear blue eye, high forehead, and thick black hair—who waited for them at the lectern, greeted them ardently, and asked them their names?

The experience only grew odder with Mütter's lecture. He began by speaking about the state of medicine, as the other professors had done before him. He was a charismatic presence from his first utterance, possessing a wonderfully musical voice, which, even in its lowest notes, could be distinctly heard throughout any of Jefferson's large lecture halls. His gestures were relaxed and comfortable, and his speech was smart and sharply prepared.

But while his speech was buoyed often by the great charm of his enthusiasm, it seemed oddly marred by long stretches of silence, when Mütter peered into the audience with a curious, expectant smile.

This behavior made no sense to the students. Mütter seemed so confident, and yet, when he came to a question in his speech—whether it was theoretical in nature, or steeped in known facts—he would stop, as if he were actually inviting the students to answer the question.

Finally, one student took the bait. From the depths of the lecture hall, a clear voice broke the silence and offered up an answer to one of Mütter's questions.

The students froze as Mütter quickly turned to locate the source of that clear voice and locked his eyes with the young man's. Mütter smiled brightly and thanked him for his contribution, before adding that he hoped more students would follow his lead and be so bold.

It was a strange beginning to what would be an equally strange year.

MÜTTER WAS THE FIRST PROFESSOR TO INTRODUCE THIS INFORmal style of teaching—referred to in Europe as the Edinburgh "quizzing" system—into the United States. While the other professors at Jefferson Medical College continued to give lectures traditionally—a one-way conversation with the students—Mütter's method was to actively engage with them. Instead of simply telling the students what he knew and leaving it at that, he engaged in an almost Socratic dialogue with them, challenging them with questions designed to tap into their instincts—and sometimes their biases—before telling them, or often demonstrating for them, the correct line of thinking. And then afterward, he would "quiz" them again to make sure they absorbed the lesson. It was something American students had never encountered before, and it proved extremely effective.

"I can well remember him in my student days, as he stood in yonder amphitheatre, beloved, nay almost worshipped, by his class," a former Jefferson student would later recall of Mütter. "His observation was quick, and he never failed to note at a glance the effect of his words, even upon the dullest listener . . . he always strove to lecture up to his highest mark, for he was conscious of his powers, and fond of that public approbation which their exertion invariably brought him."

Mütter's reputation as riveting lecturer also partly owed to his habit of bringing specimens to class, those he kept safely stored at the school's anatomical museum as well as those from his personal collection. And to his students, the volume of diagrams, models, and specimens collected from around the world seemed nearly limitless. There didn't seem to be an injury, disease, malady, or treatment for which Mütter couldn't seem to produce a relevant sample, and he would weave these specimens into his lectures mas-terfully, "so as to impress yet not confuse."

This was, perhaps, the great hallmark of Mütter's vision of what it meant to be a teacher. While many of his peers on the faculty adored the distance and superiority they felt as professors—that powerful chasm that separates the *learned* from the *learners*—Mütter was devoted to shrinking that very same gap. He was fiercely invested in presenting lectures that engaged with students, but his command of his subject matter also allowed him to change his lectures on the spot, if doing so would better follow the interests of his class.

"[Mütter's] kindness and enthusiastic devotion to the interests of the student, his brilliant eloquence, his finished and clear style, and polished, gentlemanly manners, gained for him the love, admiration and respect of the class," another former Jefferson student would write. "It has been fre-quently the case that medical teachers . . . have a distaste for the slow incul-cating of elementary matters or principles, but delight to revel before the bewildered [student] about some of the latest theories, or expatiate at length upon other complexities which are to him incomprehensible. With Dr. Mütter, the solid groundwork of the great superstructure was laid before the student in such a plain and impressive manner, as to be clearly under-stood by him, before he was led up to its more complex and ornate develop-ments."

But if Mütter's warm treatment of students—bright young men who paid for the privilege to be taught by him—seemed alarmingly odd to some of his peers, they would be even more ill-prepared for how he would treat his own patients.

CHAPTER NINE

THE RIGHT ARM OF
THE COLLEGE

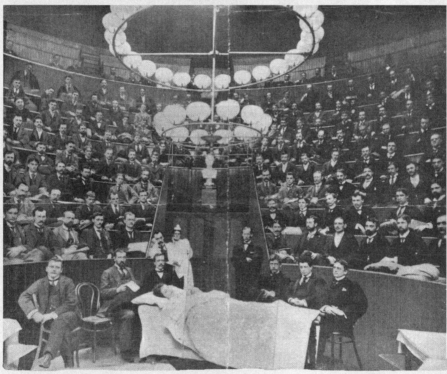

"The Pit"

GEORGE McCLELLAN FOUNDED JEFFERSON MEDICAL COLLEGE with the insistence that it include the country's first collegiate clinic, a medical facility where students could watch as their professors treated actual patients. The clinic—which accepted patients in need of both medical and surgical care—was a prominent feature in the weekly curriculum.

The people who came to the Jefferson Medical College clinic to seek treatment were mostly those who were too poor to pay for it elsewhere, but a significant number were members of the working and middle class whose complicated cases required a professor's skill. But there were no restrictions on who could add their name to the list of potential patients for use as teaching examples. And what started off as a strange idea to both the medical community and the pool of potential patients was soon embraced by both.

Within months, patients were eagerly lining up for the opportunity to receive effective treatments (even if they did have to receive those treatments in front of a room full of strangers dutifully taking notes), and the American medical community would embrace Jefferson Medical College's teaching clinic as an important and necessary advancement in the education of physicians of every stripe.

The clinic had already become an emblematic "stamp" of the school by the time Mütter first stepped into its operating room. It was often referred to as the right arm of the college, and the board that hired Mütter felt his charismatic and ambitious surgical lectures would only serve to bring the clinic to new heights.

"Brilliant as Dr. Mütter was in his didactic teachings," one of his students later wrote, "he surpassed himself in the clinical arena."

And yet almost immediately upon first stepping into that arena, Mütter saw things he wanted to change . . . and it didn't take him very long to begin taking steps to change them.

MÜTTER HAD ALREADY DEVELOPED A HEALTHY MEDICAL PRACTICE of his own by the time he became a professor at Jefferson Medical College. His reputation, his charm with his patients, and his undeniable skill had attracted a large following of his fellow Philadelphians—citizens of every class who sought out his talent and his help. But it was more than just his quick fingers and attentive eyes that drew people to him.

Mütter's methodical nature and utter focus before, during, and after the surgery was unprecedented—as was the amount of empathy and kindness he displayed for those under his care.

Many nineteenth-century physicians considered it a necessary part of their job to keep their patients in the dark about what exactly would be done to them during treatment. Surgeons especially felt that once the patient had agreed to an operation, it was their responsibility to the patient to proceed with the operation no matter what . . . no matter how loud the patient might scream in protest throughout the procedure, or how violently he or she struggled or resisted, verbally or physically.

Mütter, on the other hand, believed in transparency. Inspired by his own experiences on the other side of the doctor-patient relationship, Mütter faithfully explained to patients about their medical circumstances, and gave them their options plainly and clearly. He did not downplay the risks they might be taking, or the pain they would likely be tasked to endure.

While other members of the medical community—including some among his school's own faculty—assumed that patients would be scared away by this sort of frank dialogue, Mütter saw firsthand that his patients were grateful for it.

Furthermore, Mütter was known for putting "considerable emphasis" on the care and attention he paid to patients prior to performing the operation. He would not only develop a bond with the patient via gentle, consistent communication, but would also physically as well as mentally prepare them. He showed them the tools he would use, and he began to get the body parts slated for surgery "accustomed to manipulation," by massaging each by hand and touching the most sensitive areas with clean surgical instruments or fingers for several days prior to the operation. It was a unique approach to medicine, one that Mütter seemed to have invented out of whole cloth.

Professional distance was the standard in American medicine and elsewhere. Even the French surgeons Mütter held up as heroes were famous for the callous manner in which they treated their patients. Guillaume Dupuytren—the French surgeon whom Mütter admired most, and whose technique he studied extensively during his time as an *interne* in Paris— was accused of treating his patients worse than one would treat livestock when it came to presenting them before his students.

"If his orders are not immediately obeyed, [Dupuytren] thinks nothing of striking his patient or abusing him most harshly," remembered an American medical student studying in Paris. "A very favorite practice of his during his consultation is to make a handle of the noses of his patients. Whenever a man enters with any disease of the head, he is immediately seized by the nose and pulled down onto his knees where he remains half in sorrow and half in anger at the treatment until he is allowed to rise and describe his disease."

But it wasn't just preparing for his surgery in which Mütter invested his time. He also believed strongly in aftercare, ensuring that the difficult work he did as a surgeon would not be undone later by simple infection, the tearing of delicate stitches from careless movement, or any other preventable calamity. He examined his patients several times a day after surgery, checking and cleaning their wounds, deciding new treatment strategies and even strictly monitoring what the patient ate or drank—not just the types of foods and beverages, but their volume and frequency as well.

Because of this care, Mütter's work and reputation rose above that of his contemporaries. He took on the abysmal realities of nineteenth-century medicine—the need to perform incredibly complex surgeries on patients who were wide-awake, in unsterilized environments that were lit only by candle, lamp, or daylight—yet he was still able to heal the sick and restore the wasted and withered to strength and health. And when it came to his plastic surgery, he could transform the deformed to wholeness.

Jefferson Medical College's surgical clinic was housed in a beautiful amphitheater. It was a large, well-lit space with a sizable surgical table in its center. Students sat in rows of wooden benches, which encircled the main "stage" in increasing heights to ensure everyone had a good view. The dark wood was kept cleaned and polished. Numerous lamps cast a golden glow

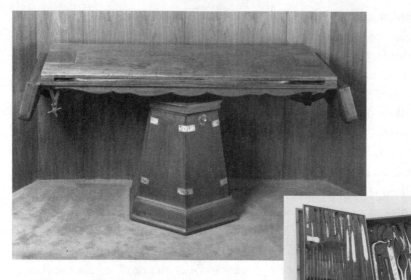

Jefferson Medical College's Operating Table and
Surgeon's Amputation Kit

over the room and its tense occupants. The clinic was a pride of the school,
a true jewel in Jefferson's crown.

Mütter saw it as incredibly lacking.

It wasn't the surgical amphitheater itself that drew his ire. Of course, he
felt honored to be performing his craft in a space that was so beautiful, so
cared for, and so well lit. Rather, he disliked the implication that the surgical experience was limited to just that one room—the operating room. It
seemed to utterly ignore the important and various facets of surgical treatment that Mütter deeply valued and which took place outside of the room's
narrow confines.

Mütter was appalled to learn that after patients underwent operations
before the students in the amphitheater of the college, they were sent immediately home in a carriage. There were no recovery beds—let alone recovery rooms—where patients who had just endured painful surgeries
could rest and receive further care and observation.

It didn't matter if the surgery was simple or complex, if the wound
was tightly sown or strained and weeping, or if the patient felt well or disori-
ented. Regardless of their condition, they would be put into a rarely cleaned
carriage whose wooden wheels would clatter and jump against Philadelphia's
uneven cobblestone streets for as long as it took to reach their destination.

Mütter could hardly imagine a more cruel follow-up to the emotional and physical trauma of surgery.

It was enough that patients had to endure the operation itself; to then subject them to the risk of infection, injury, and completely unnecessary pain by transporting them home without rest seemed needlessly brutal, in addition to being completely and medically unhelpful.

To Mütter, the solution seemed obvious. Jefferson Medical College should build its own hospital—a teaching hospital that could be the first of its kind in the country. But since that would take some time, a temporary solution would be to rent some rooms in the area to serve as the recovery rooms that were so desperately needed.

He shared his idea with his colleague, Dr. John Kearsley Mitchell, the chair of medicine, whom he thought might be a friendly ear. Mitchell was eighteen years older than Mütter, but they were both native Virginians who shared a Scottish ancestry.

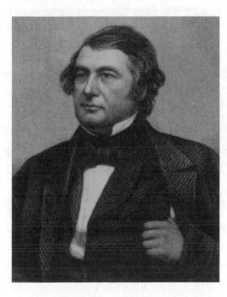

John Kearsley Mitchell

Mitchell—a handsome man, tall and portly, with a gentle, polished bearing—was born into a family of doctors. Not only were his father and grandfather doctors, he would have a son and grandson who would become physicians too.

But he was far from conventional. He wore his brown hair severely combed from left to right, which gave the unfortunate impression that he was trying to cover up a bald spot. He often wore a scarab ring on his left middle finger, a souvenir from his "oriental travels," and relished how people would "imagine the thrilled mystery centered about this ring." Indeed, Mitchell had spent several globe-trotting years on a merchant ship bound to Calcutta and Canton, before settling in Philadelphia as a practitioner.

Mütter liked how much Mitchell was invested in the lives of his students, how they often considered him their friend and not just their professor.

"In sickness and trouble, they turned to him, and they never sought his aid in vain," it would later be written of Mitchell. "Many a poor young fellow, struggling in the vortex of a great city's temptation, has he sustained by his wise counsel and kindly sympathy. Many a needy student has he helped from his own purse, and none the wiser."

Mitchell was more than just a kind teacher; he was a thoughtful and pragmatic physician. He was also among the first advocates of the germ theory of disease, the idea that some diseases were caused by organisms too small to see with the human eye which invaded humans, animals, and other living hosts, and it was the growth and reproduction of these organisms that caused disease.

This theory flew in the face of the common prevailing thoughts on the subject—especially the long-standing miasma theory, which pinned the cause of many diseases on "bad air" the infected person had breathed. When epidemics broke out, doctors did not think diseases spread because the infection was passed from person to person. Rather, it was broadly assumed that all parties infected had breathed the same poisonous vapor or mist, and doctors claimed this bad air was incredibly easy to identify—and thus avoid—because of its foul smell.

Mütter believed that Mitchell's forward-thinking philosophies might make him a fantastic ally in convincing the board to expand its one-room clinic into a decent hospital, where the patients could be protected and cared for properly . . . and Mütter was right.

Together, Mütter and Mitchell worked toward their now shared vision. Between the two of them, they were able to find a building with grounds close to the college that could easily be repurposed for a hospital and that was available for purchase at minimal cost. Mütter was elated at this development and immediately put forth a petition that the Jefferson Medical College board move forward with the plan as soon as possible.

But the petition was summarily rejected. The board felt that building a collegiate hospital was simply unnecessary, and no amount of persuasive argument from Mitchell or Mütter could change their minds. It was a crushing blow, especially to Mütter, who could not hide his frustration with the decision.

"Mütter, he of the musical voice and charming personality, Mütter, the debonair, the eloquent, the enthusiastic, the beloved of the class," a Jefferson Medical College alumnus would later write, "had wished the institution to build a hospital in 1841, but was defeated by the stupidity against which . . . even the gods fight in vain. . . .

"But that didn't diminish his love of Jefferson," he added, "and the potential he saw."

"In his love for the Jefferson College, in his pride in its present, in his faith in its future, [Mütter] was second to none," another former student wrote. "He believed that the Institution was second to none. He believed that the Institution was entering a great era."

Unable to teach the way he wanted to in Jefferson's legendary surgical clinic, Mütter simply decided to perform surgeries elsewhere.

He knew Jefferson Medical College had a relationship with the Pennsylvania Hospital and so he would take whole classes to witness surgical lectures in a space that he thought was better suited for it.

The classes at Jefferson Medical College were large; Mütter needed an equally large way to transport them. His solution was to rent the biggest omnibus he could find—pulled by three horses with seating on top as well as inside of the vehicle. Nonetheless, students often had to crowd in to ensure that everyone could fit. The sight of so many students piled into one vehicle, bustling and shouting as they made their way across the cobblestone streets, proved to be more comical than academic. "This disorderly transportation was an event of great delight to all small urchins on route," one student later recalled, "and afforded in winter, as I well recollect, inestimable chances for snowballing and boyish sharp-shooting."

Mütter's care, attentiveness, and willingness to engage made him a favorite with his students and his patients, but he was also earning the respect of some of his peers on the faculty, especially Joseph Pancoast—whose position as chair of surgery Mütter had usurped.

At first glance, Pancoast was an intimidating sight. A large man in both height and weight, his face was obscured by his thick wavy hair, which curled at his temples. His eyes were overwhelmed by heavy eyebrows, his cheeks and chin were obscured by a variety of unkempt beard and mustache combinations that he audaciously trotted out. Being an active surgeon and anatomist, Pancoast always chose to dress for ease of movement, not for style. In fact, even formal portraits of him often show his tie and clothing askew.

But while the sharply dressed, cleanly shaven Mütter and the hirsute, slovenly Pancoast may have differed in their approaches to fashion, they found ample common ground in their philosophies about teaching medicine.

Like Mütter, Pancoast took great pains to teach the very complicated subject of anatomy in a way that allowed his lessons to be absorbed easily and quickly.

"He made anatomy so plain," a peer once wrote of him, "that the dullest pupil, if at all attentive, could not fail to be enlightened."

As a physician and surgeon, it was said that Pancoast had one flaw—and it was perhaps this defect that kept him from retaining his position as Jefferson's chair of surgery: He was a poor pathologist. That is, when he was presented with an ailing patient, one could not be assured his diagnosis of the problem would be correct. It was a poor weakness to have when a person's life was at stake.

Still, once a diagnosis was correctly made, Pancoast's skills at surgically resolving the issue were nearly unrivaled.

"Pancoast, the dexterous, the dramatic," a former student gushingly wrote about watching his professor at work in the operating room, "with a hand as steady as a rock, but as light as a floating perfume; with a heart that was a stranger to fear, and with an eye as quick as a flashing sunbeam."

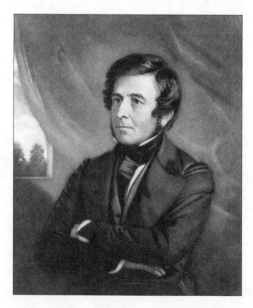

Joseph Pancoast

As the only faculty member whose chair had been usurped—let alone usurped by the faculty's youngest and most inexperienced member—it had been uncertain what relationship, if any, Pancoast and Mütter would have.

But it turned out they were admirers of each other's work and shared similar senses of humor, similar values, and similar aspirations for moving forward the art of surgery. Soon, they began to visit each other's lectures and, perhaps most amazing of all, calling upon each other for assistance in the operating room. And Pancoast began to publicly appreciate Mütter's unorthodox but crowd-pleasing style of teaching.

"You have but just now listened to a lively and instructive lecture from my friend and colleague the Professor of Surgery," Pancoast told a class of students still settling down from their latest lecture with Mütter, "and I trust you have been so well entertained and put in so good a humor as to listen at this late hour of the evening, with patience and with kindness, to that which I have now the honor to address to you."

While other doctors may have held a grudge or let awkward tension drive a wedge between them, Mütter and Pancoast chose to "work in seemingly perfect harmony" and a lifelong friendship was forged.

"Mütter and Pancoast, Pancoast and Mütter," a former student would write, "each striving to assist the other [in] the alleviation of human suffering, the welfare of the surgical clinic, and the advancement of the honor and renown of the Jefferson Medical College."

HOWEVER, NOT EVERYONE IN THE MEDICAL COMMUNITY WAS SO welcoming to the young, eccentric Mütter.

Some felt that his type of clinical instruction should be denounced and "sneered at." They accused it of being imperfect, insufficient, and unrealistic, and alleged that Mütter was conveying a false impression of what a doctor's role should be. They criticized his lectures, saying that his lessons were designed to theatrically mislead rather than instruct.

Some were openly disappointed in Jefferson Medical College for even hiring him, a neophyte who they felt was not the best surgeon, nor the best teacher, and whose contributions to surgical literature were completely lacking.

His critics would rail that the adoration of his students had more to do with "his personal attractions, features, voice and bearing" than his skill or merit, and bitterly accused him of "playing for popularity" in his lectures.

"In no period in our medical history was rivalry so marked with jealousy and unfairness," a peer noted. "Medical lore and literature contain ample evidence of the personal abuse and criticism which medical men showered upon one another and of the acrimony which characterized the discussion and unwarranted jealousy that we have in America."

And as it turns out, one of Mütter's biggest critics could be found among his fellow members of the Jefferson Medical College faculty.

CHARLES D. MEIGS HAD WAITED HIS ENTIRE CAREER TO BECOME the chair of obstetrics at a nationally renowned medical college. Twenty-five years after moving to Philadelphia as "a Varginny student"—what Philadelphians charmingly called any medical student whose accent gave away his Southern roots—he felt this appointment gave him the first opportunity of showing fully what was in him.

Meigs's original dream had been to return to the South after graduating, to serve as a glowing example of American medicine down there, but his wife, Mary, derailed those plans. Mary had always lived in what Meigs saw as the sheltered North, and she was horrified by some of the brutal scenes that were commonplace in slave states: public auctions where wailing mothers were torn from their children; freshly beaten slaves whose wounds leaked through their tattered clothing; an entire culture that was utterly comfortable in treating their fellow human beings like chattel. Unable to stomach it any longer, she insisted under no certain terms that they return to the North at once.

Her ultimatum would prove fortuitous for Meigs. Once appointed to its influential faculty, he threw himself into being a Jefferson Medical College professor with the greatest ardor, studying all the literature he could about obstetrics and women's health in all six languages that he spoke and read.

"He took great pleasure in his lectures during the first years that he occupied the chair," his son would later recall. "They were a constant and agreeable stimulus to his mind, and, being new ground for him, broke into the tedium of his daily routine work among the sick.

"Being thoroughly versed in all his subjects, and having a most active mind and lively imagination, which readily felt the stimulus of large classes and a sympathetic audience, he was roused to efforts which this new field alone served to bring forth," he continued, "and to show to himself and to others what latent powers he had."

But while Mütter and Meigs shared a passion for their new roles, their approaches to medicine and teaching could not have been more different. It didn't take long for the simplest things to cause discord between them.

While Mütter taught his students to spend days slowly desensitizing the parts of a patient's body that would be subject to surgery, through gentle touch and massage, Meigs taught that one shouldn't "bother too much" when it came to patients' comfort, instructing them to absolutely avoid "fussing about," for example, when their female patients were in labor. He encouraged students to follow his lead and simply "read and write in another room until the delivery [is] ready."

Though the concept of sepsis—the idea of diseases being spread by doctors through contaminated tools and unwashed hands—would not be widely accepted for four more decades, Mütter seemed to understand the dangers of doctors not keeping their hands, clothing, tools, and surgical areas clean.

Though *antisepsis* was not a term or concept used at the time, Mütter was known to be very "clean" in his technique and worked under "as near an aseptic technique as was possible at the time." His diligence continued after the surgery as well. At a time when the use of poultice—a moist, warm porridge of meal and seeds—to seal wounds was still very popular because doctors were unaware that they were providing a near-perfect breeding ground for bacteria, Mütter spoke out against this "filthy abomination." Instead, he encouraged his students to use a "mild, clean, and simple warm water dressing" to aid in healing open surgical wounds.

Charles D. Meigs did not share Mütter's views on the subject of doctorly fastidiousness. At his popular obstetrics practice, Meigs saw numerous women throughout the day and thought nothing of examining each one using largely unwashed equipment, including his own unwashed hands. A simple rinse with water—if he believed it was needed—was sufficient for Meigs when it came to his hands, tools, and sponges. He wore a single work frock until the end of the day, regardless of how many patients he saw and no matter how stained it might become with blood, pus, or other fluids.

He vigorously and publicly disagreed with those who believed that diseases were spread by doctors, and refused to give in to those who insisted on aggressive washing of hands and tools. Meigs felt that doing so would imply that "doctors were not gentlemen" because "all gentlemen were clean men."

It seemed an odd stance to take in a city that had been—and continued to be—terrorized by infectious diseases. But Meigs had reason to feel confident in his opinions, considering his professional history. After all, when the cholera epidemic hit Philadelphia in 1832, Meigs was one of the handful of doctors to receive a silver pitcher of recognition from the city council for the "heroic role of the medical profession in battling the infection."

And he lived in a time when the concept of medical sterilization was so unrecognized that the appearance of pus in an infected postoperative wound was "welcomed as harbinger of a successful surgical outcome."

Soon the school seemed to be dividing into two: the partnership of Thomas Dent Mütter and Joseph Pancoast on one side, and Charles D. Meigs and his longtime friend and chair of chemistry Franklin Bache on the other.

Still, that first year, Mütter and Meigs kept any disagreements private. Perhaps both of them wanted to make a good impression on the Jefferson Medical College board. If the board was so powerful it could fire George McClellan, the college's own founder, perhaps it was wise to keep their conflicts to themselves.

NEITHER MÜTTER NOR MEIGS WOULD HAVE ANY IDEA DURING the 1841–1842 session that this would be only the first of fifteen years that they would teach side by side. And not just the two of them. The entire faculty—who'd earned the nickname the Faculty of '41—would remain united in an unprecedented fifteen-year reign at Jefferson Medical College, and later would be called "one of the most illustrious faculties in the history of American medical education."

Nor could they have imagined that amid the chaos of the years to come—the infighting, the public battles, the private slights, the life-and-death issues that faced not only medicine but the entire country—that this community of doctors would usher in a period of remarkable prosperity and growth, a period of the true rise and healthy growth of the school, which later would be described as "the golden age of the second great School of Medicine in Philadelphia."

All Mütter knew was that he had survived his first year, and he wanted to at least celebrate that accomplishment.

Perhaps he would host an extravagant dinner prepared by the city's best French chef, the well-known M. Latouche, who was famous for pairing his cellar's choicest wines with such decadent meals as oyster pies made with one hundred oysters, or eight quails roasted and larded to perfection, or even a whole hog's head trimmed with jelly, which alone cost as much as an average Philadelphia weaver was paid for half a week's work.

Or perhaps Mütter would reward himself with several new silk suits—each in a brighter color than the last and trimmed in delicate ribbon.

But he suddenly knew what he wanted: to commission a portrait of himself by famed Philadelphia painter Thomas Sully.

A Sully portrait was practically a tradition among the Philadelphia elite, proof that you had made it. Despite Mütter's new income and status as a Jefferson Medical College professor, he still struggled with what he believed was a lack of respect within the larger community. In many ways, he still felt like an outsider.

"The mere acquisition of great wealth did not guarantee admission to the ranks of Philadelphia's upper class," a British writer traveling through Philadelphia observed. "The exclusive feature of American society is no where brought so broadly out as it is in the city of Philadelphia. It is, of course, readily discernible in Boston, New York, and Baltimore; but the line drawn in these places is not so distinctive or so difficult to transcend as it is in Philadelphia."

Still, Mütter felt the success of his first year was a step in the right direction, and he wanted Sully to capture that in a portrait that would be uniquely Mütter.

Unlike the stern-faced portraits popular among doctors at that time, the small oval oil painting by Sully shows Mütter as an almost romantic vision. His thick dark hair tousled from his face in an unselfconscious pompadour. His pink cheeks are flushed, his eyes bright, his mouth curled up into a sly smile.

Opting out of one of his bright-colored suits, Mütter instead wears a brown coat with high stiff white collar, black bengaline cravat tied in a flat bow in front, and a white pleated jabot. The glossy dark brown fur of his shawl collar pops against the pastel pink of the background.

It was the portrait of a man who seemed certain of his bright future. He had no idea what was to come.

PART TWO

THE PHYSICIAN SHOULD HAVE
A REVERENCE FOR HIS ART

In every village in our land, the parson, the lawyer,
and the doctor are the "great men of the place,"
and none stands higher than the doctor.
Whose friendship is more highly prized;
Whose name is so often coupled with expressions
of gratitude, and love, and confidence;
Whose visit is more anxiously expected or more warmly
received; whose cheerful smiles and kindly
expressions so readily banish gloom and sorrow;
Whose hand is so eagerly grasped by the devoted wife
when she thanks him for the care with which he has
watched over her husband, herself, or her children;
Into whose ear is the tale of private griefs, hidden
sorrows, blighted hopes, and dreadful anticipations
of the future, so readily poured forth!
Be ye sure, gentlemen, that such a position is . . .
an object worthy of the utmost desire, and
is a reward more "precious than rubies,"
for the fatigue, anxieties, and sorrows,
with which the pursuit of his calling
is almost necessarily attended.

Thomas Dent Mütter

CHAPTER TEN

DWELL NOT THEN UPON WHAT HAS BEEN DONE

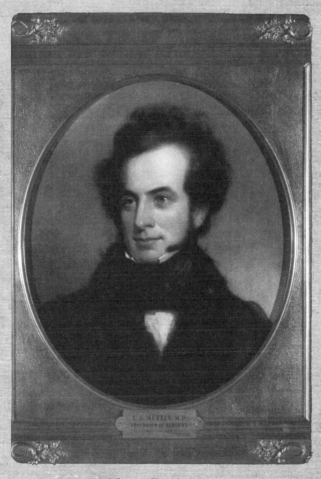

Thomas Dent Mütter,
Portrait by Thomas Sully

THE LETTER ARRIVED A FEW DAYS AFTER MÜTTER BEGAN HIS second year of teaching at Jefferson Medical College.

Philadelphia, Nov 10, 1842
To Professor Mütter.

Dear Sir,

   At a meeting of the Class of Jefferson Medical College, held on Monday the 7th instant, Thomas K. Price, of Virginia, having been called to the chair, it was resolved, unanimously, to publish your very able and eloquent Introductory Lecture to the present Class. The undersigned being appointed a Committee to solicit a copy, do earnestly add their wishes to those of the Class, that you will comply with their request, which will ever be appreciated by them, and by us individually, as a source of the most grateful remembrances.

The students closed their letter:

We have the honor to subscribe ourselves,
   Your most obedient servants

before signing their names.

IT WAS A PROMISING START FOR THE NEW SCHOOL YEAR.

Enrollment at Jefferson Medical College had increased by more than fifty percent between the Faculty of '41's first year and their second. In this watershed moment for the school, the board's decision to take the college in a new direction two years earlier had now proven triumphant. The sounds of almost 350 students settling into their wooden benches on that first day served as a comforting anthem for the school, one that seemed to portend a bright future.

Mütter, in particular, seemed to shine in this new spotlight.

"No one who attended his lectures could deny their intrinsic excellence," Joseph Pancoast would later write. "He sought diligently what was good and valuable, wherever it was to be found and, passing it through the alembic of his own mind, added to it, from his large experience, an amount of novelty which was by no means inconsiderable."

The affirming invitation from his new class of students to publish his introductory lecture was irresistible. Mütter replied to their request almost immediately.

Philadelphia, Nov 12, 1842

Gentlemen—Your note requesting a copy of my Introductory Lecture for publication, has just been received, and it will afford me pleasure to comply with the wishes of the Class. Be pleased to accept my thanks for the flattering manner in which you have conveyed the sentiments of those whom you represent, and believe me to be

VERY TRULY YOURS,

THOS. D. MÜTTER

The lecture, "a retrospective view of surgery for the last few years," would be only Mütter's second publication. His first, *The Salt Sulphur Springs, Monroe County, Va.*, had been a disaster.

THAT FIRST PUBLICATION WAS INSPIRED BY MÜTTER'S 1834 VISIT to the Virginia spa. He had made the trip with the primary hope of restoring his health, but once there, he couldn't resist slyly investigating the spa's claims of having "healing waters"—a claim not uncommon among such retreats. His charm had earned him clientele among the spa's visitors, providing him with an up-close view of the effects the salt sulphur springs were having on those who longed to be healed by them.

His conclusions, meticulously detailed in his article, were not flattering. While he gave credit to the agreeable temperature and dry atmosphere of the springs, which he stated were an advantage for those seeking treatment for lung-related issues, he asserted quite emphatically that the waters themselves did *not* have any curative properties, and especially did not cure cases of consumption (now called tuberculosis), a power the owners of the springs boldly claimed they held.

The article was published in 1840, six years after Mütter's visit, and was swiftly regarded as heresy by defenders of the springs, both within and outside the medical community.

A significant portion of the medical profession of that era recommended the therapeutic merits of such springs, and the general public had embraced them also. To take a public stand against the springs was to make all the people who believed in the springs, and the doctors who recommended them, appear foolish, uneducated, and gullible. It was not the best first impression for Mütter to make with his debut article.

Not to mention, the springs were big business. Enormously popular and well patronized, they were massively profitable, so the proprietors had a vested interest in maintaining the illusion that mineral springs could cure the sick.

Mütter's critical exposé earned him the displeasure of one specific spring owner by the name of William Burke. Burke was a physician—or at least happily claimed to be—and was less than enthusiastic about Mütter's comments on the efficacy of springs. Burke's reaction was to treat the article with scorn, and to attempt to publicly discredit Mütter.

Since Mütter had chosen to introduce climate into the argument, Burke went on to give him a proper lesson on the subject in a short book titled *The Mineral Springs of Western Virginia, with Remarks on Their Use and the Diseases to Which They Are Applicable,* published shortly after Mütter's findings went public.

"It is well known," Burke pointed out, "that an excess of oxygen in the air is detrimental to the consumptive who gains no benefit from 'pure mountain air' which actually counteracts the effects of mineral waters and other internal remedies."

This line of argument ignored the fact that many owner-proprietors bottled and sold mineral water to those unable to come to springs, and reaped considerable profits from them.

"One need look no further for confirmation on this point than the advice of the celebrated Dr. Beddoes, so eminent in consumptive cases, who recommends to his patients, thus afflicted, to sleep over cow-houses, where the proportion of oxygen in the air is less, and that of azote [i.e., nitrogen] great," Burke continued, using half-truths and quasi-science—including the above Dr. Beddoes, whose advice about the healing properties of sleeping in an unvented room above piles of fresh cow manure was apparently accepted as being medically sound—to build a public case against Mütter.

Mütter stood by the conclusions he stated in *The Salt Sulphur Springs, Monroe County, Va.*, but he also recognized the timing of this controversy was incredibly poor. His appointment to Jefferson Medical College was fresh, and he felt pressure to recant and head off any further criticism that could spring up in the face of the "overwhelming evidence" Burke provided.

Begrudgingly, Mütter wrote a public semi-apology to Burke that was dated November 9, 1841—exactly three weeks before classes started under the Faculty of '41 at Jefferson Medical College. In it, he wrote:

> I have said to many, as I would say to you or any well-informed
> physician, that the Red Sulphur never yet cured a case of tubercular
> consumption, and you know as well as I do that such is the fact, for
> there is no cure for the disease. But I have always said privately and
> publicly that the Red Sulphur was a most valuable water in many cases
> resembling consumption. Not only have I said this, but I have sent you
> many a patient, and hope to send you many more. Very truly your
> friend and well-wisher,
>
> THOS. D. MÜTTER

Whether Burke ever realized Mütter's sneaky double entendre in "well-wisher" remains unknown—but he made no mention of it when he would later publish the letter, in its entirety, in his own book on the subject. A book that, of course, praised the springs.

STILL, MÜTTER MUST HAVE BEEN HEARTENED THAT HIS SECOND publication would follow so swiftly, and under far less duress. Publishing was an important step to establishing a doctor's reputation in the mid-nineteenth century, and Mütter was extremely lacking in that area. Every other professor at Jefferson Medical College had either written or edited one or more textbooks, or had one on the way. Mütter had one highly controversial article . . . and a related public apology. This new publication of his lecture on surgery was exactly what he needed.

O N

RECENT IMPROVEMENTS IN SURGERY.

AN

INTRODUCTORY LECTURE

TO THE COURSE ON THE

PRINCIPLES AND PRACTICE OF SURGERY,

IN

JEFFERSON MEDICAL COLLEGE

OF PHILADELPHIA.

DELIVERED NOVEMBER 3, 1842.

BY THOMAS D. MÜTTER, M.D.

PUBLISHED BY THE CLASS.

PHILADELPHIA:
Merrihew & Thompson, Printers,
No. 7 Carter's Alley.

1842.

The introductory lecture—one of three Mütter lecture-speeches that Jefferson Medical College would publish in his lifetime—gives compelling insight into what surgery was like at the time, and Mütter's grandiose vision of it.

"The renown of an art, the noblest of all," Mütter theatrically wrote of his chosen field, "the first and last and only object of which is the alleviation of human suffering."

Still, Mütter seems self-conscious about his reputation as a doctor who was a little too eager to believe and share the latest medical advancements.

"This has been called the *age of progression*—the *age of advancement*," he begins, "and our profession, gentlemen, has partaken of the general excitement. It may with truth be said, that of late it has exhibited much of the 'freshness and vigor of youth.' . . . None can urge now as in former times, that we continue in a state of comparative apathy, and content ourselves with servilely following the dictates of our predecessors.

"A contrary disposition, indeed, seems to prevail, we are too anxious to be known as *active* men, and hence crude theories, senseless innovations, and not seldom injurious practical measures, have been crowded into the science."

Mütter swiftly changes direction, chastising those who reject new ideas too easily, as well as those who are aggressively critical in the hopes that it will make them look more impressive—rather than taking the risk of being seen as open-minded to ideas that could radically change medicine for the better.

"But it is a surprising as well as humiliating reflection, that even with all this energy and vigor, with all the lights of modern science to guide us, with all the accumulated facts, *false* as well as true, of the crowd of laborers in the field, there should exist such diversity of opinion on subjects of the most constant observation," Mütter wrote. "No operation, no theoretical opinion, no mode of practice is broached, but there at once springs up a controversy attended, too often, with an acrimony and harshness disgraceful to all concerned.

"And why does this obscurity arise? It may be traced, gentlemen, to our eagerness to become known as *discoverers*, as the inventors of something *new*, as the great *lights* of the age; in conclusion, ere the facts upon which these conclusions are based have been properly investigated. We have, in truth, '*Rested contented in ideal knowledge*'; we have received as perfect, theories idle as day-dreams, and the foundations of our art must crumble to the earth, unless we learn more discretion and better judgment in the selection of the materials of which they are to be constructed."

From this starting point, Mütter engages the class with a discussion of modern advancements in surgery—both European and American—but not before warning them that "the numerous operations to be discussed have been as indiscreetly puffed and eulogized, as they have been injudiciously and hastily condemned." But thanks to "patient and unprejudiced investigation, aided by experience and reason," wrote Mütter, they can now be placed "in their true light."

He then continues sharing his thoughts about the innovations of his age, including the use of microscopes ("a new field of investigation, besides throwing a flood of light upon a subject hitherto the most obscure") and the ongoing mystery of cancer ("I fear much remains to be done ere we arrive at its true origin and proper treatment"). And he gives praise to unusual but seemingly successful surgeries, including those of French surgeon Jean Zuléma Amussat, whom he credits for inventing a "most ingenious operation in certain varieties of imperforate anus" (a sorrowful condition in which a person is born without an opening to their anus, and thus is unable to defecate), in which "he cut[s] through the barrier" between the rectum and the vagina to evacuate a "rectum distended with feces."

He concludes, "No operation of modern times is more deserving your admiration, as well as imitation under similar circumstances."

Mütter affirmed some of his most lasting and important philosophies of medicine. Though obviously he understood and respected the power and potential of surgery, he implored his students to exhaust all nonsurgical options first:

"It is the boast of modern surgeons, and well may we boast, gentlemen, that a resort to painful and mutilating operations is now much less frequent than formerly," he writes. "In other words, diseases considered but a few years since as invariably indicating a resort to the knife, are now readily cured by constitutional treatment alone."

He praised the advancements without which "incurable deformity, permanent maiming by the knife of the surgeon, or the quiet of the grave, was the inevitable fate."

He also disparaged those who seek a career in medicine as a moneymaking scheme.

"Allow not then the temptings of the demon of avarice to lead you astray," he warns them, "the gains of the mercenary and hard hearted empiric though often alluring to the poor and diligent, but honest and honorable votary of his art, can in the end be productive of no comfort, no satisfaction."

He spoke with empathy about how frustrating and confusing medicine could be in a world where so much wrong information is accepted as truth, and quackery runs rampant.

"The dark clouds of ignorance, and error, and presumption do indeed gather more and more around and above us, and often the true votaries of our noble art are bowed down with despair," he wrote. "It comes not within my province to discuss the causes of this increase of the evil, but there is surely none more efficient than the facility with which a medical degree is usually obtained, and consequently the little value set upon its possession by the community at large. I trust, however, that a better state of things will sooner or later arise, and in the mean time should any among you be disheartened, let him not look to the boasted success of the lying and impudent quack, but to the brilliant examples of wisdom, and intellect, and honesty with which our profession is replete. In whatever direction we turn, the trophies of these great men are before us."

And finally and perhaps most importantly, after years of holding up European—and especially French—medicine as the pinnacle of medical achievement, he took pains to praise *American* innovation.

"It must have been obvious to you that American surgeons have been no laggards in the mighty race for professional fame," he wrote. "That they as well as their collaborators in Europe, have been steadily engaged in adding each a stone to the pyramid of modern surgery! The flame which burns so brilliantly abroad has thrown its rays across the wide Atlantic, and soon its genial warmth will be felt from one extremity of our country to the other."

He championed American doctors in Philadelphia, New York, and Boston, highlighting their recent accomplishments and even shining a spotlight specifically on an American doctor, a Professor Warren of Boston, whose surgeries he lauded for their "most daring courage, intrepid coolness, rigid anatomical knowledge, and practical experience." In that moment, Mütter could not have imagined how, in only a few years, John Collins Warren would go on to change the art of surgery—as well as Mütter's own life—forever.

In the final moments of his lecture, Mütter challenged his young students to join him in making American doctors the new medical vanguards.

"Shall [this progress] be permitted to subside?" he asked them. "Will you who are destined to be the pillars upon which the medical science of this country is to rest, fail to add fuel to this flame? Will you by slothful indulgence, wasteful sensual gratification, ignoble and puny contentedness which readily *receives* but never *gives*, let pass this golden era?

"Will you not rather 'gird up your loins' to the toil—and by your diligence, morality and laudable ambition, wreathe a new chaplet of glory for the land of liberty and equal rights? Show to the world that if in politics, religious tolerance, and social virtue, America once stood and will stand again, the foremost of nations, she may also boast of her medical science.

"There are many among you who are discouraged from entering with ardor upon the pursuit of the profession, from the supposition that nothing or next to nothing remains for them to discover," he tells his students. "Let no such idea take possession of your minds; ours as I have already told you is a progressive science and very far from perfection. . . . Let me urge upon you constant, patient, unprejudiced investigation. The harvest is rich and he who boldly thrusts in his sickle will assuredly reap an abundant reward. . . .

"Dwell not then upon what has been done," he told them, "but what remains to do."

In the ensuing years, Mütter's mettle would be tested on just that.

CHAPTER ELEVEN

THE ROOT OF
THE TROUBLE

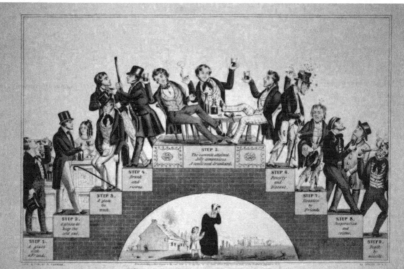

THE DRUNKARDS PROGRESS.
FROM THE FIRST GLASS TO THE GRAVE.

Despite its being home to over a thousand medical students and a plethora of doctors, hospitals, and medical schools, Philadelphia was still a place of chaos: socially, politically, and medically.

Crushing poverty had become an everyday fixture of Philadelphia life. One neighborhood (the relatively small area between 5th and 8th Streets, from Lombard to Fitzwater) had become so crammed with the city's most degraded classes that it earned the nickname the Infected District.

A reporter from *The Evening Bulletin* investigated the harrowing neighborhood and found conditions among the 4,000–5,000 people who lived there so wretched that he felt "incapable of reporting their full horrors to his readers." This area of the city—less than a mile from where Jefferson Medical College held its classes—seemed like a different world from the rarefied circles in which the doctors of the city drank imported French wine while dining on oysters, terrapin, quail, and ice cream.

In the Infected District, it was common practice for shops to charge a penny for a meal that was made up entirely of scraps begged at the back doors of the wealthy. It was a common custom for one enterprising individual unable to afford rent at even the lowliest of flophouses to secure a room at a boardinghouse for twelve and a half cents a day, and then sublet as many sleeping spaces as could fit at a bargain price of two cents a head.

The police and fire department at the time were of little help. The police were known as watchmen because the uniformed men could—and often did—lock themselves in specially constructed "watch-boxes" to protect themselves from the same criminals from which they were supposed to be protecting the community. The watch-box method would be abandoned, however, when rioting mobs realized they could simply destroy the watch-boxes and kill the police officers.

The fire department was equally troubled. The all-volunteer companies were neighborhood-based, and just like the neighborhoods they had sworn to protect, some "were very respectable" while others "were the reverse," as one doctor later observed.

"The more humble and gentle the name of the [firefighting] company, the more apt it was to be pugnacious," he recalled. "For instance, 'The Good Will' would fight *anything* at *any time*."

A watcher in the State House tower was tasked to be on the lookout for fires. When one was spotted, he would then alert all the fire departments en masse via taps on a bell. The disorder and chaos that would follow those bell taps was legendary.

"When there was a fire, hand engines and hose carriages were dragged by men, a shrieking crowd ran along the pavements, and quiet citizens got out of the way, as there was 'often a fight which would have brought joy to the heart of a Comanche or Pawnee,'" a Philadelphian recalled in harrowing detail. "Great disorders and riotous demonstrations were frequent . . . the firemen fought citizens, policemen and other firemen with scrupulous impartiality. One summer, two rival fire companies fought each other *instead of a fire* in the neighborhood of Eighth and Fitzwater Streets and the battle lasted *all day*. Two weeks later, the carriage of the Franklin Hose was thrown into the Delaware by a rival company."

One of the major challenging issues of 1840s Philadelphia was alcoholism, and the violence and death that seemed always to accompany it. By 1841, there were more than nine hundred taverns within Philadelphia County. In the Infected District, rum was commonly sold for a penny a glass, which might explain why the phrase "Rum is at the root of the trouble" was so commonly used when discussing the city's problems.

The threat that alcoholism posed to Philadelphia was so real that, by the early 1840s, the county supported nineteen temperance societies, which proudly claimed a total of seven thousand members. Total-abstinence societies—groups that forbade their members from consuming any alcohol whatsoever—topped them with more than ten thousand members.

Still, rampant alcoholism was an issue. When it came to the lower classes, alcohol-related crimes, injuries, and deaths only served to feed the popular belief that the poor had earned their lot in life and thus deserved no charity.

Some took this idea even further, espousing the notion that there were people who were simply born to be poor, and who were actually quite happy living as they did. "He that is down needs fear no fall," one clergyman of the time helpfully offered to explain why he thought the lower classes should be "of good cheer."

But it wasn't just the poor that suffered in this overflowing city. Philadelphia's working classes were consistently brutalized under the yoke of the free market.

Men of all ages and backgrounds arrived in Philadelphia daily—from Europe, Asia, and the American South—all looking for work. The population of the city exploded from less than 140,000 people in 1820 to more than 250,000 by 1842, and significant credit could be given to the city's industrial output.

Foundries, factories, and mills of all kinds could be found within the city's borders. There were mills for spinning cotton and weaving wool. Factories that built locomotives, fire engines, and chandeliers. The factories of Philadelphia produced, at their height, nearly one-fourth of the nation's steel, and the city's twelve sugar refineries made it the country's largest single supplier of commercial sugar.

To keep this extraordinary confluence of businesses going, these factories, mills, and foundries needed workers, but the city's exploding population always seemed to contain more eager workers than were needed. Philadelphians were often forced by circumstance to accept abysmal wages for what inevitably proved to be long hours of relentlessly grueling work.

Unskilled factory operatives, coal heavers, shipyard workers, and carpenters were paid less than a dollar a day to work fourteen hours a day, six days a week. Most factories recognized only the Fourth of July as a holiday, and vacation and sick time were, of course, nonexistent.

Men had to compete not only with each other for these backbreaking jobs, but with children as well. In a time before laws prohibited child labor, factory and mill owners were happy to put even the youngest children to work. In one dramatic case, the Dyottville Glass Works near Kensington employed 300 people in its industrial plant. Of those 300 employees, 225 were boys, "some not yet eight years of age."

Young girls were not exempt from the furious maw of factory work. The area's matchstick factories in particular sought them out, paying a wage of $2.50 a week. The girls happily took the work to help keep food on their families' tables, having no idea, of course, that they were being slowly poisoned by the factories' dangerous chemicals. The girls worked long hours in poorly ventilated rooms, licking their own chemical-coated fingers often to help in processing so many small slivers of wood, so difficult to see and keep track of in the dark factory setting. And what would start out as simply toothache and painful swollen gums would swiftly evolve into rotting tissue. Soon the girls' jaws were covered with large weeping abscesses so deep, the bone could be seen and the wound would unremittingly leak a foul-smelling discharge.

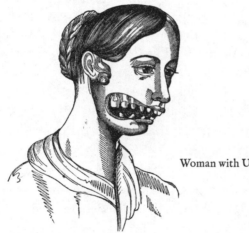

Woman with Ulcer of the Cheek

The condition became so common it would eventually earn a nickname: phossy jaw (phosphorus being the active ingredient in matches during the mid to late nineteenth century). And if the slow disfigurement (with accompanying brain damage and inevitable organ failure) weren't horrific enough, the chemicals the workers ingested daily caused the exposed jawbones of these now-deformed girls to glow greenish white in the dark.

Despite all the advancements of the time, the medical profession simply could not keep up with the increasingly deadly health challenges that this newly industrialized city presented. And one of its largest failings was in women's health.

CHAPTER TWELVE

THE WORLD TO COME

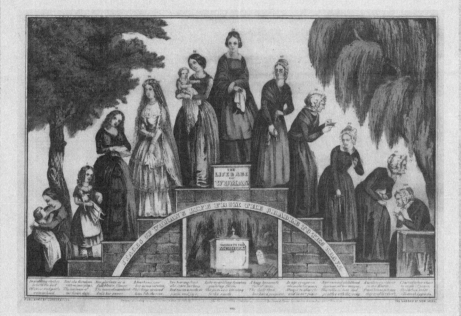

THE PHYSICIAN MUST BE
A CHARITABLE MAN

Every practitioner will tell you that he daily gives up
a large portion of his time to cases from which he
cannot possibly derive the slightest pecuniary reward.
But I would not confine the charity of a physician
to the mere giving of alms; no, there is a charity far
more precious than this, the charity of the heart.
The kind expression, the sympathizing tear, will often
convey more solace, more heartfelt and permanent
satisfaction, than if we poured all the gold of Ophir
into the lap of our suffering patient.
It is this charity which "covereth a multitude of
ills," which will secure to him the widow's love,
the orphan's prayer, the poor man's blessing,
that the physician should chiefly cultivate.

Thomas Dent Mütter

E
VEN IN A BRUTAL CITY LIKE PHILADELPHIA, WHERE YOUNG MEN were killed daily under the crushing boot heels of the industrial age, women could still be expected to die first. And the reason for their shorter life expectancy was as common as it was heartbreaking: childbirth.

Babies were delivered at home, with or without the help of trained midwives or doctors, with or without clean water or heat. Bringing life into the world was a dangerous prospect, and one that American woman entered into often: Women gave birth to an average of seven children in their lifetime. The statistics only get more sobering from there: One in every two hundred births resulted in the death of the mother; one in every four births resulted in the death of the infant.

In the mid-nineteenth century, women had almost no reliable way of avoiding getting pregnant barring complete abstinence. It is no wonder that the religious group known as the Shakers—which prohibited all sexual activity among its congregation and had been led by "Mother Ann" Lee, a woman whose youth was plagued by difficult pregnancies and who lost every single one of her children shortly after giving birth to them—was steadily growing in popularity.

The only forms of birth control available at the time, such as animal-skin condoms, which were rinsed and reused, were primitive and largely ineffective. It would be over a century before hormonal birth control would be invented.

During this time in history, menstrual cycles were often irregular, or absent altogether, thanks to any number of factors, including attacks of common diseases, periods of malnutrition, physical stresses on the body, and/or a recent pregnancy. Oftentimes, the earliest moment a woman could be certain she was pregnant was the first time she could feel the baby stirring in her womb—an event called the quickening.

The importance of the concept of the quickening during this era cannot be overstated. Nineteenth-century philosophers and theologians who followed the beliefs of the Christian West accepted the concept of "delayed animation" as the absolute truth about conception. It was a common and widely accepted belief that the unborn were not fully alive, or at least not fully human, until several months after conception, when those first movements were felt.

Therefore, the quickening was not just the unborn child becoming animated but the moment the unborn child received its *rational soul*.

Even doctors from this era—who were still early into their studies of embryology—gave credence to this idea, explaining that the womb "seemed capable of producing growths that mimicked fetuses so persuasively that only the absence of fetal movement gave them away as mere 'moles' or 'false conceptions.'"

Or as one nineteenth-century physician bluntly put it, "Not everything which comes from the birth parts of a woman is a human being."

So while it was generally understood that pregnancy was a nine- to ten-month process, the quickening became the main determining factor for pregnancy as well as the beginning of human life and, perhaps more importantly, the mother's moral responsibility to that life.

In part because of the moral loophole that the concept of the quickening provided, abortion that took place before the quickening wouldn't technically be a crime in America for another seventy years. An estimated one in every thirty pregnancies was terminated in the nineteenth century.

Poor women did it by drinking mild poisons, or thrusting certain plants or crude tools into their bodies. Some would endure being struck repeatedly in the abdomen until the desired effect was achieved.

For those with more money, abortifacient drugs and surgical abortions were becoming commercially available in America, particularly along the Eastern Seaboard, where advertisements for abortion services ran in the local papers.

Abortions were so popular and common that one woman in New York City—born with the name Ann Trow Lohman but publicly known as Madame Restell—made a fortune by boldly and shamelessly offering abortions commercially in the late 1830s. Her New York City–based abortion business, which included pills and surgery, grew so popular that she opened additional storefronts in Boston and Philadelphia.

But the tide was changing in America. Physicians were moving toward the view that human life began at conception rather than at the quickening, and medical testimony in nineteenth-century criminal cases had a growing influence on both law and popular opinion. One of the earliest cases to challenge and ultimately change abortion law in America called to the stand as its medical expert one Dr. Charles D. Meigs.

BY THE TIME MEIGS EXAMINED ELIZA SOWERS, SHE HAD ALREADY been dead for some time. Evidence of her final pain-racked days could be found all over her small, pale corpse, "mute testimony to medicine gone wrong," as Meigs's friend Dr. James Rush had warned.

Eliza—a former paper mill worker who had recently seen her station in life improve when she was hired to be a maid and was asked for her hand in marriage—had tried everything to end her terribly timed pregnancy. She swallowed magnesia, and tansy, and pennyroyal. She was bled. She consumed cups of tea made from powdered roots. She drank down one and a half bottles of an unknown wine-colored "medicine" she got from a local doctor with the promise that it would "make her regular," gagging on the liquid, which she said was "sharp to the taste." When it didn't work, she desperately did the whole routine again a few weeks later. At night, she begged her sister, with whom she shared a bed, to help her, but no matter what they did, she couldn't, as they said at the time, "get to rights."

When Eliza finally began to show, her new boss referred her to Henry Chauncey, a self-described "botanical physician" who assured the young woman and her boss that this situation could easily be remedied.

Chauncey secured Eliza a room in a boardinghouse far from her home and place of employment. Its main selling point was that it was known for not asking questions. Chauncey then gave Eliza a new round of tinctures and formulas to drink—a black-powder tea, ergot, savin oil—and left, assuring her that nature would take its course.

Unfortunately for Eliza, nothing changed except her level of suffering, which grew and grew until the woman in charge of the boardinghouse hunted down the "doctor" to fix the situation. Witnesses later would testify that when Chauncey reentered Eliza's room, he carried something that "shined and looked like a knitting needle" to finish what he believed his "medicine" had started. Eliza's piercing screams rattled the closed boardinghouse door, and almost immediately after, Chauncey left the boardinghouse again.

Eliza bled alone and heavily into the night and through the next day. And the next. And the next. Finally, after a week, a nervous Chauncey moved the girl's pale, tortured body to a different boardinghouse—this one frequented by prostitutes. Regrettably for Chauncey, the landlady at this boardinghouse knew exactly what was happening, and the severity of the situation. After a night of watching Eliza moan in pain, and constantly replacing the hot bricks at her feet to keep her warm, the landlady called in Dr. James Rush, a well-known and respected doctor in Philadelphia. He would later testify that he knew at first glance she was going to die.

"I found her with a livid face [and] wild staring eye," he told the court at Chauncey's trial, "sighing, moaning and excla[iming] of agony; her abdomen was very much swollen, and hard and tender to the touch; her extremities cold and she was pulseless."

Rush shared his ultimate conclusion with Chauncey: There was no saving her. Chauncey agreed, and together, they fed her six or seven glasses of wine, which would serve as the only treatment she received while Rush was there. Rush convinced Chauncey to move her to his house so she wouldn't have to die in such disreputable lodgings, and he did. But the next day, either in transit or soon after arriving at Chauncey's house, Eliza Sowers died. She was twenty-one years of age.

And now, Dr. Charles D. Meigs was staring at her lifeless body, having been asked to testify at the trial of her murder. This wasn't the first time Meigs had been called to such a harrowing scene, but it had been a while.

After his wife demanded that they return to Philadelphia (being unable to stomach the relentless presence of slavery in her husband's native South), Meigs found his first patients among the poor and destitute. While the position of his wife's family in society provided him with an introduction to several esteemed circles, his relatives and their friends did not, and indeed they could not be expected to employ him in so delicate a position as that of their family obstetrician until he had proven himself fit to be trusted and sufficiently skilled. Meigs had no choice but to start at the bottom. But through hard work and persistence, he was able to secure patients of higher and increasingly more impressive social rank.

Meigs didn't have an easy time at first. Early in his career, he had several very difficult cases of childbirth, which "greatly disturbed and tried his strength and nerves." In one of the cases, he made a wrong diagnosis and though the mother and child survived, relatively unharmed, the mistake haunted him. He eventually became "so disgusted" with himself for the error that he quit practicing obstetrics to relieve himself of "the painful responsibility which belongs to that branch."

For two straight years, he worked purely as a general physician and sent all such obstetric and gynecological cases to his friends. But he found it impossible to maintain a practice without obstetrics. With his family growing and his expenses increasing, he admitted that he "began to fancy that the wolf was approaching his door." For the sake of his family and his finances, Meigs returned to obstetrics but this time with a new steely boldness, perhaps born from his discomfort at being forced to practice it at all.

From that day forward, Meigs's vision for women's health was clear and plainly stated: A physician for women must be "endowed with a clear perceptive power; a sound judgment; a proper degree of intelligence; and a familiarity with the doctrines of a good medical school." And once a physician had obtained this high level of competency, he must be somewhat ruthless in his firmness about what should be done. Once Meigs embraced this philosophy, his business and reputation only increased.

WHEN MEIGS WAS ASKED TO TESTIFY IN THE ELIZA SOWERS trial, it was an important moment in his career. The trial had already attracted much attention. It had a tragic figure at its center: Eliza, the type of working-class girl trying to live a better life, with whom many in Philadelphia could identify. And it had its villain, Chauncey, who at first denied that Eliza was even pregnant when he began treating her. He told Rush that it was a simple case of inflammation brought on by excess food and drink as well as exposure to a damp draft in Sowers's room.

And to make matters worse, he attempted to paint Eliza's last hours alive not as a time of unimaginable suffering, but rather a "period of religious ecstasy." He claimed that in her last moments, she was whispering prayers with a placid smile, utterly joyful at the "blissful immortality in the world to come."

It was only after a friend of Eliza's demanded her body be disinterred, and three separate physicians confirmed she was pregnant—using as evidence the fact that her uterus was twice the size of a non-pregnant woman's, and the fact that when they sliced into her ashen left breast, "the milk flowed freely"—that Chauncey finally admitted she had been pregnant. He explained that he had lied only "to spare the feeling of the family." The physician estimated that she was at least five months pregnant when she died, and the cause of death was an infection "resulting from a laceration of the uterus caused by an instrumental abortion."

WHEN CHAUNCEY WAS ARRESTED AND INDICTED FOR THE MURDER of Eliza Sowers, the American medical world took notice, and not just because of the drama of the distressing tale. Rather, they were deeply invested in the outcome of the case because they knew it would affect their practices.

Chauncey had four distinct charges lodged against him. The first two charges—murder by simple assault, and murder by means of poison—were less important to the medical community than the last two: murder by means of assault and abortion, and murder by means of mere abortion.

The Eliza Sowers case proved to be a turning point in how America viewed abortion—or at least how the American legal system would begin to view it. When Chauncey was initially being charged and held for murder, he attempted to get bail through a loophole regarding how the law defined murder. He demanded that he be released on bail on the grounds "that it was a defendant's right in murder cases where 'intent to take life' was not present. But with intent absent, how could this be considered a murder case at all?"

The release was refused. It was plainly explained: "The death of the mother following criminal abortion is murder, not because the agent accomplishing the act intended to kill the female, but because, the act being unlawful in itself, he is held responsible for all its results."

With this statement and its resulting act, abortion was being formally criminalized. But an important distinction was made. The court described the criminality of abortions as being "necessarily attended with great danger to the persons on whom they are practiced," implying that the ground of its unlawfulness was its tendency to injure the woman (which was often cited as the reason abortions could be considered unlawful). Now new language was also added, and the court formally termed abortion the "destruction of [the] offspring" and an act "feloniously to destroy the fruit of [the woman's] womb."

Therefore, for the first time, abortion was legally viewed as something that could bring harm to the mother *as well as* the death of the unborn.

When bail was denied and details of the case were released, the trial became a citywide obsession. After an intense jury selection process, more
than seventy witnesses (most of them for the defense) testified for nearly a
week before a crowded courtroom.

The prosecution likely hoped that the esteemed Dr. Meigs would help
shine a light into the dark areas of reproductive science. But instead, Meigs
unwittingly showed just how little nineteenth-century doctors could admit
to knowing about the reproductive process in women.

When Meigs took the stand as one of the three physicians who examined Eliza Sowers's body, he openly admitted that he did not clearly understand how conception took place. He did say that he understood it enough
to reject the whole idea of the quickening as worthless, and declared that
making it a demarcation point for whether or not a woman could legally get
an abortion was "very great nonsense on the part of the lawyers."

Furthermore, knowing that the media's spotlight was upon him, Meigs
took the opportunity to chastise any woman—including the late Eliza
Sowers—who approached physicians requesting an abortion. After all,
"did they not know their own duty as well as their physicians?"

It was not uncommon for Meigs to use his position as a doctor as a sort
of pulpit from which he could condemn anyone he thought was being disobedient.

"I love my profession as a ministry, not as a trade," he would later be
quoted as saying. "Can any human avocation have a stronger tendency to
elevate and purify the mind than the physician's? What other? In what light
shall he see the nature of man so clearly and so plainly?"

WHEN CHAUNCEY WAS LATER FOUND GUILTY, IT PROVED TO BE A
watershed moment. In the twelve years after his sentencing, the courts of
Pennsylvania issued some of the strictest laws against abortion in the entire
United States, expressly prohibiting the procedure no matter what stage of
pregnancy a woman found herself in.

Life had been hard for women in America up until then, and it was
about to get even harder.

But for one segment of women—a desperate population kept largely
hidden from view—there was a growing reason to hope that their lives
could one day improve. And that hope came in the form of Thomas Dent
Mütter.

CHAPTER THIRTEEN

THE WOMEN WHO WERE SWALLOWED BY FIRE

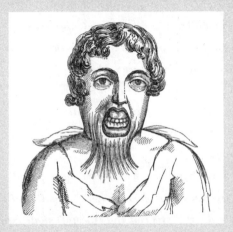

THE PHYSICIAN MUST BE
A MAN OF STRICT INTEGRITY AND VIRTUE

It is with much gratification I can assert that
    no profession, not even that of our holy religion,
    boasts a higher code of morality than ours.
How edifying, and how eminently calculated to direct
    the thoughts of the medical man into the noblest
    channel, are the daily instances with which
    he meets, of exalting and touching fortitude,
    of sublime patience, of heavenly faith.
Yes, yours is truly a moral, yea, a religious
    profession.
And be assured that when, with tottering step and
    sinking frame, you grope through the "valley of the
    shadow of death," His rod and His staff shall support
    you; and at the last, when the frail barrier which
    separates our fleeting world from that whose duration
    is eternity is passed, you will be greeted with cheering
    welcome:
"Well done, thou good and faithful servant;
I was sick, and ye comforted me."

Thomas Dent Mütter

Many of the women who came to Mütter were monsters. That is how they were seen on the streets, how strangers would describe them, and how they saw themselves when they were confronted with the horror of their own reflections.

In the nineteenth century, women were largely dependent on men. While there were always exceptions to this rule, for the most part, to have a roof over her head, food in her stomach, or a life worth living, a woman needed a man to provide it—in one way or another. And for a woman to find a husband and leave her father's house, it was said she needed to be beautiful and pure, modest and obedient.

So what could the future hold for a woman whom the world saw as a monster?

To understand how these "monsters" were created, it is important to understand how women were forced to dress at this time: an imposed modesty that could literally kill them. Every morning, women began the process of dressing themselves for the day in the era's notoriously restrictive clothing. Layer upon layers of cotton, wool, and silk, and these pieces of clothing held snugly to the body with tightly bound ribbons and laces. When this routine was finally complete, her movement was, of course, severely limited.

The way women walked, moved, or even stood up in the 1800s was dictated in part by these restrictive layers of clothing. And yet, household chores—cooking, cleaning, minding children—were expected to be performed while wearing these restraining frocks.

Now imagine the typical nineteenth-century kitchen, where cooking was often still done over an open flame. Pans were placed on grates, and pots hung from swinging arms that could be pulled out of and pushed into the fire.

It was in this horrible concurrence of troubles—a veritable death trap of early domesticity—that these monsters were born.

HOW EASILY IT COULD HAPPEN—A PIECE OF HOT EMBER LOOSENS itself from its pack and rolls to the floor, its orange flame licking the fine lace of a petticoat; or a splatter of hot oil hops from a swinging pot and leaps—flame-touched—onto a woolen apron; or even something as basic as a child running toward his mother to hug her legs and accidentally pushing her into the flames. Once started, these types of fires were devastatingly difficult to stop.

Within moments, more of the woman's clothing would begin to catch fire, layer after layer, building intensity. Restricted in her movements and impeded by that easy flammability of the natural fibers, she would help-lessly flail, trying to reach the flame and beat it out.

However, the air would only serve to fan the flames, making them grow larger, stronger, and more powerful. And in her bending over, the fire would often hit the neck of the dress, a virtual powder keg in its combina-tion of air, restrictive dense fabrics, and light airy layers of decorative cloth.

And this is where the real damage was done. The woman's face would soon be consumed with flame—burning, blistering, turning skin to liquid, and tearing flesh from bone. It was said the lucky ones died. The ones who did survive were cursed to live half a life, as monsters.

OF COURSE, MÜTTER KNEW OF THESE WOMEN. SURVIVORS OF SUCH horrible burns often sought the help of plastic surgeons, hoping there was something that could be done. Those who had been burned as children had never known a normal life.

Very little could be done. Typically, years would have passed, and the scar tissue would have grown painfully tight around the women's faces. Some of the skin was thick and tough; other parts were stretched impossi-bly thin. The landscape covered by the disfigurement was often large: Hor-rific scarring commonly reached from the woman's chest up to her eyes. Because of the alarming aftermath of their gruesome burns, these women— hidden from society by their shame-filled families—frequently couldn't close their mouths, blink their eyes, or turn their heads.

The older they got, the more they realized their already small world was only going to shrink: Who would take care of them once their siblings left the family home to start their own lives, and their parents grew old and thin from age and failing health?

Too often, death by their own hands seemed their only solution. And by the time they grew desperate enough to find their way into Mütter's office, they would tell him that is exactly what they would be prepared to do if he did not help them.

THE MOST OBVIOUS SOLUTION—TO CUT AWAY THE DAMAGED SKIN and replace it with healthy skin from another person or even another area of the victim's own body—was assumed to be impossible. In fact, experiments in this area had halted progress in plastic surgery for centuries.

"It is now generally admitted that 'plastic surgery' originated in India," Mütter would tell his class. Earlier in the millennium, Indian criminals earned "peculiar punishments" for their crimes—noses sliced off, ears, lips, limbs. The natural result of this practice was the creation of a black market for doctors who claimed to be able to replace missing body parts.

"And what the knife of the executioner called forth in India," Mütter would tell them, "disease and accident have excited in Europe and America."

Mütter continued his far-reaching investigation of the genesis of plastic surgery, telling the story of Gaspar Taliacotius of Bologna, whose fame depended on his having practiced the art of restoring lost parts of the body by grafting and who tried but ultimately abandoned attempts to make noses from the skins of other people.

Mütter told how Taliacotius attempted to transplant the skin from the arm of a porter onto the noseless face of his patient.

"All went well for the space of thirteen months," he explained, "but at the end of that period the borrowed organ gradually lost its temperature, and in a few days became gangrenous; upon inquiring, it was found that at the self same period the original owner of the nose had died!"

The students would laugh at this obvious tall tale, but Mütter continued.

"The sympathy between the nose and its parent was indeed most extraordinary," Mütter told them. "Not only did the former die with the latter, but during life it was effected by the pains of the original proprietor." He then told them another artful story about "three Spaniards, whose noses were all cut from [the skin of] the same porter" and who were shocked to discover their noses swelling enormously in size. In an effort to get to the source of the problem, the Spaniards tried to locate the porter, only to hear that he was bruised and swollen himself, and recovering in bed after being severely kicked by a horse. The Spaniards, in retaliation, went and kicked the horse!

The students would again laugh, as Mütter smiled and rolled his eyes. But his expression turned stern when he brought home his point: As preposterous as these stories were, the chief consequence of this ridicule was that there was "no attempt to perform these operations made after this period until the latter end of the last century."

The fear of being seen as foolish had prevented progress; "an art nearly lost, yet of the greatest value to mankind" was a grim consequence indeed.

"Even now *plastic surgery* must be considered in its infancy, for although much has been done, much remains to do, in order that the true value of the principle may be fully established," he told his students.

And Mütter was now attempting to put into action what he had been teaching his students: He was going to move the science and art of plastic surgery forward.

IT WAS A KNOWN FACT THAT TRANSPLANTING A PIECE OF SKIN—from either the same person or a different one—would result in the body's rejecting it. What might at first seem pink and hopeful would slowly turn yellow, then green, then black, as the skin flaked off what inevitably was, at this point, a festering pus-filled wound.

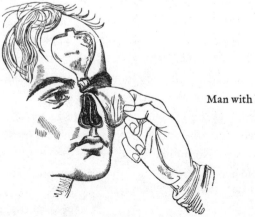

Man with Nose Being Reconstructed
from Forehead

However, the French doctors popularizing plastic surgery in Paris introduced Mütter to what was, for him, a revolutionary concept. While moving the skin completely from one area to another did not seem possible at that time, surgeons realized that if one section of a patient's skin remained attached to the body, and that skin was simply twisted over an open wound, it had a higher probability of attaching, slowly grafting itself onto the new area, becoming healthy and growing as if it had always been there. It was how French surgeons were able to construct a whole nose from the twisted skin of a person's forehead.

It was this new approach to plastic surgery that inspired Mütter to try and help these women. His vision was ambitious in its scope. Any woman who agreed to it would have to endure a long, painful operation while wide awake, followed by a lengthy recovery time. But it promised a miracle: It promised to unmake the monster.

Mütter had no idea that the surgery he was planning would one day carry his name—the Mütter flap—and that it was so visionary and ahead of his time that it would still be performed more than a century and a half after his death.

All he knew in that moment was that he had formulated a plan to help these tragic, fate-struck women, and now he needed to see if it would work.

WHEN THE TREMBLING WOMAN ENTERED HIS OFFICE, MÜTTER greeted her severely deformed face with the same warmth with which he greeted friends on the street; his glittering blue eyes locked directly onto her misshapen ones.

It was disarming to the twenty-eight-year-old woman, who—in the twenty-three years since she received her life-changing injuries—had grown used to people avoiding eye contact with her, often even turning away from her in revulsion. She, in turn, was used to avoiding eye contact as well.

Even though Mütter positioned himself directly in front of her, the woman kept lowering her head out of his eye line, from pure habit. But Mütter persisted, dipping his head down to maintain their connection and smiling confidently. It was important that she trust him, and vital that he ascertain the task that lay ahead of him, not unlike a general surveying a battlefield before planning his maneuvers.

"I received a burn when five years old by my clothes taking fire," she told him, her words slurred and slow. "My grandmother being a great doctress nursed me. . . . As they wished me to remain in as comfortable a position as possible, my life being entirely despaired of by the family, medical aid was not called. . . ."

As she spoke, Mütter let his eyes wander over her. Her lower eyelids were drawn down by her shocking scars. It made it difficult for her to blink, and her face grew wet with the persistent flow of tears.

"Dr. Burns, a neighboring physician, hearing of my circumstances, could not refrain from calling to see me," she continued. "He called twice as a friend, and was then forbidden to come again until sent for, which was never done."

The angles of her lower jaw were completely altered by the burns, so much so that her teeth were nearly horizontal. Her tongue, with no barrier to press against, developed chronic hypertrophy (swelling to abnormal proportions) and she was unable to close her mouth for more than a few seconds at a time.

"When I was eleven years of age, an attempt was made by Dr. Cook, of Bordentown, to afford some relief," she told him. "Being young, I was much alarmed, and opposed him. My near relations, being unwilling to see me suffer, united with me; and he was obliged to desist before completing his design. I therefore did not experience any relief."

The clavicle on her right side was also so completely embedded in scar tissue and thickened skin that it could scarcely be felt, and there was no external indication of its location. Her chin was drawn down to within an inch and a half of the top of her sternum, making her unable to turn her head left or backward. There was so much thick roping scar tissue covering her from chin to chest that she appeared not to have any neck at all.

"My condition has been most humiliating and made my life a burden," she whispered to him. "Death is preferable to a life of such misery as mine."

Mütter took in what she said and nodded, before giving her a brief, steady smile.

"Do I have your permission to examine your back?" he asked. She looked at him strangely, but nodded her assent and began to undress.

When finally she was able to lower the fabric from her shoulder, Mütter saw her back for the first time: It was perfect. Healthy, pink, and free of the burn scars to which the front of her body was yoked. He broke into a wide bright grin, almost laughing with joy. She, of course, would have no idea, but this sorrowful woman was indeed a perfect candidate for his new surgery.

Once she had re-dressed, he invited her family to join them in the room.

He fully explained to them what he had learned from his examination. He told them what other surgeons would likely suggest, and how futile any of the usual operations for such deformities would be. Instead, he asked if he could perform a surgery on her that was entirely different from any previously conducted.

"Although [the surgery would be] severe, as well as somewhat hazardous," he explained, "[it] promised partial, if not entire relief."

It was an enormous promise to make. The woman agreed, and Mütter immediately placed her in "preparatory treatment."

CHAPTER FOURTEEN

TO UNMAKE MONSTERS

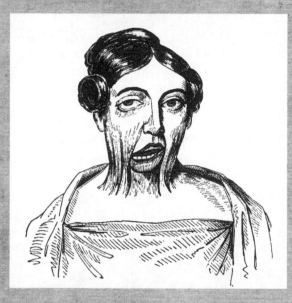

MÜTTER HAD TO WAIT UNTIL HIS PATIENT WAS READY. IT WAS going to be a long, multistage surgery, and once the procedure had started, there was no turning back. If Mütter wasn't allowed to perform his envisioned operations—swiftly and fully—there was a strong possibility that the patient would bleed out on the table. Mütter had walked the young woman through every step of the surgery, being clear and frank about what was to come and what was expected of her despite the pain she would feel. Once Mütter felt she was sufficiently prepared, mentally and physically, he scheduled the surgery. In the room would be six other men—two doctors whom Mütter had asked to assist him and four medical students who had begged to witness the procedure.

Mütter sat the young woman down on a low chair and placed her in the strongest light possible. He asked her to throw her head back as far as she could, farther than was likely comfortable for her. She strained her neck, wincing, as one of the doctors stood behind, holding her head firmly and gently to maintain this difficult angle.

Mütter sat himself in front of her and washed her neck one last time, feeling through the cloth the rough landscape of scars that had become so familiar to him. He asked the young woman if she was ready. She nodded, her body already restrained by another doctor's arms. Mütter took a final look at this woman, trembling and vulnerable before him, her neck bared for his knife. He took a deep breath, and began.

THE FIRST INCISION WAS A LONG ONE. IT BEGAN IN THE "SOUND" unscarred skin, outside of the most heavily scarred area on one side of her throat, and continued until it passed into sound skin on its opposite side. His goal was to cut through the dead center of the most scarred area of her throat—"the most vital part of the neck."

Mütter was sure to handle the scalpel lightly but firmly, the scalpel cutting uniformly through the skin, deep enough to get through the heavy scar tissue, but light enough to, hopefully, avoid the delicate muscles of the neck and the heavily trafficked arteries and veins. It seemed to work. There was blood, but it was not much.

He kept cutting through the skin—swiftly and confidently but deeper and deeper—as he moved strips of the scarred skin from her neck and placed them in a basin out of her field of vision. When he thought he had cleared all the scarred skin he could afford, he told the assisting doctor holding her head to help to raise it into its proper position.

Despite the throbbing, shocking pain the young woman experienced, Mütter could see the gratification on her face. Without the thick webbing of scar tissue dragging her face down, she was able to blink her eyes easily and painlessly. She was able to close her mouth. She could turn her head for the first time in more than two decades.

But, of course, Mütter had to remind her that the surgery was not over. There was more she would need to endure.

After instructing her not to look down, Mütter made "a most shocking wound six inches in length by five and a half in width."

The next step in the operation was Mütter's most daring innovation: the manipulation of skin to form the flap, which would give name to Mütter flap surgery.

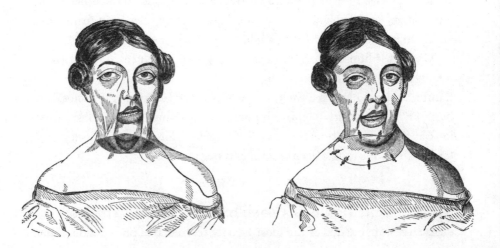

Mütter knew that in order for this change to be permanent, he could not leave the wound to heal as it was, writing "for I knew very well, that if permitted to heal by granulation only, the patient, so far from being benefited, would be made worse than before." He would need to find skin to fill in the wound he had just opened, and this is where the untouched skin on her back would prove most useful.

Mütter asked the woman to sit perfectly straight as he washed the skin on her back. Neither the front or the back of her body could be leaned against any fabric or wood because of the wounds. He positioned his two assistants to either side of the woman, there in case she needed to reach out and hold something to keep from collapsing.

He acted quickly, carrying the scalpel downward and outward over the deltoid muscle. The woman tried to stifle her cry as Mütter carved out a piece of skin from her back—six and a half inches in length, by six in width, slightly larger but the same shape as the wound on the front of her neck—making sure to leave the flap attached by a thin strip of skin that traveled up the upper part of her neck.

As with his work on the front of her neck, he was mindful not to cut too deeply. But despite his best efforts, one small vessel was opened. For the rest of the surgery, a steady stream of blood dripped onto the floor, ticking like an insistent clock.

Mütter carefully loosened this flap of healthy skin, lifting it entirely off her back and bringing it around to the front of her body. As he lifted the skin over her shoulder, the thin strip of skin connecting it to her body folded over itself, but did not tear. He placed the skin in the gap that the front wound had created. It fit nearly perfectly, and with strong sutures he immediately began securing the edges of the wound to the edges of the fresh flap of skin.

Once he saw that the edges of the wounds on the front of her neck were secured, Mütter then applied several clean cloth straps to support the sutures, but determined that no other dressing at this stage was advisable.

Working his way back, he sewed up the wound left by the strip of skin on her neck, using straps and sutures as best he could, and fusing completely together the parts of her neck that he could without strain.

Finally, all he was left with was the large wound on her back, the one making the floor slick with her blood. It was too large to seal, so Mütter unrolled a clean, damp compress made of fine lint across the raw surface of the wound. He carefully wrapped a bandage around both wounds, and then, realizing what needed to be done, applied a bandage around the woman's head to hold her head tilted backward. Mütter realized that scars, by nature, contract, and that for the best chance at full mobility, her neck would need to heal in a stretched position.

It was done. Of course, the true test was whether the new skin would take hold, making permanent the changes the patient felt. Mütter had given her the best possible chance he could. And while the doctors and students in attendance were left in awe of the work Mütter had done and the innovation it showed, Mütter redirected all praise to his patient.

"The fortitude with which this truly severe operation was borne excited the admiration of all present," he wrote. "Scarcely a groan escaped the patient, nor was it necessary to give her more than a mouthful or two of wine and water during the whole period of its duration."

With that, the patient was put to bed.

"Rest and quietude were enjoined," he wrote of the recovery process. It was all the woman could do, for eating or drinking of any kind had been strictly prohibited by Mütter.

Mütter kept careful watch over her the first night, but other than a slightly raised pulse and understandable complaints of stiff neck and sore back, she seemed perfectly well. The next day was much the same; his notes read: "A little nervous, but no fever; no swelling or pain in the wound; some thirst and hunger, but willing to go another day without sustenance."

But Mütter's luck seemed to have run out by the third day. The woman suddenly developed a fever, soaking the thin sheets with sweat. There was increased pain at the wound sites, and she was uncomfortable no matter what position she took. Restless, anxious, and unable to relieve herself, she was prescribed by Mütter "an enema to be administered at once" (the constipation that commonly followed surgery was often the source of numerous problems if left untreated) and "spoonfuls of cool barley water to be taken every hour or two."

The treatment, thankfully, worked. On the fourth day after the operation, Mütter finally had his opportunity to see if his vision was right. Had the surgery been successful?

As the woman nervously sat in front of him, Mütter removed the bandages that were holding together the skin of her tender throat. As he loosened the straps, he steeled himself for what he might see: Would he be greeted with the sight of healing skin or the putrid scent and sight of a blackening, infected wound?

When the last piece of fabric was removed, he saw what he had helped create. He smiled.

"The wound united along the edges, with the exception of here and there a point," he wrote, "a small pouch of pus at the most dependent part of the flap."

It had worked. Or rather it was working. Now Mütter just had to continue the good process that was already on its way.

He evacuated the pus through a small opening in its vicinity; took out some of the pins; reapplied the straps; dressed the shoulder; and immediately ordered that the patient be fed for the first time in almost a week: "a little mutton broth" followed by an enema of salt and water to ensure against bowel toxicity.

When he noticed a "troublesome circumstance" where "a band of tissue, certainly not thicker or wider than a small wire" was contracting, Mütter immediately brought the patient back into the surgical room to fix it.

He also located a good dentist who could straighten her lower teeth—including the removal of one—allowing the angles of the lower jaw to change.

After several long days and restless nights, Mütter felt the patient was ready to move about and "enjoy the full benefit of the operation." When the woman was brought to a mirror, she could barely believe what she saw.

"The whole appearance of the patient is so much altered," he wrote, "that persons who saw her before the operation, scarcely recognize her as the same individual."

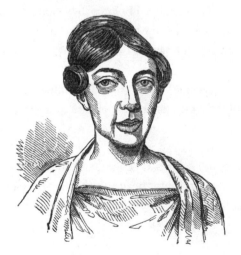

Mütter modestly wrote later, "It will be sufficient to state that no unfavourable symptom made its appearance."

The woman was less conservative in her praise.

"The comfort and satisfaction I feel, cannot be expressed," she wrote in a letter to Mütter. "Your exertions in my behalf have been blessed far beyond my most sanguine expectations. You have set my head at liberty, so that I can turn it any way, at pleasure, and without pain; you have relieved the drawing of my eye; and I am also enabled to close my mouth with comfort, a blessing that cannot be described!"

The Mütter flap surgery was a success, and as news of it spread, patients came out of the shadows to seek his help.

In June of that year, Mütter performed a surgery on a twelve-year-old girl who was severely burned when she was just four. "For nearly eight years she had been unable to turn her head to the left side, the lower lip was inverted, and the chin drawn down nearly in contact with the sternum," he wrote, and though he would remark that "this case was even more unfavourable" than the previous one in the severity of the condition and age of the patient, he was "determined to perform the operation which had proved so successful."

Though the operation was a success, he did note that perhaps one of the hardest parts was keeping a twelve-year-old girl from "speaking, swallowing, or motions of the neck of any kind."

Six months later, Mütter was brought an even younger patient, a nine-year-old boy who had "a deformity of the mouth and throat" as the result of his clothes having accidentally taken fire years earlier. The appearance presented by this boy was shocking: His mouth was kept permanently open, his incisor teeth were losing their perpendicular position, his chin was drawn to within an inch or two of his sternum, and a strong band of the scar tissue passed along the center of his throat from chin to sternum.

This time, not only did Mütter rise to the challenge of performing a delicate and painful surgery on a fully awake nine-year-old child, but he did so in front of a full classroom of Jefferson Medical College students.

He would later write: "The operation . . . was performed before the medical class on the second Wednesday in January, and on the first Wednesday in February he was brought into the amphitheatre with scarcely a vestige of the deformity remaining. . . . Here, in three weeks time, a cure of a deformity hitherto considered hopeless, was effected."

Finally, after two years of successful surgeries, Mütter was asked to publish his findings in *The American Journal of the Medical Sciences.*

"Two years and more have elapsed since the first of the operations reported was performed," he wrote in his introduction, "and the patient still continues relieved. No contraction has taken place, and the success of the experiment may therefore be considered complete: the other cases are also doing well."

Mütter was thrilled at the article's release and the reaction to it. He realized how important publication was to having his vision for medicine be understood and adopted. But he also felt that every moment behind the quill and inkpot was a moment he couldn't spend in the surgical room.

"[Mütter] felt it a glorious thing to be able to rescue a patient from present suffering or impending danger, when everything else had failed, by the achievement of a successful surgical operation," Pancoast wrote. "He had before him a beau ideal of the art and science of surgery, which he was striving first to reach before he made his final record, but which, with advancing knowledge and deepening insight, kept ever assuming higher and higher grounds."

But Mütter knew that if he wanted his work to effect real change in the field of medicine, there was only one thing he could do. Somehow, between his hours of lectures and his intense surgical workload—which included lengthy preoperative and postoperative care—Mütter would have to write his own textbook.

CHAPTER FIFTEEN

TO REMEDY EVILS

3

JEFFERSON MEDICAL COLLEGE.
SESSION OF 1846—7.

The regular Course of Lectures will commence on Monday the 2d day of November, and end on the last day of February.

ROBLEY DUNGLISON, M. D., Professor of Institutes of Medicine.
ROBERT M. HUSTON, M. D., Professor of Materia Medica and General Therapeutics.
JOSEPH PANCOAST, M. D., Professor of General, Descriptive and Surgical Anatomy.
JOHN K. MITCHELL, M. D., Professor of Practice of Medicine.
THOMAS D. MUTTER, M. D., Professor of Institutes and Practice of Surgery.
CHARLES D. MEIGS, M. D., Professor of Obstetrics and Diseases of Women and Children.
FRANKLIN BACHE, M. D., Professor of Chemistry.

Every Wednesday and Saturday during the course, Medical and Surgical cases are investigated and prescribed for before the class During the past year not fewer than 1,000 cases were treated, and upwards of 172 were operated on. The Clinical Lectures are so arranged as to permit the student, should he desire it, to attend the Medical and Surgical practice and lectures at the Pennsylvania Hospital.

On and after the 1st of October, the dissecting rooms of the College will be open under the direction of the Professor of Anatomy and the Demonstrator.

Owing to the large size of the class, which numbered 469 during the last session, it became expedient to make extensive and important alterations in the college edifice. These will be completed by the 1st of September.

R. M. HUSTON, M. D., Dean of the Faculty.
No. 1 Girard Street.

GEO. W. CARPENTER & CO.,
WHOLESALE DRUGGISTS,
No. 301 Market Street.

Have always on hand a large and general assortment of choice Drugs and Medicines, Surgical Instruments, Anatomical preparations, Chemical and Philosophical apparatus, and everything appertaining to the Profession. They give especial attention to the orders of Physicians in the country and in distant States, and will extend to such as furnish satisfactory references a liberal credit, and furnish them with articles of the best quality at as low prices as those of like character can be had elsewhere in the United States.

A UNIFORM AND CHEAP EDITION OF

DICKENS' NOVELS AND TALES.
IN THREE LARGE VOLUMES.

LEA & BLANCHARD HAVE NOW READY,

THE NOVELS AND TALES
OF
CHARLES DICKENS,
(BOZ.)

In Three Large and Beautiful
CONTAINING ABOUT

Price

The frequent
to prepare one,
printed on fine
and fifty pages
Some of the work

ENC

Thirteen years hav
and the numerous imp
and arts, and the num
supplement necessary
Professor Vethake, thi
Encyclopædia, will be

Any of the books in
Druggists of Philadelp

THE PHYSICIAN SHOULD BE
A SELF-RELYING MAN

The physician should be one who,

    while he treats authority with all due deference,

    yet has the spirit to feel that he is no man's man

    who knows that he can trust himself . . .

Who feels that, when called to combat with the "King

    of Terrors" himself, he is fully armed at all points;

Who is assured that the shield, which he boldly thrusts

    forward to screen his suffering patient, is polished,

    strong, unyielding; so that, however sharp or well

    directed the dart, it must glance or be broken.

Such a man is indeed a treasure to the community

    in which he lives, and an honor to the noble profession

    of which he is a member.

Thomas Dent Mütter

J EFFERSON MEDICAL COLLEGE KNEW WITHIN THE FIRST YEAR that their ambitious experiment with this new faculty had succeeded. The popularity of the new faculty caused the student population to double after one year. And in two years, it tripled. It affirmed the ever-growing prestige of the college and it solidified its stature as an American institution.

Students eagerly signed up by the hundreds for lectures on how to best mix their own medicines, the quickest way to amputate a limb, and the most effective ways to bleed and leech patients.

Leeching—attaching leeches (a type of blood-sucking worm) to a patient's body—was an important part of medicine at that time. Doctors kept their ample jars of medicinal leeches in their offices. Mütter shared with his students how Paris's Hôtel-Dieu's need for leeches was so great that a full-time "keeper-of-leeches" was a part of the hospital staff. Leeches were used in a variety of ways, but mostly to draw blood either *to* or *from* a specific area, in an attempt to relieve pain or inflammation. But doctors in that time period found a variety of novel ways to use leeches in their practices. John Kearsley Mitchell recommended that his students apply one hundred leeches to the stomach of anyone who was suffering from typhoid. And Charles D. Meigs advocated the use of leeches to cure several common gynecological problems, and made sure to eke out time each year to teach his students the best ways to apply wriggling black leeches directly into a woman's uterus, using a sleek wooden speculum.

Meanwhile, Mütter's surgical clinics had grown so popular that he was finally able to demand the recovery rooms for which he had petitioned so heavily in his first year. The college refused to buy an entire building but agreed to rent floors above the two stores next to the college and remodel them to accommodate fifteen patients.

It was not ideal for Mütter by any stretch, but this miniature surgical facility would serve as the place where he would perform his art for the next decade of his life, and would serve as the college's only hospital for another thirty years.

Mütter was thrilled that his patients—many of whom had traveled so far and would suffer so greatly in their quest to be made new—were now able to receive round-the-clock care. Students eagerly volunteered to provide nursing care to the patients in the recovery ward, and Mütter doled out the spots as rewards.

With the students monitoring the patients—keeping their wounds clean and dry, strictly following the aftercare instructions, and feeding them meals brought from a nearby restaurant—Mütter could focus on his newest task: his textbook.

MÜTTER HOPED THE TEXTBOOK MIGHT HELP HIM GAIN MORE influence and respect so that he could be a more effective advocate for the opinions and philosophies that were so important to him. While his position at Jefferson gifted him with a tremendous platform to share his ideas with the incoming generation of physicians, he still felt a disconnect when it came to having his perspective respected by his peers. He was aware that this was in some ways his own doing: his name-dropping, his flamboyant dress, his open frustration with those in his community who, he felt, failed to live up to the standard the medical profession demands were all qualities that often ruffled the delicate sensibilities of many of Philadelphia's medical elite.

"Mütter's fancy was full and free, and in its brilliant play, was sometimes hard to govern," Pancoast would later explain. "He had a desire for the possession of personal influence and position, which less ardent and more philosophic minds might deem *excessive*."

However, Pancoast was swift to clarify Mütter's intentions.

"These advantages were not coveted by him, however, for personal aggrandizement solely," he said, "but rather that he might be able to promote the interests of those who were dependent upon him or courted his support."

However, no matter how much time Mütter spent in the service of self-improvement, he was also painfully aware that some of the factors that eased others into positions of power were utterly beyond his control. The significant income he was now earning would ultimately prove unhelpful in climbing the ranks of Philadelphia's social hierarchy; in Philadelphia, family had always been valued above wealth.

In the years before he became a professor at Jefferson, Mütter had met and married Mary Alsop, a quiet, pious young woman from the elite Connecticut Alsops. However, her esteemed family did not mean much in Philadelphia. The influence of the Alsop family name was felt most strongly in Connecticut and to some extent Washington, DC—where Mary's aunts were persistent and successful in their goal to marry politicians—but carried much less weight in the City of Brotherly Love.

Still, Mütter had held hope that the combination of his wife's pedigree, his eminent position at the college, and the fashion and lifestyle that his new career allowed him could secure his entrance to the parties and social circles that even dull Franklin Bache could find invitation to just for having issued from the womb of Benjamin Franklin's granddaughter.

After all, it was not entirely unheard of that the upper class would accept some members of the "natural aristocracy" who had proved their right of entry by demonstrating talent and what was considered to be virtue. But it was rare.

Even the new industrial and financial leaders and successful speculators in real estate found it hard to gain admittance to the upper social stratum in Philadelphia and indeed were generally seen as "vulgar."

"The lines of demarcation in [Philadelphia] 'society' were as strongly drawn as in Europe, or more so," Philadelphia humorist Charles Godfrey Leland would later recall, "with the enormous difference [being] that there was not the slightest perceptible shade of difference in the intellects, culture, or character of the people on either side of the line. . . . Very trifling points of difference, not perceptible to an outsider, made the whole difference between the exclusives and the excluded."

And the upper echelons of Philadelphia society were tempting places to want to be accepted.

"How am I able to communicate a just notion of the intelligence, the refinement, the enterprise of Philadelphians?" another British tourist would write of his time among the Philadelphia elite. "Their agreeable and hospitable society, their pleasant evening-parties, their love of literature, their happy blending of the industrial habits of the north with the social usages of the south? All this must be left to conjecture, as well as the Oriental luxury of their dwellings, and the delicate beauty of their ladies."

Mütter was told to be patient and to keep working hard, but it only served to make him more frustrated. Especially when he took into account how Charles D. Meigs was treated.

MEIGS HAD NOT BEEN BORN INTO THE PHILADELPHIA ELITE. FAR from it, in fact. He was born on the island of St. George's in Bermuda, but his father Josiah's legendary temper forced them to leave. It was an unfortunate trend, and the family found themselves relocating across the United States—first in New England, then in the South—for much of Meigs's early life.

The vagabond life was not easy for the large and growing family. Meigs's parents already had four children when Meigs was born—Henry, Clara, and Samuel, who were still living, and little Julia, who died when she was just over six months old—and continued to have children despite the family's habit of packing up and moving on. Juliana, Ezra Stiles, and John Benjamin were born after Meigs and lived, but a little brother died shortly after his birth on a ship while the family was traveling from Bermuda back to the mainland. They named the infant Sea, and then buried him there.

It must have been a relief to Meigs's mother, Clara, when the family decided to settle permanently in Georgia, in a little frontier town whose population numbered "only two hundred and seventy souls." Josiah was hired to be president of a new school currently being built there, and felt secure that his family could finally lay down some real roots in this semi-wild, sparsely inhabited country surrounded on all sides by a great forest.

The American frontier was an ever-shifting landscape at the time, and the land within twenty-eight miles of young Meigs's front door was still occupied by Native Americans—the various tribes of the Cherokee, Creek, Choctaw, and Chickasaw. It was also a short distance from Hiwassee, Tennessee, where Meigs's uncle, Colonel Return J. Meigs—his father's elder and best-beloved brother—lived.

Colonel Meigs was a legend in the family. He had fought so bravely all through the Revolutionary War that the United States Congress itself gave him a sword for gallant conduct. Now he served as the government's Indian agent in Tennessee, overseeing numerous tribes in the area. Over six feet tall and as "erect as a tree," he commanded the respect of all around him. So much so that the Native Americans in his area referred to him as the White Chief.

It was in this land "of law and lawlessness, of wild nature and of cultivated humanity, of education and refinement, of ignorance and downright barbarism" that Charles D. Meigs spent his formative years.

"Here was a spot, a climate—forest and stream, hill and dale—well calculated to tempt a hardy, active and most restless child to the pursuits best fitted to develop a strong and vigorous body," Meigs's son would later write of his father's childhood. "Not only so, but the basis of that decision of character, which, under the various terms of courage, pluck, grit, endurance, constitutes, it seems to me, the chiefest element in the mental constitution of most of our ablest and most successful men—that predominance of will which comes of a sound, robust body, and which we ought all to endeavor to evolve in our children—must have here been laid in my father, broad and deep."

The combination of the wilderness of this area surrounding his home and the refinement of the college being built proved to be the defining element of Meigs's childhood. His father made sure that all of his boys were highly educated: multilingual and well-versed in a variety of subjects. But living in the frontier country meant that young Meigs couldn't help but also become familiar with what it meant to live "a truly savage life."

"He had made the acquaintance of a certain Jim Vann, a well-known and conspicuous Indian of the Cherokee tribe, who had a store on the frontier," his son would write. "On one occasion, when on his way down to the coast, Vann said to my father: *Now, Charlie, if your mother will let you, I will take you back to the Indian country when I return, where you can see how we live, and I will give you the finest Indian (Injin) pony in the country.*"

While Meigs thrilled at the offer, it wasn't easy to convince his family to allow the young Meigs to take this trip. While many knew Vann to be a generous and kind man, no one could escape the fact that when he was in his moods, he became "a most violent and brutal fellow."

And indeed, Meigs's mother at first flatly "and with high indignation" refused even to listen to such a project. But Meigs persisted and "never ceased to beg and entreat and knock, until finally, in a very despair of escape from his knockings, she yielded."

Having received his mother's blessing, he waited for Vann's return. And waited. And waited. And just when all hope was about to die, Vann arrived, riding a powerful black stallion, looking the very picture of adventure. Meigs climbed on the back of the horse and off they went. Meigs would live "in the Nation" for over a month. He was twelve years old.

Meigs spoke often of this time in his life, and especially of Vann's savagery and wildness.

"As I grew older, I came to think that some of his stories about that time have been exaggerations," Meigs's son would later confess, "but when I found my grandfather writing to his brother, the government agent to the very tribe to which Vann belonged . . . I can well believe that all my father's stories may have been quite within the truth."

The letter, written just four years after Meigs's extended trip with Vann, reads: "Poor Vann has *ceased from troubling*, and the circumstances must be pleasing to you, for his death was a public blessing."

So how was it that Meigs, who was so brutish in his interactions with people and had such an unconventional past, could be accepted into Philadelphia's highest social strata while Mütter still struggled to be seen and heard?

BY THE MID-1840S, MEIGS WAS WILDLY POPULAR IN PHILADELPHIA medical circles, a man of great versatility and personal magnetism, and he was an extremely rapid writer.

Meigs was swiftly creating an extensive literary work, starting with his translation in 1831 of Velpeau's *Traité Élémentaire de l'Art des Accouchemens, ou Principes de Tokologie et d'Embryologie,* under the title, *An Elementary Treatise on Midwifery, or Principles of Tokology and Embryology.* For the next thirty years, one book after another flowed in rapid succession from his hand. He prepared many of his books within a few months, and even composed one of his bestselling textbooks, *Females and Their Diseases, a Series of Letters to His Class,* in the interval between two teaching sessions. Meigs's 1838 textbook, *The Philadelphia Practice of Midwifery,* was so hugely popular that a second edition was already necessary by 1842. This despite the fact that critics had called it "a meager book," noting that the author had not only made no attempt to classify the several varieties of deformities in his chapter on deformed pelvises, but actually stated that "the task would be useless." They also criticized him for his views on embryology—which they called "very misty" and confusingly lost in "a haze of words"—and for his strongly held belief, which was incorrect, that the placenta was entirely fetal in origin and that no vascular connections existed between it and the uterine wall.

But students and readers in the medical community loved his textbooks, which were theatrically written and often studded with harrowing dialogue-filled scenes between doctor and patient. In the chapter about the muscular structure of the womb, he wrote about a physician who, upon introducing his hand to remove a retained placenta, "found his arm so firmly grasped by the cervix that he was unable to withdraw it until the spasm had relaxed by copious bloodletting."

Bloodletting and leeching were commonly prescribed forms of treatment by Meigs, who was an eloquent advocate of the use of the lancet in a variety of circumstances, including the threat of miscarriage, to overcome the rigidity of the birth canal, and as his cure of eclampsia (a sometimes fatal condition caused by dangerously high blood pressure found in laboring women).

EVEN MÜTTER HAD AGREED THAT MEIGS WAS AN ENGAGING AND highly readable author with the enviable ability to vividly impress into the minds of his readers whatever views he wanted to promote. Unfortunately, Mütter disagreed with many of those views. He found many of Meigs's ideas lazy, others inaccurate, and some to be outright harmful, especially his tendency not only to positively *deny* the contagious nature of diseases he came across in his practice (such as childbed fever), but to take a step further and ridicule anyone who opposed with him.

It was this bravado and colorful showmanship that earned him a devoted following within the Jefferson Medical College student body, including the future Class of 1845 graduate Edward Robinson Squibb.

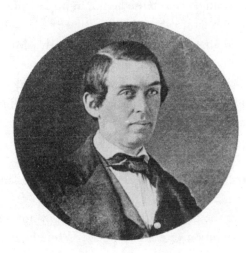

Edward Robinson Squibb

Squibb was a local boy, born on the Fourth of July of 1819, whose attraction to medicine seemed eerily similar to Mütter's. At age twelve, Squibb watched his mother and all three of his sisters die within a year of each other. His father suffered a stroke soon after, and though the elder Squibb survived, he was an "ineffectual invalid for the rest of his days." And being from poorer circumstances than his classmates, Squibb paid his tuition at Jefferson Medical College by working as an apprentice for a Philadelphia pharmacist—where he learned the art of grinding crude drugs, mixing elixirs, and compounding powders—and then by working at the pharmaceutical house of J. H. Sprague, between attending classes full-time.

But of all the members of the Jefferson faculty, it was Drs. Meigs and Bache who were Squibb's "unqualified favorites."

"Dr. Bache, with his patriarchal white beard and distinguished lineage," Squibb wrote in the journal he kept his entire life, "with his clear, playing, logical and unforgettable definition of chemistry, is the most forcible teacher I have ever known. . . . He contrasts strongly with some of the rest."

Meanwhile, Squibb described "the clean-shaven, dramatic, Bermuda born" Meigs as having "the originality of idea, and erratic, familiar manner, curious postures and gestures which would not fit well elsewhere."

"He and Bache are wildly different as good and bad," Squibb said appraisingly. "And yet both are capital teachers."

While he admired both men, Squibb's praise for Meigs echoed over more pages. Squibb saw Meigs as "a striking figure as he stood before his class, his sharp features animated, his long dark hair brushed back over his ears, his spectacles pushed up on his high forehead," noting his skill and knowledge of obstetrics, and how unafraid he was to use humor in his lectures.

For instance, a charmed Squibb wrote about how one day in class—to illustrate how little women knew about the realities of childbirth—Meigs recounted his experience of aiding a young French woman in the birth of her child. Peals of laughter filled the lecture hall as Meigs described the doleful expression on the young woman's face as he attempted to examine her post-labor, and through her shock she could only tell him, *"Ah, mon pauvre docteur, c'est tout gâté pour jamais!"* ("Ah, my dear doctor, it's all spoiled forever!").

Squibb's opinions of the other faculty members, especially Mütter and Pancoast, were not as favorable.

Squibb wrote about watching the duo—with an admiring but not uncritical eye—during a public exhibition of plastic surgery. While he gave credit to the "small, blue-eyed Mütter with his dark curly hair graying prematurely, and his finely chiseled features" for explaining every move in his clear, musical voice, he was critical of the "round faced Pancoast, bald except for a monastic fringe, a spot of his full red lower lip showing below the twists of his sandy handlebar mustache," who throughout the delicate surgery could be seen wiping his bloody fingers on his pocket handkerchief and his instruments "on whatever was handy."

Squibb was an outspoken student and did not hide his opinions of his professors, even openly discussed his differences with them. They, in turn, would invite him to sit in the best seats in the amphitheater for their lectures, and he earned invitation to parties at the professors' homes. Bache invited Squibb to his "medical-club meeting," where, ironically, strictly professional conversation was prohibited by rule, and Squibb even went to back-to-back student parties held by Pancoast and Meigs. The menus at both parties—chicken salad and ice cream at Pancoast's; chicken salad, oysters, and ice cream at Meigs's—resulted in the young medical student finding himself and his fellows students in a tavern at night's end, where they collectively hoped that a little brandy would "keep down the rebellion in [their] stomachs."

But Mütter was absent from many of these festivities, and the reason his time was so fully occupied during this period could be traced back to Europe.

WHILE MÜTTER OFTEN FELT MISUNDERSTOOD AND DISMISSED IN America, he remained a darling of Europe. In July 1844, *The British and Foreign Medical Review* published a rapturous write-up of Mütter's surgeries, especially those on the severely burned—a population that many had been led to believe was "beyond any real medical help."

They wrote:

> There are few, if any, deformities consequent on accident, short of the irreparable loss of limbs, which have so successfully set at defiance the *art* of surgery for their removal, as those occasioned by burns; indeed the surgeon has felt that, in the production of the deformity which he could fully anticipate and had ample leisure to watch, nature's antagonising powers have overmatched him. . . .
>
> We, therefore, hail with satisfaction any attempt to remedy evils which have been either from neglect or unavoidably produced; and we cordially congratulate Dr. Mütter on the success which seems to have attended his operations. . . .

We shall have great pleasure in resuming a more intimate acquaintance with Dr. Mütter's present productions; and shall be pleased, as we have reason to expect, if they lead to an introduction to some more comprehensive work, by which we may judge of the present state of transatlantic surgery.

Mütter eventually caught the attention of a British publishing house, which was releasing what they hoped would be the definitive surgical textbook of the famous British surgeon Robert Liston, known as the fastest knife in the West End.

Liston, like Mütter, was a colorful figure in surgery. He was tall, ambitious, and charismatic, often yelling, "Time me, gentlemen, time me!" to his students before beginning his amputations.

Although Liston was renowned for his success stories—such as the removal of a forty-five-pound scrotal tumor in four minutes; prior to the operation, the poor patient had been forced to carry his scrotum around in a wheelbarrow—he also developed a reputation for the flamboyancy of his surgical failures. For instance, his joy at amputating a patient's leg at the thigh in less than three minutes was hindered greatly when he realized he had also inadvertently sawed off the patient's testicles.

And perhaps, most famously, another leg amputation performed in less than three minutes had the unfortunate result of killing three people: the patient (who survived the surgery but died of gangrene several days later); his young assistant (whose fingers he accidentally sawed off during surgery and who would also later succumb to gangrene); and "a distinguished surgical spectator" whose coattails Liston also slashed. The man, who found himself surrounded by geysers of blood, was so convinced that the knife had pierced his vitals that he immediately "dropped dead from fright." It was later described as "the only operation in history with a 300 percent mortality [rate]."

But those luckless cases were, of course, rare for Liston.

And if anything, Liston was far more likely to enrage and alienate the medical community with his thoughts on surgical hygiene than with tales of his darkly comical surgical mishaps.

Like Mütter, Liston inherently understood that there was a connection between the cleanliness of a doctor and the rate of infection among his patients. It was an unpopular line of thinking during a time when "surgeons operated in blood-stiffened frock coats" and "the stiffer the coat, the prouder the busy surgeon."

"There was no object in being clean," a medical historian would later note of this era in surgery. "Indeed, cleanliness was out of place. It was

considered to be finicking and affected. An executioner might as well manicure his nails before chopping off a head."

Liston was unafraid to challenge the thoughts of the day, which he considered fundamentally wrong. It was even written that his suggestions for
hygiene improvement to reduce obstetric infections and mortality from puerperal fever had crossed the ocean and "outraged obstetricians, particularly in Philadelphia."

But despite his "abrupt, abrasive, argumentative" nature, he was also
known as a man who was "charitable to the poor and tender to the sick."

"He relished operating successfully in the reeking tenements of [Edin-
burgh, Scotland's] Grassmarket and Lawnmarket on patients [whom his
peers] had discharged as hopelessly incurable," a historian later wrote.
"They conspired to bar him from the wards, banished him south, where he
became professor of surgery at University College Hospital in London and
made a fortune."

To the publisher, it seemed a perfect pairing to combine these two controversial, rising stars of surgery, and create a textbook that would bridge
the gap between Europe and America.

Mütter was invited to edit an American edition of Liston's textbook, the
lengthily titled *Lectures on the Operations of Surgery, and on Diseases and Accidents Requiring Operations.*

All Mütter was tasked to do was to read the tome and then add his own
thoughts and ideas to the material. To be clear, the text of Liston's book
would not and could not be largely changed, but Mütter would be free to
clarify points for an American audience of readers and add his own anecdotes and illustrations as needed.

Mütter tackled the project with a dark glee, and between his full teaching load and his demanding surgical practice, he found time to add more
than two hundred additional pages of anecdotes and opinion, and several
fearsome illustrations, increasing the size of the book—much to the surprise of his publisher—by over half. The American edition, with Mütter's
additions, came out in 1846, two years after Liston published the original.

The book would teach medical students the best ways to tackle the basics, such as incisions, hemorrhage, and the dressing and union of wounds.
It covered injuries of the scalp, the cranium, and the brain, including the
most effective trephining techniques—that is, the use of small circle-
shaped saws to drill into the skull for eventual bone removal. Tumors of all
kinds were discussed—tumors of the eye, tumors of the throat, tumors of

the ear—including methods of swiftest and safest removal, since of course all patients would be awake during surgery. And Mütter was sure to extensively cover the burgeoning field of plastic surgery.

Mütter made sure to push forward his theories on presurgical care—how hours, days, or even weeks spent working with the patient prior to a surgery could be instrumental in a successful outcome. While the speed of the surgeon's hands was certainly helpful, Mütter strongly believed that working with the patient was equally important—a somewhat radical idea.

In his preface, he proudly spoke about the book and about himself in the third person:

> In presenting to the profession in this country these lectures of Mr. Liston, I feel fully assured that no apology is necessary; like everything emanating from that excellent surgeon, they teem with practical and judicious advice, and their perusal will amply repay even the veterans of our art.
>
> It will be observed that this volume contains all the lectures published up to the present date, but does not conclude the course. It is simply a collection of much valuable matter, delivered in 1844 at the University College, London, and furnished the profession through the pages of the "London Lancet." It must prove a most valuable *addition* to the other works of Mr. Liston, republished in this country, and which should be in the hands of every surgeon.
>
> The additional matter furnished by the editor is included within brackets [ ], and amounts to near two hundred and fifty pages, a much larger quantity than he at first expected to add, but he trusts it may not be without its advantages as illustrating some points of surgery but slightly or not at all referred to by the author. Another volume will be issued hereafter, should the publication of the lectures be continued.

Mütter felt confident that the book would be a breakthrough for him. In preparation of this, he began to change his demeanor slightly, dulling his personality and downplaying the perceptions that people had of him, even with his own students.

In fact, for the 1845–1846 semester, Mütter's own introductory lecture began, "I fear that some among you will be disappointed at the turn I have given this discourse, but my aim, gentlemen, is to *instruct*, not to *amuse*."

That year, Jefferson Medical College could not only claim the largest enrollment of students in its entire history (469 students), but also the largest enrollment of students of any institution of its kind in the entire United States.

The college celebrated by renovating its main lecture hall. The upper and lower lecture rooms were enlarged to seat 600 students (up from 450) and the upper lecture hall—known as the pit—was reserved for Mütter and was

LECTURES

ON THE

OPERATIONS OF SURGERY,

AND ON

DISEASES AND ACCIDENTS REQUIRING OPERATIONS.

BY ROBERT LISTON, ESQ., F. R. S.,

SENIOR SURGEON TO THE UNIVERSITY COLLEGE HOSPITAL, AND PROFESSOR OF CLINICAL
SURGERY IN THE COLLEGE.

WITH

NUMEROUS ADDITIONS

BY THOMAS D. MÜTTER, M. D.,

Professor of Surgery in Jefferson Medical College, Philadelphia; Fellow of the Royal Medical and
Chirurgical Society of London; Foreign Honorary and Corresponding Member of the Provin-
cial Medical Association of Great Britain; Corresponding Member of the National
Institute at Washington; Fellow of the College of Physicians, Philadelphia;
Member of the Academy of Natural Sciences, Philadelphia; Corresponding Member of the New York Medical Society;
Honorary Member of the Medical Societies
of Philadelphia, of Virginia,
&c. &c. &c.

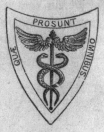

PHILADELPHIA:
LEA AND BLANCHARD.
1846.

where he would perform all of his surgical lectures. Mütter insisted that a connection be made between the pit and the upper floors being rented as recovery rooms in the building next door. This "miniature hospital" would represent a precursor of Jefferson Medical College's subsequent formal teaching hospital, which would be built nearly thirty years later.

Even the exterior of the college changed. Now when the nearly five hundred students came pushing toward the building doors, they would climb a fine set of marble stairs and negotiate the six Corinthian columns that graced the facade, evoking the form of a Grecian temple.

"In every respect, the comfort and advantage of the students have been consulted," the college would later state in its annual report, "and the outward form has been devised and executed in a style, which, lest it does credit to the architect, is an ornament to the city. Nowhere, perhaps, at home or abroad is there an edifice more admirably adapted for its important objects—none where more facilities are offered for successful teaching."

MÜTTER'S PRESTIGE, TOO, CONTINUED TO BLOSSOM. FORMER U.S. vice president John C. Calhoun even brought in his own daughter to Mütter to see if he could help fix her various curious ailments.

"[We] expected . . . to be back yesterday," Calhoun wrote in a letter home, "but the Doctor spoke with such confidence of restoring her hearing & befitting her in relations to the curve of the spine, that she has been induced to remain some time longer."

(It was only a few months later that former president Andrew Jackson, under whom Calhoun had served as vice president, died, sending the whole country into deep mourning. In honor of "the irreparable loss our Nation has sustained by the death of the illustrious Andrew Jackson," the entire faculty, staff, and board of Jefferson Medical College wore crepe on the left arm for sixty straight days, and the building itself was shrouded in black mourning bunting for six months.)

Mütter's reputation had grown enough that the medical community was slowly warming to him too. He held charming parties often at his own home, where his wife and their servants (five free men) lived. It was a large home, filled with elegant and expensive furniture ("Mütter has no children and makes a good income by his profession," a peer would offer as an excuse for such opulence, though no reason was given—nor would one ever be— for why Mary and Mütter's union remained a childless one).

At Mütter's parties, he attempted to blend all strata of people, though he still struggled with not offending others when he expressed what he considered to be obvious facts and theories about the future of medicine.

When a visiting doctor came through Philadelphia, he was delighted to have received an invitation to one of Mütter's famous dinners. When he arrived, he found a motley group called together to dine: local doctors, British consuls, University of Pennsylvania professors, ministers of France, a former Virginia governor, and the most recent mayor of Philadelphia, and of course Mütter himself, who left a memorable but unfortunately less than charming impression on the man.

The doctor later wrote in his diary, "At so large a dinner conversation is never general, but the company collect in little sets. Everything was very handsome. [Mütter] is, however, a good deal of a humbug, and has to great excess the bad habit of puffing himself. To this, however, I imagine he chiefly owes his success."

Still, Mütter felt his life was now on the right track and that this book would only serve to fortify the obvious: that he was a major force in the future of American medicine and that his life as a surgeon was about to change.

He was right on one count: His life as a surgeon *was* about to change, but not for the reasons he imagined.

ON OCTOBER 16, 1846, THE SAME YEAR THAT MÜTTER'S TEXTBOOK was published, a dentist named William T. G. Morton and a professor of surgery named John Collins Warren stepped into a Harvard University lecture hall and gave a demonstration that would change the face of surgery forever . . . and render Mütter's just-released textbook on surgery almost instantly obsolete.

CHAPTER SIXTEEN

GENTLEMEN, THIS IS NO HUMBUG

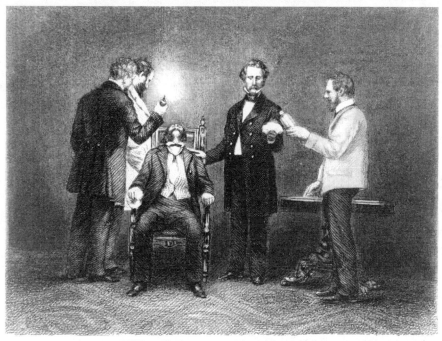

William T. G. Morton, Administering Ether

IN 1844, A CONNECTICUT DENTIST NAMED HORACE WELLS CAME to Harvard to share an astonishing discovery: If a person inhales the right quantity of the chemical nitrous oxide, the result is that they will feel no pain during medical or surgical procedures. It was hard to believe—a game-changing discovery that could instantly and permanently alter the practice of surgery.

AND IT WAS, AS WAS MADE EVIDENT TO THE ELITE HARVARD CLASS, a total fraud.

After all, when Wells proudly gave a demonstration of it in front of an eager class of Harvard Medical School students and faculty, the poor boy he selected as his patient continuously screamed out in wretched pain whenever Wells tried to extract his rotten tooth. They called Wells a swindler and said his discovery was a humbug. Wells was crushed, and his career never recovered.

But as it turned out, Wells was not a fraud. It was an "incident of history gone awry." The young man with the rotten tooth would later admit that he actually felt no pain and didn't even know the extraction had happened until he saw the bloody tooth in the dentist's hands. But as no one at the time knew, his screaming was simply one of the most common side effects of inhaling nitrous oxide gas. For reasons that were unknown, individuals who had recently inhaled nitrous oxide gas were known to scream, groan, or show agitated behavior—despite the fact that they were feeling absolutely no pain.

Unfortunately for Wells, he was not aware of this side effect, and neither was his audience at Harvard. So it happened that a medical breakthrough was showcased at one of the country's leading medical schools, and no one even knew it.

And even stranger, this wasn't the first time.

THE PAIN-ERASING EFFECTS OF NITROUS OXIDE WERE DISCOVERED almost a half century earlier by a chemist named Humphry Davy, who began his experiments with the chemical at England's Pneumatic Institution. However, these experiments were largely performed on himself and sometimes his friends. He became so fixated on the high he felt when inhaling the gas—addicted, some would later say—that he risked his life more than once in his attempts to inhale larger and larger quantities, and even had a colleague build him a portable gas chamber so he could have access to the gas wherever and whenever he wanted.

Although Davy was clearly very impressed with nitrous oxide's ability to seemingly stop the body from feeling pain, it seems that he never thought to promote it as an anesthetic for surgery. Instead, he promoted it as a cure for hangovers, and proceeded to perform detailed experiments—on himself, of course—to see just how many bottles of wine he could drink in a night and still have the effects "erased."

But Davy was not alone in missing the enormous potential of nitrous oxide, despite frequent interaction with it. In the early 1830s, sulphuric ether and nitrous oxide were both used as recreational drugs. In America, the fashionable and the young found themselves at "laughing gas parties" or "ether frolics," a popular traveling amusement.

In the 1830s and 1840s, it was not uncommon for a showman claiming to be a "professor of chemistry" to set up shop in towns, villages, and cities throughout the United States with the express intent of showcasing these amazing gases and their "exhilarating features." Of course, the most crowd-pleasing moments of the night were when the "professor" invited members of the audience to the stage to inhale the gases themselves. The sudden loss of equilibrium and inhibition would delight and shock the roaring crowds.

It was at one of these "laughing gas" demonstrations in 1844 that dentist Horace Wells realized the potential of sulphuric ether and nitrous oxide. The morning after witnessing the spectacle, he convinced a colleague to extract one of his teeth after he himself had inhaled some nitrous oxide. After the tooth was successfully removed, an elated Wells shouted out, "It is the greatest discovery ever made! I didn't feel as much as the prick of a pin!"

But if Wells's disastrous experience at Harvard had a bright spot, it was that he met John Collins Warren, the influential professor of surgery at the Massachusetts General Hospital.

Warren was already familiar with the idea of using nitrous oxide as an anesthetic through his acquaintanceship with Charles Thomas Jackson, "one of the most eccentric and bizarre of all personalities connected with the discovery of surgical anesthesia."

Jackson, a graduate of Harvard Medical School, began inhaling nitrous in 1841, and by 1844, he had persuaded several local dentists that the gas could be helpful in relieving the pain of their patients' toothaches. And it was Jackson who suggested in September 1846—nine months after Wells's embarrassing incident at Harvard—that another Boston-area dentist, William T. G. Morton, use sulphuric ether mixed with air, believing it might prove to be an even better anesthetic than nitrous oxide. Morton tried it out and found the results astonishing. He then asked John Collins Warren if he might share this latest innovation with his class.

And that is how on October 16, 1846, in the same surgical amphitheater as Wells's fiasco, Warren and Morton gave the first-ever public demonstration of the effects of this "anonymous" liquid on a patient.

It was an incredible sight.

Morton served as the esthetician—who both prepared the anesthesia mixture and administered it by tipping the jug of gas into the patient's face. The confident Morton looked out into the audience as the young patient slowly seemed to lose complete consciousness. Once the patient appeared fully out, Warren stepped in to skillfully remove a small tumor from the young man's neck. The patient seemed peacefully asleep during the whole procedure, even as the scalpel sliced through his flesh and the suture needles repeatedly pierced his skin.

After the surgery was over, the duo patiently waited for the grand finale. Finally, the patient appeared to wake up from this man-made slumber and told the slack-jawed audience that he felt no pain.

It was then that Warren—who had not spoken during the entire surgery—finally uttered his iconic words about the dawn of a new era in surgery:

"Gentlemen, this is no humbug."

CHAPTER SEVENTEEN

ADVENT

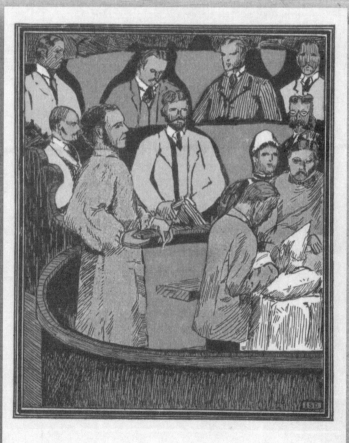

December 23, 1846 . . . Thomas Mütter
in clinic demonstrates ether anæsthesia for
the first time in Philadelphia.

THE PHYSICIAN MUST BE
A DETERMINED, PERSEVERING MAN;
A MAN OF STEADY PURPOSE

There is scarcely a quality which so much dignifies
human nature as consistency of conduct—and
no weakness more deplorable than that of instability.
Examine, choose, compare, reject, but having once made
your selection of profession, stand by your decision.
Difficulties, and privations, and hardships, must be
encountered; but determination will overcome them all.
And not only sloth and folly, but even genius
will be outdone by perseverance.
It often is the case that he who can endure the most
is in the end the most successful.

Thomas Dent Mütter

T HE EARLIEST DEMONSTRATIONS OF ETHER ANESTHESIA WERE performed during painful yet somewhat minor surgeries—tooth extractions and small tumors—but each one was an "unqualified triumph." As people clamored to know more about this amazing new discovery, Morton realized that his unique combination of sulphuric ether and nitrous oxide could be a potential moneymaking opportunity. He not only refused to tell people the makeup of this transformative gas, but he also stopped all public trials of the anesthesia—which he called Letheon, after Lethe, Greek mythology's mythical river of forgetfulness.

But the medical community wouldn't stand for it, and an enterprising young surgeon named Henry J. Bigelow specifically called out Morton to give a more ambitious demonstration. Bigelow explained that while toothaches and small tumor removals were all well and good, he wanted to know if this promising surgical tool would work in "capital" (or major) surgery.

Bigelow—who already imagined that Letheon contained sulphuric ether—challenged Morton to use his "preparation" in a leg amputation he was slated to perform. The amputation was one of the most dangerous, deadly, and painful kinds of this type of surgery: full amputation at the thigh.

This was a true test of the new anesthesia, and one that medical men were all familiar with: the image of the man held down on the table as the doctor approaches with his kit of amputation tools; the first jolt and yelp of pain as the long, curved blade of the amputation knife slashes the man's skin, ripping into it violently; as the saw makes its way through veins and arteries and on to muscle, everyone's clothing becomes dark, wet, and heavy with sweat and the eruptive spurts of salty blood; as the doctor pauses to switch tools, the man might receive a surge of adrenaline like an electrical shock, and the men tasked with holding him down redouble their efforts as he bucks wildly, his skin now hard to grab because of the slick coating of his own blood; and then everyone hears it, the sound of the amputation saw's blade hitting the bone; minutes pass as the room fills with the slow growl of the saw, the cracking of bone, and the screams of the poor man tasked to endure it all.

Now imagine being the surgeons who had to face this scenario so often, and who—because of the calling of their profession—had to be the traumatizing source of so much agony, even as a deep desire to *relieve* the pain of others was the reason so many of them wanted to become physicians in the first place.

It is no mystery why surgeons often prized the speed of a surgery over its precision. Warren himself described how difficult these types of surgeries were to perform in the early to middle nineteenth century, writing:

> It was the custom to bring the patient into the operation room and place him upon the table. The surgeon would stand with both hands behind his back and say to the patient,
> "Will you have your leg off, or will you not have it off?"
> If the patient lost courage and said, "No," he had decided not to have the leg amputated, he was at once carried back to his bed in the ward.
> If, however, he said, "Yes," he was immediately taken firmly in hand by a number of strong assistants and the operation went on regardless of whatever he might say thereafter.
> If his courage failed him after this crucial moment, it was too late and no attention was paid to his cries of protest.
> It was found to be the only practicable method by which an operation could be performed under the gruesome conditions which prevailed before the advent of anesthesia.

Having been publicly called out, Morton felt forced to accept the challenge. In front of Bigelow's watchful eyes, Morton was able to render the patient "unconscious and insensitive to pain." And the amputation surgery was a complete success. Not only that, but Bigelow was able to convince Morton to share his recipe of how to create Letheon simply and cheaply and to give authorization to Bigelow to write the first truly detailed public announcement of his discovery. The Bigelow-penned paper would be read before the Boston Society for Medical Improvement in early November and published as a report in *The Boston Medical and Surgical Journal* a week later.

Though all would agree that Bigelow's actions represent the first formal announcement of the discovery of surgical anesthesia to the medical profession, there was considerable controversy at the time about whether Morton should be credited with the first *use* of ether anesthesia.

As it turned out, a rural physician named Dr. Crawford W. Long, who ran a practice in Jefferson, Georgia, had been using ether anesthesia for minor procedures as early as 1842. But unlike Morton and Wells, Long did not share the news of this breakthrough, and therefore, his works on his own history with ether anesthesia were not published until well after Morton's demonstrations.

REGARDLESS OF THE LONG AND CROOKED ROAD IT TOOK, WHEN news of ether anesthesia reached Thomas Dent Mütter, he immediately saw its vast potential and knew he had to try it for himself.

Not everyone in the community shared Mütter's enthusiasm for the potential of ether anesthesia, and some even advised him not to do the surgery, but he was determined.

Two days before Christmas in 1846—just two months after Morton and Warren performed the first public ether anesthesia demonstration—Mütter brought a young man with a large cheek tumor into the pit of Jefferson Medical College. Having read everything he could on the subject, Mütter carefully administered the anesthesia himself and performed the surgery.

It was . . . effortless.

Mütter—about whom it was said that he "appeared often at operations to be painfully sympathetic with the suffering of the patient"—became the first surgeon in Philadelphia to administer anesthesia and soon became consumed with the idea of harnessing its incredible promise . . . never imagining the resistance he would face.

CHAPTER EIGHTEEN

ALL THE FAIR DAUGHTERS OF EVE

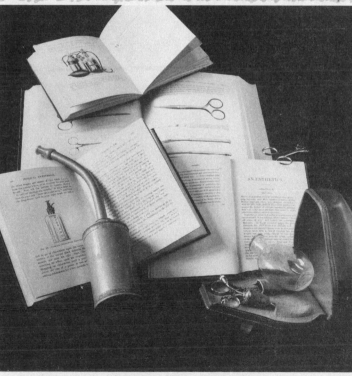

Early Tools and Texts on Anesthesia

MUCH TO MÜTTER'S SHOCK, THE MEDICAL COMMUNITY'S OPPO-
sition to ether anesthesia was immediate and widespread, especially in
Philadelphia.

"We are persuaded that the surgeons of Philadelphia will not be seduced
from the high professional path of duty into the quagmire of quackery by
this will-o'-the-wisp," the editor of the powerful *Medical Examiner* noted
when speaking about the subject of anesthesia. "We . . . regret that the eminent men of . . . Boston should have . . . set so bad an example to their
younger brethren."

In their defense, when "inhalation anesthesia" was introduced into the
medical community, not all the surgeries were successful. As doctors and
dentists began their own experiments with the imperfect chemicals and
dosages, there was a great number of deaths. Many in the community
would begin to see ether anesthesia as no more than a passing fad, yet another dangerous medical novelty in a century that seemed rife with them.

"The last special wonder has already arrived at the natural term of its existence, and the interest created by its first advent has in a great measure
subsided," the New York City medical journal *The Annalist* wrote in January
1847—just three months after ether anesthesia made its Harvard debut. "It
has descended to the bottom of that great abyss which has already engulfed
so many of its predecessor novelties."

And Philadelphia—"the medical Athens of America"—was perhaps the
most resistant to the idea of it. The first medical textbook to mention anesthesia was *On Bandaging and Other Operations of Minor Surgery*, written by
a Philadelphia surgeon named Fitzwilliam Sargent, and in it he wrote:

> These agents have been employed to relieve pain in all sorts of opera-
> tions . . . they have been administered by the ignorant as well as by the
> learned, and without any discrimination of cases.
>
> It is not at all surprising, therefore, that in many instances injurious, and
> sometimes fatal, consequences have ensued. . . .
>
> It should be recollected that the mere performance of an operation, with
> comparative freedom from suffering to the patient and with satisfaction to
> the surgeon, is but one step towards the cure of the affection for which the op-
> eration is performed: the treatment of the patient subsequently is a matter of
> equal importance; and with reference to this part of the surgeon's duty, any
> cause which disturbs the healthy play of important functions, whether it be
> the impression of too intense pain, or of too powerful narcotic agents, is to be
> regarded as an evil.

Mütter was dismayed that something he considered a gift from God
could be seen as an evil by his peers and contemporaries. The strong feelings against the use of anesthesia went much deeper than just a gentleman's disagreement about its use. Institutions began to take public stances
against it. The board of Philadelphia's Pennsylvania Hospital—the main
hospital with which Jefferson Medical College had a working relationship— successfully voted to ban all use of the surgical anesthesia for seven
years.

Even worse for Mütter, one of anesthesia's most outspoken critics would
emerge among his own faculty: Charles D. Meigs.

IN HIS 1846 INTRODUCTORY LECTURE, MEIGS EXPLAINED TO A
packed lecture hall what he perceived to be his responsibilities as both a
professor and a physician.

"I acknowledge that I am an enthusiastic admirer of my profession.
My speech declares it, and my whole past life is perpetual proof of it.
But I love that profession as a ministry, not as a trade . . . ," he told
them. "In what light shall he see the nature of man so clearly and so
plainly?"

Meigs truly saw his role as God-given, and thus his opinions as actual
absolutes.

"He taught in his lectures not only the absolute duty of the student to be
always a student, in order that he might personally command the use of all
that the observation and experience of the world were constantly discovering
in the way of remedies and cures . . . ," his own son would later write of him,
"but he also ever taught that there was in medicine a moral element, which

did not enter so deeply into any other human vocation except that of the preacher.

"He always held that there was in the practice of medicine what he sometimes called a missionary element, a high flavor of charity," he continued, "which no man could, and no good man would, desire to escape from."

After examining what he saw as the facts of this new discovery, Meigs believed it was his responsibility to take "great pains to demonstrate the dangers of ether inhalation." It should come as no surprise that Meigs, a professor who was not afraid to be theatrical in his lessons, would take this particular lesson to the extreme.

And what could be more effective in showing how easily a life might be destroyed by this, in his opinion, "dangerous agent" than by etherizing a sheep *to death* in the classroom?

Sometimes it would be just one sheep; other times, Meigs would bring up to four—forcing the class to watch each one die in succession in order to afford his students, as he alleged, "a practical illustration of its dangers."

"Prejudice was an element deeply rooted in his character," his future colleague Samuel D. Gross later wrote of Meigs. "His opposition to [anesthesia] was founded, not upon personal experiences, but upon the reports of medical journalists, who inconsiderably exaggerated its evil effects."

Meigs didn't care if the lesson he was teaching was in direct opposition to the work and passions of peers such as Mütter. In fact, he seemed to delight in being their foil, so certain was he of himself.

One professor recalled how Meigs even got into the habit of interrogating other surgeons as to whether or not they were planning to use anesthesia during their next clinic day.

"Certainly, my dear friend" was the invariable answer.

"Then, by God, I hope you will kill your patient!" was the invariable rejoinder, the professor remembered.

Once this same professor grew so upset that Meigs would say such a thing that he shouted at Meigs, "You will find it hard when you die to pass the gates of St. Peter, opposed as you will be by the vast flocks of sheep, the family, friends, and descendants of those you so unceremoniously and unkindly immolated upon the altar of science."

Meigs simply responded with a hearty laugh.

HOWEVER, MEIGS WASN'T ALWAYS TRIUMPHANT WITH HIS RABID evangelism against ether. A favorite story shared by those who resented his disdainful position on anesthesia was about one of the days when he brought a sheep into the amphitheater to be "heroically etherized" to death.

In every way, it was the standard demonstration he loved to give. The animal, ears nervously flitting, was dragged into the center of the lecture as hundreds of students looked on.

Ellerslie Wallace, Meigs and Mütter's former student, now serving as Meigs's dutiful assistant, poured the freshly prepared ether from a demijohn as Meigs gave his speech.

"Pain," Meigs began, "what is *pain*? Is pain something temporary? Is pain something necessary? What is pain *worth*?"

With a nod from Meigs, the fat sheep was hefted onto the examination table. Meigs lowered his glasses and read the directions clearly and loudly. Wallace, following the instruction as best he could, began the sloppy process of etherizing the sheep, tilting the heavy jug of ether into the hastily constructed mask held firmly on the animal's face. The sheep bucked and struggled against its handler as its feet flailed on the wooden surface. The poor animal's plaintive bleating sounded not unlike the shrieks of a woman as it echoed against the lecture walls.

Meigs stepped away from the table, pushed his glasses onto his forehead, and looked out into the sea of students as the ether took effect and the sheep's body relaxed. Its breathing slowed. With another gesture from Meigs, the assistant removed the mask. The sheep remained motionless. Meigs placed his ear on the sheep's body and listened.

"Genesis 3:16," Meigs finally said, straightening up, "*In sorrow thou shalt bring forth children.*"

This was a lecture Meigs loved to give: Pain, and what we can learn from it. Pain, and how it was sometimes necessary. And, with this cherry-picked Bible quote: Pain, and how it was something women *must* endure, how it was God's will that they should suffer in labor for all time as penance for original sin.

Other obstetricians had begun to use ether in labor, Meigs explained, and word was spreading. Now women had begun to ask for it, to *beg* for it, this gas that promised to take all the pain away. There were stories of women so desperate for relief that they clawed at the eyes of the doctors who tried to remove the ether-soaked sponge from their faces. Meigs recounted to his students how his own laboring patients now pleaded with

him for ether, and how they wept and tore at their clothes when he refused—
which he did every single time.

The sheep had been lying on the table for about twenty minutes and it
was then that Meigs called forward one of the nearly five hundred students
who were packed into the lecture hall and asked him to come to the center
of the room and inspect the etherized sheep. The student complied and
gingerly began examining the animal, gently at first, and then more and
more roughly.

Finally, the student said what Meigs already knew: "The animal is
dead, sir."

Meigs's assistant carefully examined the sheep and confirmed the diagnosis.

"The animal is dead," Meigs repeated. "Healthy when he entered. Given
ether, exactly—*exactly*—as directed, and now, as a result, it is dead. *Dead.*"

Meigs instructed Wallace to remove the sheep, and the students watched
as the animal was dragged by its feet to the lying-in room at the back of the
amphitheater. Meigs noticed how their eyes trailed the animal.

"Imagine if that was your patient," he said, without turning his eyes
away from his audience.

"What is death?" he asked after a pause. "Should it be natural, or unnatural? What should we *fear* more of, pain or death? What should we try
to *prevent*, pain or death?

"My long and extensive practice of midwifery has rendered me a familiar
witness of pain and its various forms," Meigs continued. "And now, I have
grown accustomed to looking upon labor pain as a most *desirable, salutary*,
and *conservative* manifestation of life force. And I have found that women,
provided they were sustained by cheering counsel and promises, are freed
from terror and able to endure *without great complaint*, those labor pains
which the friends of the anesthesia desire so earnestly to abolish and nullify
for all the fair daughters of Eve.

"Perhaps, I am cruel in taking so dispassionate a view of the case," Meigs
confessed. "I know what you have heard. That a *hundred thousand* have
taken it without accident! I am a witness that it is attended," Meigs insisted,
gesturing to the sheep, "with alarming accidents, however rarely.

"So I ask you? Should I exhibit a remedy for pain to a thousand patients
in labor—merely to prevent the physiological pain and for no other motive—
and risk *destroying* one of them? Is relief from natural pain, decreed pain, for
even a thousand patients worth the risk of *killing* one woman?

"My *God*," he whispered, "if that were to happen, I ask that you clothe me in sack-cloth. I ask that you cast ashes on my head for the remainder of my days. What motive could I have had to risk the life or the death of one in a thousand? What motive should any of us?"

Meigs rapped his thin knuckles on the wooden railing that separated the students from the lecture floor. Meigs's style of lecturing was described by a colleague as being "conversational, not at all rhetorical. His habit was to walk around the arena of the amphitheatre, when he was not engaged in demonstrating, with one hand in his pocket and the other on the railing, earnestly talking as it were to the group of young men immediately before him, apparently forgetting that he was in the presence of anybody else."

Some of his critics had written that Meigs's lectures were often too melodramatic, or too conversational for a scholarly audience. A fellow professor even wrote that in the lecture room, Meigs was the best actor he had ever seen, for he "possessed all the requisites for success upon the stage— remarkable powers of mimicry, great enthusiasm, and a strong perception of the ludicrous."

But Meigs paid them no mind. He knew his lectures were persuasive and effective, and that he got his point across. And as he looked into the faces of his students and saw them enraptured, he felt the power of his position—a position he deserved and had *earned*.

And it was in that moment that it happened: a slight moan, barely audible, rose from the back of the amphitheater. It was low and almost human.

Meigs froze as he tried to place the sound and trace it to its origin. The only movements in the room were Meigs's eyebrows slowly gathering at the center of his face.

The sound filled the lecture hall again, grew louder, gained clarity. *Baaaa* . . .

The collective eyes of his students immediately found the source: the once-dead sheep was now rising, groggy and confused.

The students paused in their note-taking. Pens wet with ink dried in the air. Meigs stood silent and stiff before them, refusing to turn.

The sheep announced itself once more—*Baaa!*—before it attempted to stumble to its feet. It promptly fell over, a loud clatter in the suddenly uncomfortably quiet room. Soon after, the students couldn't help but erupt in deafening laughter as the sheep stumbled inelegantly out of the room, taking Meigs's boastful dignity with it.

CHAPTER NINETEEN

IF I MAY BUT TOUCH HIS GARMENT, I SHALL BE WHOLE

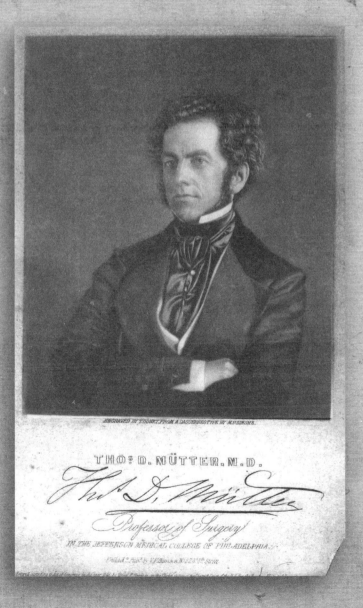

ENGRAVED BY TOOMEY FROM A DAGUERREOTYPE BY M.P.SIMONS.

THOS D. MÜTTER. M.D.

Thos D. Mütter

Professor of Surgery

IN THE JEFFERSON MEDICAL COLLEGE OF PHILADELPHIA.

THE PHYSICIAN SHOULD BE
A DISCREET MAN

It seems scarcely possible

that one possessed of the ordinary attributes

of a gentleman could ever forget

the sacred character of confidence . . .

"Whoso keepeth his mouth and his tongue,

keepeth his soul from troubles."

Thomas Dent Mütter

MÜTTER'S FIGHT FOR ANESTHESIA TO BE WIDELY ACCEPTED—TO be adopted by doctors and surgeons as swiftly as possible in order to end what he saw as unnecessary human suffering—proved to be a turning point in his career. Those who had trouble taking the young, boastful doctor seriously were now finding themselves watching him carefully. Those who once gossiped about his method of getting out of an overlong Mass—by having his students rush into church and falsely claim there was an emergency— were the same doctors who now doggedly tracked his surgeries, praised his successes, and even adopted his positions, becoming his ally.

Among the former critics who looked at Mütter with fresh eyes was Edward Robinson Squibb. The Jefferson Medical College alumnus, after spending several years as a naval surgeon, decided to return to his old school to "rub up" on the latest medical developments.

Squibb was deeply impressed with the Mütter flap surgery and wrote about watching Pancoast and Mütter perform together on a young man whose entire neck and chin were heavily scarred.

"The operation was an extensive one," he noted in his journal. "Pancoast assisted Mütter throughout . . . and it was independently remarked by the gentlemen who sat on either side of me that it was a beautiful sight to see two great surgeons working so amicably and so harmoniously together, without any exhibition of envy or rivalry. . . . Whether as an exhibition of perfect good feeling, or of self-control, or a mixture of the two as is most probable, I must tell them of this circumstance, for such things have good effect."

Yet when Squibb had the opportunity to watch each man give a solo surgical lecture, his past critical view of Pancoast was not swayed. He wrote that Dr. Pancoast's lecture on the anatomy of the abdomen was "the most bungling demonstration I ever saw," and he was unnerved when Pancoast performed a difficult operation without aid of an anesthetic, and the shrieking patient's "blood and tears detracted from the artistic effect."

Squibb seemed awed, however, by Mütter's now-famous ether surgeries. He described in detail Mütter's amputation of a forty-five-to-fifty-year-old man's leg just below the right knee.

"The patient was not easily etherized," Squibb noted—a common problem during a time when the chemical makeup of ether anesthesia solutions was not standardized or entirely reliable—"but was finally brought under the full effect. . . . The double flap operation was performed just above-the-knee with the bone being sawed through at its middle. . . . At the end, just before the dressing, the patient was asked if he felt the operation and replied he did not know it was done."

Indeed, Squibb wrote that there had been no groaning or noise during the operation at all, except when the anesthetic effect would diminish—a signal for Mütter to swiftly renew the patient's supply of ether. But despite the fact that ether anesthesia helped the operation to be "very well and prettily and quickly done," it was still a gruesome sight to behold. "Some notable bleeding from the end of the bone but probably not serious," Squibb wrote. "A large audience and only one case of fainting."

Still, he was deeply impressed with Mütter's thrilling showmanship and his dedication to promoting the use of anesthesia. He described the operation as a grand performance—"Barnum by Dr. Mütter," he jotted into his journal, comparing Mütter to P. T. Barnum, the wildly popular showman and famous fun house promoter.

Mütter's ability to use his surgeries to funnel the natural curiosity about anesthesia surgeries toward a faster and broader acceptance of them was no accident. Mütter found any resistance to anesthesia maddening. While even he would admit that it was far from a perfect discovery, there was no escaping the fact that having the ability to anesthetize a patient could alter, evolve, and improve the practice of surgery, and that these improvements outweighed the drawbacks of its "growing pains."

Mütter's desire to experiment even more with this wonder drug was hampered by the constant need to find ways to do so without upsetting any of his peers, many of whom were undecided about anesthesia.

Mütter had fought hard to make sure Jefferson Medical College provided recovery rooms to all patients who offered themselves up to the knife at the school's surgical clinic. It proved to be a success with students, who visited and volunteered.

Mütter's fellow Jefferson Medical College professors Joseph Pancoast and John Kearsley Mitchell encouraged this development by offering to keep their clinics—the anatomical dissection room and medical clinic—open whenever the surgical clinic was open. Both Pancoast and Mitchell publicly supported anesthesia surgeries but did not perform them nearly as often as Mütter did.

Together, Mitchell, Mütter, and Pancoast decided to make an even larger push and ask that all four areas—the surgical clinic, medical clinic, dissection room, and recovery rooms—open a full month before classes began each year and remain open for another full month after graduation. They argued that this would allow students to give "zealous and enduring attention" to the clinical medicine and surgery as well as give them "ample opportunities . . . for pursuits in practical anatomy" when "the student has much more leisure than during the session." The college assented, under the strict understanding that the professors—and not the school—were responsible for the clinics when the school was not in session. The professors agreed.

When the college was forced to halt all activities to undertake a thorough renovation of the building, the trio pushed for an even more ambitious vision: that the Jefferson Medical College hospital remain open year-round. This time the board agreed without any debate.

"So satisfied are the faculty of the value to the students of clinical instruction," they would later explain in their announcement, "that the clinic is open on appropriate days, not merely during the session, but throughout the year; and the medical and surgical practice is superintended and directed by the professors themselves, so that the faculty are, in truth, occupied incessantly through the year in the business of instruction."

With this news, Mütter now had unrestricted access to the school's surgical clinic, where he could perform whatever surgeries he wished on whomever he wished, using whatever tools, innovations, and chemical agents he wanted. It was, for Mütter, an utter dream come true, and his work blossomed even more because of it.

IN THE 1846–1847 SESSION—THE ACADEMIC YEAR WHEN MÜTTER first began working with inhalation ether—the Jefferson Medical College clinics treated 796 patients.

The renovations of the school were being finished when the academic year began, so this number doesn't even reflect a full year of clinical treatment—only eight months. Comparatively, the much larger Pennsylvania Hospital, with its full staff of doctors and nurses, treated 1,391 patients in its *twelve*-month period.

"The Clinic enables the professors to exhibit to the class the mode of applying principles taught . . . to immediate practice," the school advertised in its annual announcement. "It is most richly supplied with medical and surgical cases. . . . The patient is examined, prescribed for, and—if surgical aid be demanded—is operated on before the class."

Now that the evolved, year-round clinic was swiftly becoming the pride of the school, the board kept strict accounts of all the patients who came through the clinic's doors, and those records show the diverse types of people that Mütter, Mitchell, and Pancoast attended.

Of the 796 patients who sought medical attention that year, over half—an impressive 409 people—came to be treated in Mütter's surgical ward. The majority of these patients were adult, but a significant number were children: 176 of the 796 patients were under the age of ten, and 82 of those were under the age of three. When it came to the sex of the patients, the split was much more even: 399 males and 397 females.

Mitchell and the students who volunteered to help at the medical clinic saw a variety of ailments common to the nineteenth century: diseases of the

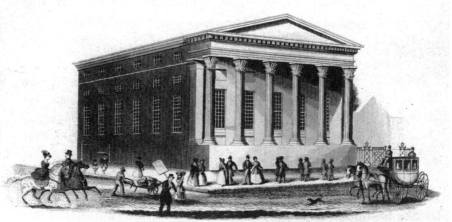

Jefferson Medical College after the Renovations

mouth, the stomach, and the intestines. They treated chronic enlargement of the spleen, herpes, psoriasis, scabies, lumbago, scrofula (tuberculosis of the neck), and impetigo (a highly contagious skin infection with painful, bursting facial sores). They treated tougher cases, like lupus, cholera, epilepsy, and gonorrhea, and even tried their best to help patients whom they would eventually diagnose with "idiocy" or "insanity" or "hypochondria."

But if the medical department could claim a colorful range of ailments, the diversity of the surgical department's patients was even more astonishing.

They arrived with mangled fingers that had been crushed between train cars, dangling thumbs that had been sliced almost completely off their hands, eyes blasted nearly to pulp by gunpowder, and broken bones of every shape, size, and position.

There were countless cases of clubfoot. Mütter's reputation for curing it had become so great that he asked Pancoast to help with the workload.

Both Mütter and Pancoast were performing the most common operations: removals of tonsils, operations on glaucoma and cataracts, removal of foreign bodies from all types of flesh (including and especially the eye), and amputations of both arms and legs (though Mütter and Pancoast shied away from using the term *amputation*, which seemed pejorative to them, and instead referred to the surgery as the creation of "conical stumps").

They devoted themselves to delicate surgeries on the joints of the shoulder, the elbow, the wrist, the knee, and the neck—ailments created by injury or from disease.

Mütter swiftly and cleanly removed tumors from every inch of the body: the eyelid, the lip, the cheek, the jaw, the ear, the forehead, the scalp, the neck, the temple, the chin, and even the eyeball itself.

He removed fatty tumors from the breast, the chest, the shoulder, and the shoulder blade, and cut them from limbs, spines, and labia.

"Multitudes of surgical patients, as attested by the register, came under treatment in the clinic . . . ," Pancoast would later boast. "This list included almost every variety of surgical disease, and more than the usual proportion of the more serious and important cases known in surgery. . . . [A] very large number of them were sent by practitioners from different and often distant places, and on which most of the resources of the art had been previously employed in vain."

BUT WHAT MADE THE JEFFERSON MEDICAL COLLEGE SURGICAL clinic so unique was the class of surgeries that Mütter listed as *deformities*.

Of course, Mütter performed his namesake surgery—stitching back together the faces and bodies of burn victims—as well as his nearly equally famous surgeries on those who suffered from cleft lips and cleft palates of varying degrees of severity.

He performed surgeries because of "spontaneous contraction of hands and feet," "relaxation of ligaments of the ankle," "loss of nose from fight," "deformity of legs from Rachitis" (commonly known now as rickets), and a "deformed chest from a diseased sternum." He even treated a man who suffered horribly from elephantiasis and, immediately afterward, took up a collection for the man, reminding the students that compassion for someone like this does not stop at the operating room door.

Mütter tried to fix them all and, more often than not, was successful. Of the 796 patients who sought medical attention at the Jefferson Medical College clinics that year, the college recorded among them only three deaths—a stunningly small number.

"He loved . . . to match himself with the most difficult cases," Pancoast would say of Mütter. "He carefully prepared himself, even in the minutest points, for the difficulties he had to encounter, and then, with equal skill and firmness, with a sparkling eye and dilating faculties, advanced to his task, more like (than anything else with which I can compare him) to a warrior . . . his courage aroused with the danger and his pulse stirred with the energy of the strife."

As his reputation and popularity grew, patients—rich and poor, old and young—came from great distances just to be examined by this strange but compassionate genius.

"His office was thronged with patients from every part of the Union, waiting patiently their turn, for hours, to consult him," a student would later recall.

"At the clinic of the College, on his entrance into the receiving rooms, crowded with patients attracted by his fame, they gathered around him with a confidence and infatuation which seemed almost to say, *If I may but touch his garment, I shall be whole*," he continued, quoting a line from the New Testament (Matthew 9:21) about Jesus healing the sick.

"At no time had the ample resources of Philadelphia for medical instruction been so diligently fostered," the board said of the clinics, "or more triumphantly exhibited."

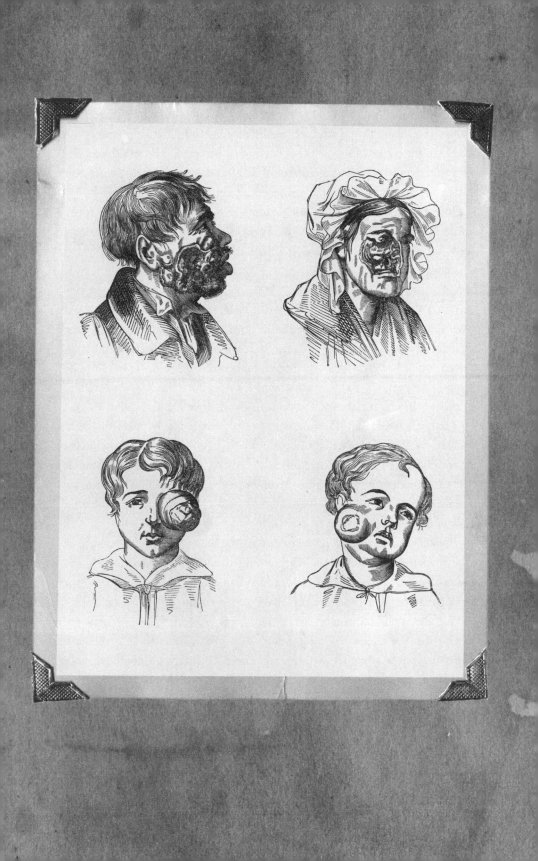

"In no hospital which I have visited, abroad or at home, could [students], in the same space of time, have witnessed so much or profited so richly," Pancoast would later say in praise of the clinic Mütter had fought so hard to expand, "and [his students] must frequently recall to mind the ardor, the energy, the zeal, the soul, with which this portion of Professor Mütter's duties were performed, whether in the treatment of surgical diseases by medical measures only, or by the severer, but not less necessary, application of instruments."

It was from this platform that Mütter wanted to help direct the future of medicine in a more compassionate direction—and to him, that meant more aggressively promoting the use of anesthesia.

HOWEVER, MÜTTER HAD TO FACE ONE HARD FACT: DESPITE HIS own surgical successes, anesthesia did not largely decrease the percentage of deaths that resulted from operations. It was true that the patients experienced much less pain if under the influence of ether during surgery, but overall, they still died at the same rate as surgical patients who endured operations without anesthesia. The reasons for this were complicated.

First, inhalation anesthesia was not an exact science. In this time before standardization of medicine, the patient couldn't always rely on the quality or consistency of the sulphuric ether he received. There were discrepancies among providers, among regions, even between the years in which the sulphuric ether was produced, all of which served to hinder doctors from being able to use it effectively.

It was often a guessing game to determine how much was needed to sedate the patient . . . and how little could be used to kill them. However, accidentally killing a patient by overuse was a larger problem for the other inhalant some surgeons were exploring: chloroform.

The use of chloroform as an anesthetic was introduced in 1847 (the year after ether anesthesia made its debut) by a professor at the University of Edinburgh in Scotland. The discovery was met initially with enthusiasm by American anesthesia supporters; however, that excitement was soon tempered by news of a surge in deaths on the operating table whenever chloroform was used.

Afraid that the deaths caused by chloroform anesthesia would color public opinion about ether anesthesia, John Collins Warren wrote a second monograph, *Effects of Chloroform and of Strong Chloric Ether as Narcotic Agents*, in an attempt to educate the public on the subject.

"The introduction of chloroform produced an excitement scarcely less than that of the discovery of the narcotic effect of ether . . . ," Warren wrote. "We were soon awakened from our dreams of the delightful influence of the new agent by the occurrence of unfortunate and painful consequences, which had not followed in this country on the practice of etherization. . . . Now it appears that no less than ten well-authenticated fatal cases have presented themselves to the public eye within little more than a year."

Still, it is impossible to know how many surgeons and doctors who saw the troubling and fatal consequences of chloroform swore off the use of *any* form of anesthesia in their practice as a result.

ANOTHER REASON FOR THE MEDICAL COMMUNITY'S INITIAL RE-sistance to anesthesia was that it threatened to upset what had always been considered "normal" surgical procedures.

Surgery was traditionally performed on a conscious patient, one who was able to communicate and express pain to his or her surgeon. Surgeons and doctors would use their patients' reactions—either by asking them questions or listening carefully to their wails and cries—to help guide their surgeries. Removing this element from the act of surgery seemed strange and unnatural to some—like removing one of their senses.

Additionally, some doctors believed that using anesthesia hampered the patient's ability to heal and recover postsurgery. In an article in *The American Journal of the Medical Sciences*, army surgeon John B. Porter disparaged the use of ether anesthesia, explaining that "the blood is poisoned, the nervous influence and muscular contractility is destroyed or diminished, and the wound is put in an unfavourable state for recovery . . . in consequence . . . hemorrhage is much more apt to occur, and union by adhesion is prevented."

In his book *A System of Operative Surgery: Based upon the Practice of Surgeons in the United States*, future University of Pennsylvania professor Henry H. Smith attempted to address and dismiss those notions—especially the concept that preventing the patient from feeling the torturous pain of surgery could somehow be seen as a negative. He wrote, "In the majority of cases, the creation of pain by any operation can only be regarded, at the present time, as both unnecessary and injurious. The surgeon should therefore prevent it, and endeavor to save his patient the excitement arising from suffering, by resorting to the use of Anesthetics . . . and as its safety

has been widely tested, philanthropy and that desire to ameliorate the sufferings of mankind, which is the true basis of sound practice, demand that
neither prejudice nor ignorance of its effects should longer prevent its employment by every operator."

Still, it would be some time before this opinion was widely accepted.

AND LAST, MANY SURGEONS WHO WERE EXCITED ABOUT THE
surgical possibilities of using anesthesia—thinking they might finally have
the opportunity to perform elaborate procedures they had previously only
dreamed of doing—were crestfallen when these ambitious, well-thought-
out operations still ended with the death of the patient.

It might be thought that the increased complexity of these operations
was the major cause for the rise in "operative mortality" associated with anesthesia surgeries, but that wasn't entirely true. It was not the *ambitiousness*
of the surgery that proved to be the killer, but rather the uncleanliness,
since many physicians did not yet employ antiseptic or aseptic measures.

Surgeons could spend weeks or months planning a procedure, then ex-
ecute the operation swiftly and perfectly, and still be forced to watch help-
lessly as their "successful" surgery turned fatal when the patients died of
common postoperative problems such as infection, wound sepsis, and
shock. Indeed, Mütter's success with anesthesia surgery likely had as much
to do with his well-documented fastidiousness as it did with the swift and
planned preciseness of his hands and tools.

BECAUSE OF THESE FACTORS, A SIGNIFICANT NUMBER OF DOCTORS
of the mid-nineteenth century thought the use of anesthesia in surgery was
simply not worth the risk.

Henry J. Bigelow also tried to change the tide of opinion by writing a
series of articles outlining "the supposed dangers of anesthetic agents"
(later released as an authoritative monograph) and by giving presentations
across the country, including to the Committee on Surgery of the American Medical Association, which was based in Philadelphia at the time.

But despite all the benefits ether anesthesia provided and all the solutions to its perceived problems Bigelow and other advocates offered, there
was still resistance.

"I think anesthesia is of the devil," William Henry Atkinson, a physician and the first president of the American Dental Association went on record saying, "and I cannot give my sanction to any Satanic influence which deprives a man of the capacity to recognize law! I wish there were no such thing as anesthesia! I do not think men should be prevented from passing through what God intended them to endure!"

But Mütter didn't care what anyone said, nor did he seem to mind that this new invention made the textbook he'd spent years writing nearly obsolete within weeks of its release. What mattered was that he felt his entire world had been opened up—and by an *American* invention, to boot! What mattered was that he had earned his place of privilege and influence, and now had the glorious opportunity to use it for the greater good.

What he didn't know, but could have guessed, was that he was about to enter the "golden age" of his life. What he didn't know, and might never have guessed, was that it would be over all too soon.

PART THREE

CHAPTER TWENTY

THESE DEEDS OF BLOOD

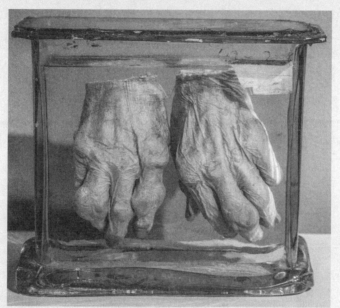

Hands Deformed by Gout

To anyone who saw him in the early 1850s, Mütter still seemed the picture of health. Now entering his early forties, he remained "a singularly handsome man": youthful, slender, and graceful with a clear sweet voice of remarkable strength and carrying power. Years after he was reprimanded at his school for wearing "a style of dress not altogether proper for a boy his age," Mütter's style remained scrupulously neat. He was "in fact, almost a dandy," one of his colleagues later recalled.

When his schedule allowed him to attend parties or gatherings, he continued to be praised, by men and women alike, for being both "a delightful conversationalist and an admirable raconteur."

Few outside his close circle of friends knew that Mütter was not a well man.

Mütter was never able to fully shake the ailments that had plagued him since boyhood, but recently, they had grown much worse. What had always been frustrating, painful, and draining was now wholly unmanageable.

Mütter's lungs never fully recovered from that brutal winter he spent at Yale. He was constantly overtaxing them—both by giving lengthy lectures in bustling, overcrowded lecture halls and by exposing himself daily to the harsh chemicals of the surgical room. His weak lungs couldn't help but be irritated by the fumes of that confined space: alcohol, ether, even burning lamp oil. He caught colds easily, fought draining fatigue, and sometimes had trouble catching his breath. But recently, his lungs had begun to shudder and ache in his chest, and when an agonizingly long coughing fit finally subsided, he would look down and see his handkerchief stained with splashes of his own bright red blood.

Meanwhile, the gout he seemed to have inherited from his grandmother preyed endlessly upon him, making him "inconceivably sensitive to pain." Without warning and seemingly without reason, the joints of his hands and feet would grow hot and red, painfully swollen to the point that even air passing over the affected part would cause searing pain, as if he were being poked by a dozen blistering needles. No matter what treatment he sought or to what preventive care he devoted himself, nothing helped.

As he was a surgeon, Mütter's hands were one of his most valuable tools. Swift and nimble, quick and precise, they were one of the reasons he was able to do the work he did. It was rare blessing enough to be ambidextrous. But to be as skilled as Mütter was with *both* his hands was seen as near miraculous ("Few can boast of [being ambidextrous] . . . and often, many who can have in fact *only two left hands*," a fellow doctor once quipped).

So when gout would temporarily cripple his hands, it would ruin days and sometimes weeks of effort and preparation, since he would be absolutely unable to perform any of the delicate surgeries he promised he would.

But Mütter knew he had to keep working. The famed clinic of Jefferson College was only becoming more popular as the Faculty of '41 celebrated an unbroken decade together. His office was flooded with the ill and injured, the desperate and damaged, all happy to wait hours or days if needed to consult with him. Meanwhile, students and doctors from all over the country came to watch Mütter perform what would later be called "some of the greatest achievements of American surgery."

Mütter could not step away from these incredible responsibilities, so instead he humbly asked Joseph Pancoast, his friend and colleague, if he could help him with his more difficult surgeries. Pancoast agreed.

"In the every-day surgical operations Mütter was careful and adroit," a student would later write of him during this time, "in the performance of those of great magnitude he leaned a little, yet always gracefully, upon the strong arm of his Colleague in Anatomy, his co-worker in the Surgical Clinic."

Indeed, Mütter and Pancoast made for a fantastic team: Pancoast's steady hand and careful eye, and Mütter's ever-ambitious forward-thinking innovations. Mütter realized that while his body might fail him on occasion, his mind was still as sharp as ever, and he began to offer his advice and aid in consultation to any doctor asking his help for as long as "his feeble physical abilities enabled him to."

Mütter changed in other ways too. After years of having his students call him out of Mass for ersatz emergencies, Mütter became a devoted member of Philadelphia's Protestant Episcopal Church, and he even spoke about working with the church to found a ward for incurables at its hospital.

"The consolations of religion supported him through his long sufferings," a peer wrote about his turn toward religion, "which he bore with patience and hopefulness."

Mütter had every reason to feel hopeful: Every attack of illness, from his boyhood to the present, had always passed . . . eventually. Although now it seemed the attacks were happening more frequently and severely, and his recovery was taking longer each time he fell ill, he still was happy to adapt and push through. He had a life to live, after all, and a very important one at that. His students and his patients depended on him, and he did whatever it took to keep moving forward.

THE MEDICAL COMMUNITY IN PHILADELPHIA—STILL SEEN AS the country's medical mecca—was learning how to adapt too.

In an effort to standardize the profession (and not just the education portion of it), the American Medical Association was founded in Philadelphia in 1847, and the following year, the Philadelphia County Medical Society.

These organizations aimed to create a forum where all "respectable physicians" could meet, debate, and exchange experiences and ideas. It was envisioned as an association that would bind the profession together: Rules of gentlemanly conduct and honorable dealing would be observed, and each member physician would feel he owed a duty to his fellow doctors and to the greater public.

And in direct opposition to the insular medical societies that fractured the local medical community, membership in the newly formed county medical society was open to any Philadelphia doctor who graduated from a respectable school, was of good moral and professional standing, and was an active practitioner. However, wary of how this might bring an influx of "quacks" into their ranks, the society expressly forbade membership to anyone who "prescribes a remedy without knowing its composition."

These societies were not only successful but influential. Here, finally, were professional organizations in which it didn't matter how rich your grandfather was, or if the school from which you graduated was impressive enough to the gatekeepers. As long as you shared a passion and focus to push the profession forward, you were in.

To Mütter, it was hopeful progress compared to what he experienced during his earliest years in the city.

In addition to the new medical societies, a variety of other medical institutions were also popping up throughout Philadelphia as the community tried to keep up with the city's voracious expansion.

The 1850s saw the founding of several new medical schools and hospitals, including the Children's Hospital of Philadelphia, the Philadelphia Municipal Hospital, and Pennsylvania College of Dental Surgery. Medical institutions founded for the benefit of society also began to spring up, including some with odd names such as the Howard Hospital and Infirmary for Incurables, the Philadelphia Society for the Employment and Instruction of the Poor, and the Northern Home for Friendless Children (which the founder felt was a tactful way to describe what was essentially an orphanage).

But for all its progress, the Philadelphia medical community was still largely unwilling to concede one point: It was "long violently opposed to [the idea of] the female doctor."

AFTER NUMEROUS DESERVING AND AMBITIOUS WOMEN WERE denied admittance to the lecture halls of the University of Pennsylvania, Jefferson Medical College, and every other educational institution serving the medical profession in Philadelphia, a group of Quakers (whose religious doctrines included complete equality of the sexes) founded the Female Medical College of Pennsylvania within the city limits in 1850. For the next decade and a half, the school grew more and more popular as hundreds of women flocked to the city to finally learn in its lecture halls.

When its board decided to change the institution's name to the more striking and official-sounding Woman's Medical College of Pennsylvania in 1867, the Pennsylvania Medical Society finally decided to take action and issued a scathing and definitive statement *against* women practitioners.

The statement declared that women should not practice medicine because women "cannot stand the strain of practice"; because "their physiological necessities forbid the attempt"; because "if married they will neglect home

duties"; and because it was offensive that at the very least these women physicians would "not consent to only attend women"; and, finally, simply because women's "nerves are too delicate for the work."

The statement had no effect on the school, which still surged with new
female students each year.

A year later, the society decided to push the issue even further by expelling any of its members who dared to teach at a women's college, and furthermore to expel any member who was found to have consulted with
women physicians in any medical capacity.

Still, these actions did nothing to stem the growing tide of women who
were actively pursuing a career in medicine.

Soon, even larger institutions were being asked to allow women to attend lectures and witness surgeries. A high-ranking physician at the Pennsylvania Hospital was so appalled at the idea of having to lecture to "mixed
classes" that he resigned his position to avoid the "indignity" of having to
teach even one single woman.

Not every male physician held this opinion. And thanks to these allies,
and especially to the persistence and bravery of those early groundbreaking
women who insisted on their right to be physicians, the first female doctor
was elected to the same Pennsylvania Medical Society that had just two decades earlier sought to end her role in the profession entirely. The decision
was met with much relief and rejoicing from the younger members of the
community.

"Woman, as usual, finally had her way," a male member would later slyly
write about the election. "And yet the earth did not rock, the sea did not
overflow its banks, the stars did not fall."

IN OTHER WAYS, MEDICINE IN PHILADELPHIA WAS UNAMBIGUOUSLY
moving forward. Mütter constantly marveled at his good fortune at being
part of such a revolutionary time in medicine, which was largely fueled by,
of all things, *American* discoveries.

He spoke with a youthful excitement about this progress in an introductory lecture that was later published in the *Medical Examiner*. He opened
his speech by fiercely advocating for his favorite recent discovery:

"Anesthesia . . . I need not, on this occasion, enter upon the history of this
purely *American* discovery. I repeat purely *American discovery*," he stated
emphatically, "for, notwithstanding the attempts made by some, to give the

credit of this most valuable of all modern improvements in surgery to Europeans, we have yet positive evidence of its being in truth *an offspring of the New World.*

"In England, Scotland and Ireland, and on every portion of the continent of Europe . . . no surgeon of any grade, high or low, pretends to practice his profession without the constant use of some anesthetic agent," he continued, unabashedly countering all anesthesia critics around him, including those of his own faculty. "When I asked my distinguished friends in London and Paris, if they employed the measure with the same degree of confidence as at first, they seemed surprised at the question and unhesitatingly declared, that *no surgeon would presume to perform a serious operation without first bringing his patient into a state of anesthesia,* provided always, there was nothing present to contraindicate the production of this condition. While there exists some difference of opinion as to the *best* agent to be used, there is *none* upon the great point of the *value* of the measure in the practice of surgery."

Mütter didn't waste time defending anesthesia, but instead spoke passionately about the new and ever-evolving possibilities that anesthesia could bring to the art of plastic surgery.

"You will be anxious, I doubt not, to learn the estimation in which European Surgeons, generally, hold what is called *Plastic Surgery,*" he said. "This department of our science, although in reality 'old enough to speak for itself,' may be considered a comparatively modern invention, for certainly the beautiful and perfect results attained in our time through its agency, far surpass anything that emanated from the hands of its original advocates and inventors. . . .

"These operations were for many years considered almost as fabulous, and have excited the ridicule of the wits of every age . . . ," he stated. "But, gentlemen, both wit and opposition have been tried in vain, and the most distinguished men in Europe unite in awarding to the measure a high and commanding position among the most useful improvements of the age. . . . *Plastic Surgery* may be considered as having fought its battles, and will soon rest under the aegis of an established operation."

This stand—and this open admiration of plastic surgery—had become increasingly important. While anesthesia provided an opportunity for surgical breakthroughs that previous generations could only dream about, it also had the potential to be grossly misused. Members of the larger medical community were beginning to voice their concern over what they considered to be "the exploitation of the manual art of surgery."

A rift in the community was developing, and it divided those doctors who some fearfully felt had a "seemingly boundless enthusiasm for questionably appropriate surgical intervention" (a category in which Mütter would most definitely be placed, despite his constant appeals to his students that surgery be their last resort) from those doctors who felt surgery was used too often. From this rift, two new phrases were popularized in the jargon of American medicine: *conservative surgery* and *radical surgery*.

DEFINING WHAT *RADICAL* AND *CONSERVATIVE* MEANT IN REFERence to surgery was always difficult, as the art and practice of it were forever evolving. The words took on different meanings at different times. But in this period in history, the words were used to articulate a sharp philosophic difference between what surgeons considered to be appropriate and acceptable operations and those that could be seen as risky, unnecessary, and bordering on dangerous.

Earlier surgeons would define *conservative surgery* as operations that were absolutely necessary to perform, mostly after a traumatic and often life-endangering injury—amputations of mangled or useless limbs, surgeries to correct dislocations or fractures, the removal of lodged items (bullets, broken glass) from the body or its organs, and so on.

But as medicine entered the 1850s, the concept of "conservative surgery" took on new meanings. Some in the community felt that the relative ease of performing surgeries with anesthesia—no patients to hold down, no screams, no wails, no thrashing—made it so that surgery was suggested too liberally and too often.

Conservative surgery therefore was defined as any surgery "devised solely within the context of the growing science of surgery" and "not used indiscriminately on anyone who would hold still."

If earlier generations feared surgeons because they viewed them as sadists who delighted in their patients' pain, the new vision of surgeons in a postanesthesia world was as ghouls—fiendish men who sought to knock you out and then revel in slicing you open in a variety of disturbing new ways when you are unable to defend yourself.

This dark vision of surgeons is clearly apparent in an anonymous editorial printed in a New York City medical journal:

"The more bloody, and even the more uniformly fatal, the higher the huzza of the ignorant and vulgar multitude for the surgeon, so called, who figures in 'deeds of blood,'" the vitriolic piece stated. "Students and junior practitioners will often run miles to witness a capital operation, and ransack neighborhoods and cities to find patients whose surgical diseases will furnish them opportunities to cut, or to witness cutting performed by others.

"And they too become partakers in the popular idolatry of the mere operators, whose frenzy for the use of the scalpel and saw, mallet and chisel, and even the red hot iron, upon the living bodies of their victims, becomes a passion, which too often degrades surgery into human butchery."

Although the hyperbole and dramatics painted a nastier picture of surgery than he saw, it was true that Mütter shared some of the sentiments of those who criticized "radical surgery."

Many of the surgeries he performed—especially the ones he did on the severely deformed—would most definitely fall under the category of radical, but Mütter had long preached that surgical intervention wasn't needed for all cases that came to his doorstep.

This was a sentiment he felt especially strongly when it came to women, who—because of the enforced modesty of the time period—were more likely to come to doctors after it was already too late for treatment to be helpful.

In fact, Mütter was criticized for being cruel and inhumane for his opinion on the treatment of breast tumors, which he firmly believed should *not* be operated on, except in very specific circumstances. He simply didn't believe there were nearly enough benefits to the surgical removal of a breast to outweigh the enormous negatives: the wretched pain of surgery and recovery; the inevitable infection that would turn the woman's chest into a painful, throbbing wound leaking with foul pus; the days, weeks, months that the woman would be unable to leave her bed, to hug her children, or to sleep, eat, or love without searing, ceaseless pain.

But a woman is seeking your help, his critics would say. *How merciless and cold must you be to refuse to aid her?*

"To answer this question in a satisfactory manner," he would reply, "it is necessary to investigate, *first,* the results of the disease when left to itself; and *secondly,* the benefits likely to accrue from the performance of an operation, its effects upon the progress of the disease, and its dangers. It is a melancholy truth that when left to itself this disease usually advances steadily, but with an unequal pace in different cases."

He would then explain how, often by the time a lump in a woman's breast has become so large, troubling, and painful that she would show it to her doctor, the cancer in the breast has likely progressed to all adjacent tissues, and—regardless of whether the tumor itself is surgically removed—would ultimately end in the death of the patient, who likely would see death at this point as "a welcome messenger," having been for months of her brutal recovery "a martyr to unspeakable sufferings, and a loathsome object to her friends."

"It is true, that some of the French, who adopt the view that cancer is invariably in its commencement a local disease, operate in cases where the English and American surgeons would hesitate to use the knife," he would tell them, "but, as a general rule, they advise an *early* operation, before the system becomes involved, or *none at all.*"

But while this philosophy was grounded in rational and logical thought, even Mütter could not escape how difficult this decision inevitably is when faced with the distressed and frantic face of a woman who doesn't know she will be dead soon anyway.

"It is urged by some, that we are justified [in performing surgery on] desperate cases, [to] escape the horrors of ulcerated or open cancer," he said. "This is certainly a humane motive . . . where the patient is young, or has some especial reason for wishing the nature of her disease concealed, and is willing to take all the responsibility of the result upon herself, after having been made aware of the almost certain failure of the operation . . . and that she must die in a few months. . . ."

"But, gentlemen," he confessed to them, "whenever I have done so, it has been with an aching heart, and a most fervent wish that my patient had spared her surgeon and herself the terrible ordeal to which she is voluntarily subjected."

To those who thought Mütter was of the camp that believed a surgeon's knife could solve every problem, his opinion came as a surprise.

But Mütter's students knew the truth. He had always taught them that "the knife promises nothing" and should be used only if the disease is caught early enough or if "it will serve to satisfy the patient in part, and prevent, to a certain degree, that terrible sickness of heart that overwhelms a poor sufferer when utterly abandoned by the surgeon."

He shared the opinion of John Watson, an influential New York City surgeon who simply said: "Surgery . . . is a good thing, a useful thing, an excellent thing in its way; but too much of it is a great evil. And the sooner you find this out for yourselves, the better for your patients."

THE EARLY YEARS OF THE 1850S WERE A TRANSFORMATIVE TIME in Philadelphia—for its people, for its industry, and for its politics.

For Mütter, it was a time when, in so many respects, he was at the height of his power: a decade into his chair at one of the most prestigious medical colleges in the country; peerless in his ability to perform complex and visionary new surgeries; and an emerging yet powerful voice within the community whose opinions—though maybe not embraced by those around him—were at least heard.

But there was another side to this life, a painful truth Mütter could not escape: the increasing failure of his own body.

"The old axiom, *mens sana in corpore sano* ('a healthy mind in a healthy body') is full of wisdom," he had told a class during a period of good health in the late 1840s, "and if there is one among you so unfortunate as to possess a feeble constitution, let me counsel him—as one who has dearly proven the misery of such a possession—to *abandon* the study of medicine at once, or at least until *vigor* and *tone* have been imparted to his frame.

"Without health," he said bluntly, "the professional life of a man is one, long dreary night of suffering and disappointment."

For the past year, Mütter had felt trapped in that "long dreary night." There were more bad days now than good. He began to worry about how strained his body was becoming. His frame felt constantly fatigued. When his joints weren't swollen with gout, they were stiff and painful to bend. In surgeries, his hands struggled to do what they once did so easily; movements that had been swift and light were now uncertain and laborious.

Mütter had trouble sleeping, trouble breathing, trouble putting on weight. His pale skin grew sallow, and his hair began to gray prematurely. He was spending a fortune on handkerchiefs because he had to constantly replace the ones that became irreparably stained by the blood he so frequently coughed up.

Mütter knew what he had to do: *Go to Europe.*

Throughout his career, Mütter had made professional visits to Europe—mostly to Paris and London, where he spent time with "numerous eminent friends." It was his way of "rubbing up" on the latest medical innovations. He would visit hospitals, sit in on surgeries, and study and observe all he joyfully could. Mütter sometimes brought former students with him on these trips, allowing those young men he saw as being the most industrious and the most forward thinking to benefit from his reputation and stature.

One student who accompanied him on a European visit was amazed at how many doors were opened to him by Mütter, how he "was greeted warmly by the most eminent medical men of London and Paris, often meeting them socially, and attending, by invitation, their operations and consultations."

To the European medical societies, Mütter was a bit of a celebrity: a dashing, outspoken, idiosyncratic American visionary. Even established American doctors would ask Mütter to be "favored by him with letters of introduction to distinguished medical men" and, after receiving such letters, "found them passports at once to the society and attentions of the recipients."

And when in residence in a foreign city, his presence seemed "at once known among the numerous American health or pleasure seekers in Paris." So though he was thousands of miles from his home, there were still throngs of people who both sought his company socially as well as wanted to be consulted by him professionally.

But Mütter knew this trip would have to be different. He had begun to feel a creeping fear about what was happening with his body. He wanted to address it—fully, boldly, and transparently—before it was too late and the damage became permanent. Or, worse—a thought he strove to chase from his troubled mind and from his devoted wife's frightened lips—before it killed him.

This time, Mütter would arrive in Europe largely unannounced, and endeavor only to be among his most "distinguished and attentive friends," esteemed doctors whom he trusted the most. In the confidence of their small offices, he would share with them the extent of the damage caused by the severe attacks of his "frequently recurring malady." He would ask them for their advice, for their guidance, and, most importantly, for the truth.

STILL, IT WAS DIFFICULT FOR HIM TO LEAVE PHILADELPHIA AND the clinic he cherished so much.

He worried about the patients he wouldn't be able to see, and whether, in his absence, their painful infirmities would be properly treated. He worried about his students, and whether their skills would slack or regress without his watchful eye. And he worried that the influence of doctors like Meigs might strengthen in his absence, stifling progress he had worked so hard to achieve.

While the sharply dressed yet ailing Mütter was tireless in his efforts to inspire Jefferson Medical College students, encouraging them to push further, dream larger, and move the profession forward, the grimly dressed yet robustly healthy Meigs would lecture them to instead stay "in the middle."

In the speech he gave to the 1852 graduating class, Meigs proffered the following advice:

"You ought to conceive, therefore, of the tenor of a medical life as one *subdued*, and brought into *conformity* . . . ," he told them. "I am far from recommending . . . habits of moping and dullness, but would have you shun all trifling and all frivolities, incommensurate with the dignity of your station, and the gravity of your concerns.

"You must go, in and out, before the people, daily; the boisterous laugh, the stormy carouse, and the discreditable spree are but evil antecedents of that visit . . . ," he explained. "There is a *just medium*," he flatly added, "and he is safest who touches neither extreme in anything.

"Therefore, we charge you: be good men, and learned men; join yourselves to every good work and purpose: oppose all evil; let your examples shine before all worthy men to encourage them," he said, before adding this threatening conclusion: "Check and reprove whatsoever tends to the subversion of religion, of morals, of the public welfare in short."

BUT WHAT MEIGS SAID OR DID DIDN'T MATTER—IT COULDN'T. Mütter felt he had no choice; he knew what he had to do. And shortly after graduation, he quietly left for Europe because he saw it as his "only means of securing relaxation and escaping the incessant calls for his services at home" and "his only hope for healing the same painful infirmities which always oppressed him."

He was determined, now more than ever, to return a healthier, stronger man and continue the work he needed to do.

CHAPTER TWENTY-ONE

THAT BOURNE FROM WHICH
NO TRAVELER RETURNS

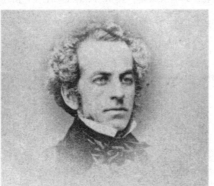

Mütter, after Illness Had Set In

THE PHYSICIAN
SHOULD BE AN HONEST MAN

Much injury is inflicted upon the profession

by its members claiming too much for its power

in controlling disease; we have taught the public

to look upon medicine with a feeling near akin

to superstition and awe; to rely upon our dicta

as infallible, to suppose us in some way

the positive arbiters of their fate; the dispensers

of health and vigor, and even life itself. . . .

Let us hasten to disabuse them of this error.

Let us tell them candidly that, although our resources

are in reality great, and that often, by their proper

administration, dangers are diminished; yet without

the help and blessing of Him who gives knowledge

to the physician, and health to the sick,

these resources are feeble and powerless!

How modest, and yet how true, was the reply of good old

Ambrose Paré when complimented upon his skill

in curing the Duke de Guise of his terrific wound:

"I dressed him, but God healed him."

Thomas Dent Mütter

WHEN MÜTTER HAD FIRST ARRIVED IN PARIS TWENTY YEARS earlier, he was wet and hungry and dashing about the streets madly trying to absorb all he could in the limited time he had. Now here he was returning again in his mid-forties, and he couldn't help but reflect on how much things had changed—how much *he* had changed.

Thankfully, he no longer had to charm his way into naval ships to afford to visit Europe. There had been considerable improvement in ocean travel in recent decades, and Mütter now preferred to travel on luxurious ships managed by the Collins Line, which in 1850 began offering the country's first transatlantic expeditions, connecting ports directly between the British Isles and the United States. The Collins Line could also boast that their ships were the biggest and fastest steamers afloat. But this luxury didn't come cheap. A solo trip cost Mütter a thousand dollars, and that number would be bumped up to three thousand dollars if he needed accommodation for both himself and his wife.

The sea was now a comforting place to Mütter. The fresh, salty ocean air made his breathing easier and his joints feel more relaxed. Though his body still felt weakened and "at the point of breaking down completely," his mind remained bright and alert and his ambition remained strong.

He had already decided on his next great project: "a full and systematic work on surgery." This time, he would be the book's sole author, and it would contain everything he had learned in his long career, as well as all the new innovations that had come to light in the years since he published his textbook with Robert Liston.

As soon as his health issues were resolved, he would spend the additional time in Paris gathering and arranging material for his new book. He felt buoyed just by the idea of it, and looked forward to the energizing beauty and sweet *joie de vivre* to be found only in the bustling streets of Paris.

LIKE MÜTTER HIMSELF, PARIS HAD CHANGED OVER THE LAST two decades. It still filled him with the same awe, but he was reminded of how much those early experiences in Paris had formed him.

"Merely to have breathed a concentrated scientific atmosphere like that of Paris," a peer of Mütter's once wrote, "must have an effect on anyone who has lived where *stupidity* is tolerated, where *mediocrity* is applauded and where excellence is *defied*."

It was a different Paris now, of course. Many of the physicians he'd seen as absolute masters had died, and his opinions of them—now seasoned with his own experiences as a doctor and a surgeon—had changed.

He was grateful for the sparks of inspiration these men had struck within him and for blazing the innovative paths that allowed him to do so much of the work on which he had built his whole career. But he was now harshly critical of how often these same visionaries seemed to treat their patients as *cases* instead of *human beings*. How they seemed to spend more time thrilling at conquering a difficult case or a particular ravaging condition than they did considering the impact—both emotional and physical—their treatments would have on their patients.

Mütter was eager to meet up with the circle of friends and doctors he had cultivated in the years since his first trip: smart, clear-eyed men who shared his compassion-based vision for transparency in medicine. It was such a relief to finally be back in their company, and he was hoping the advice he received from these men would help speed his recovery and get him back in solid health in time for the fall term at Jefferson Medical College.

But it didn't take long to see that his ambitious hopes for the summer would not come to fruition.

He could see it in their faces—their expressions becoming more tense and concerned as the examinations continued. He tried his best to lighten the mood—cracking jokes and smiling through what was obviously painful. But it was no good.

He knew how difficult it was for them to tell him the news. He had been in their shoes many times, and always tried to remember what he had learned from his maternal grandfather's friends in Alexandria: that above all else, truth is what the patient needs to hear . . . no matter how difficult it is to be the one who must say it.

"Be *honest* at the *bedside* . . . In cases of great danger, when life is really at stake, unless some cogent reason forbids, it is the duty of the medical attendant to deal *candidly* and *honestly* with the friends of the patient or the patient himself," Mütter would tell his students frankly. "Each one of us has some preparation to make, some kind word to utter, some fond embrace to exchange, ere he quits this 'earthly tabernacle,' and passes to that 'bourne from which no traveler returns.'

"If the physician fails under these circumstances to discharge his duty, painful and heart-rending though it may be," he explained to them, "the worldly affairs of his patient may, by his negligence, be left in irretrievable confusion; the happiness of a whole community may be destroyed; but, above all, he may become the direct agent by which an immortal soul is lost."

Mütter taught that lesson so easily and often, without ever realizing just how soon he would be on the receiving end of it.

His physician friends told him what perhaps in his heart he already knew—his face thinning in the mirror before him, his hair slowly turning white, his once graceful hands now becoming gnarled and bent with disease, his lungs raw and rattling.

Mütter was dying.

Regardless of the pedigree or background of the doctors he saw, or how dutiful he was in following their optimistic treatments to the letter, or how many humble prayers he offered up in church, his body would still decline.

Death, it was explained to him, wasn't a far-off *if*; it was a humbling and inevitable *when*.

PARIS WAS STILL BEAUTIFUL, DESPITE THE CRUSHING NEWS HE had just received. It was still bustling and lively and loud. Its brilliant splendor didn't dim at all in the heavy shadow of Mütter's diagnosis. In fact, it seemed even more beautiful: the enormous stained-glass windows of the impossibly old cathedrals; the exquisite women of all ages glittering in new dresses as they glided along the promenade; the singular taste of a freshly made café au lait; the cleansing smell of summer rain hitting a sweltering street; the sight of young lovers, their whole future ahead of them, kissing hard in dark corners where they were sure no one could see them.

His friends in Paris had asked him to stay.

They assured him that the treatment he could receive with them was still much, much better than any he could receive in Philadelphia.

Here, in Paris, he could extend his life and do so in luxury: eating the best foods, enjoying Europe's modern comforts, and conserving his energy—the same energy he had always devoted to fighting battles with willful Philadelphia doctors and teaching teeming waves of medical students—to, instead, heal himself.

HIS THOUGHTS WANDERED BACK TO THE MAN WHO HAD SO earned his admiration during his first trip to Paris: Baron Guillaume Dupuytren, the Emperor of Surgery.

Dupuytren had died just a few years after Mütter studied under him, marveling at Dupuytren's singular skills, his hard-won knowledge, and his unusual collection of anatomical specimens that he used in his teaching, which inspired Mütter to start one of his own.

Before he died, Dupuytren had asked a former student, Mathieu Orfila, to help him create a permanent home for this strange collection he had built for decades. And so in 1835, the same year that Dupuytren died at the age of fifty-seven, the museum now known as Musée Dupuytren was opened as the Museum of Pathological Anatomy of the Medicine Faculty of the University of Paris.

The museum, located at what had been the old dining hall of the Cordeliers Convent, included almost one thousand hand-selected specimens donated by Dupuytren. Generations of students and doctors who missed the opportunity to study under the man himself could at least learn from the anatomical pathology materials Dupuytren had collected and had used to teach over his lifetime, now organized and displayed en masse.

Skeletons, wax castings, deformed or defective organs preserved in jars, and various other "monstrosities," as well as an abundant supply of anatomical paintings, drawings, prints, and instruments.

In this way, Dupuytren ensured that his legacy would live beyond the surgeries he taught and performed. Here was a monument to a great man, the difficult work he did, and the challenging world in which he had lived.

Mütter wondered what sort of legacy he himself would leave behind.

———————

His friends' proposal to stay in Paris was extremely tempting.

Here, his work was respected; his style, appreciated; and his personality, celebrated. And it would not be difficult at all for Jefferson Medical College to find a replacement for him—the chair he was vacating was one of the most prestigious in the country; competition would inevitably be fierce—but even the best candidate would never truly fill the void created by Mütter's absence. No one did the caliber of work Mütter did—let alone at the level and the volume he was able to do it.

Still, he wondered, what responsibility did he have to Philadelphia, or to Jefferson Medical College? Hadn't he done enough? What could be worth returning for, if it would shorten his own life?

Mütter had already done so much. He had authored some of the country's earliest articles on plastic surgery—surgeries for burns, for cleft palate, for clubfoot.

He had become one of the country's leading masters of plastic surgery, helping hundreds and hundreds of people to live better, longer, more fulfilling lives.

He had brought about lasting changes for the treatment of his patients: recovery rooms, meticulously clean surgical areas, and twenty-four-hour care before and after surgery. He helped in the construction of Jefferson Medical College's first small hospital, and performed the city's first ether surgery within its walls.

He had taught more than one thousand young minds. Had he not earned the right to rest, especially now when his own health was failing him?

But there was still one concern that plagued Mütter as he wrestled with his impending mortality.

In the years that followed his discovery of ether, he had published very little. Excited by the potential of this new innovation, he had kept himself extraordinarily busy putting it to use at the surgical clinic at Jefferson Medical College. He had successfully fought to have the clinic be open year round, though this had the unfortunate side effect of severely limiting his opportunity to share his knowledge beyond the Corinthian-columned lecture halls of Jefferson.

His earlier publications had been praised for their "very explicit descriptions, including drawings" and for giving "an accurate idea of what was involved from the surgeon's point of view." He had hoped to have an opportunity to do so again in the new surgical textbook he wanted so badly to write (but knew, with this latest diagnosis, he would surely be forced to abandon when his health hopelessly failed).

What would happen to the patients who filled his waiting rooms, these men, women, and children with burned bodies, or split faces, or deformities that were so grotesque he still caught his students listing their condition as "monster"—those people who felt that Mütter was their only hope?

With so much of his amassed knowledge still left to pass along, it begged the question of who would help them when he was gone.

Sitting among the silks and fine wines and golden lights of Paris, surrounded by people who loved him and wanted nothing more than to care for him, Mütter's heart and conscience told him what he must do.

He would return to freezing Philadelphia and finish the work he was meant to do.

CHAPTER TWENTY-TWO

THE RICH FRUITS OF
LIFE'S LABORS

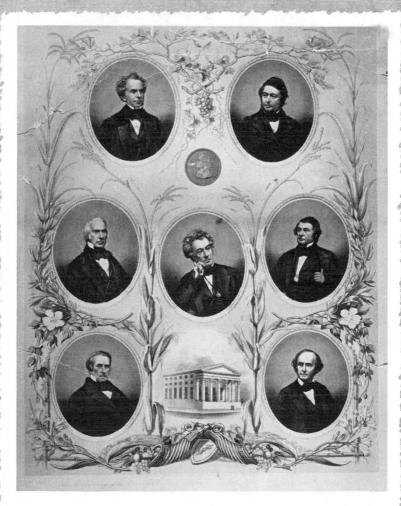

Advertisement for Jefferson Medical College, 1855–1856 Session,
Featuring "the Famous Faculty of '41"

THE PHYSICIAN
MUST POSSESS MORAL COURAGE

What profession, what art, what calling demands
    a courage so unyielding, so self-sacrificing
    as that of medicine?
He must be a brave man who can meet, without
    flinching, "the pestilence that walketh at noonday."
He must be a brave man who can remain at his post,
    when the "plague-spot" breaks every link of
    affection . . .
Oh, tell me not of a warrior's courage, brilliant
    though it may be. . . . He advances with hope, and
    is sustained, admired, and seconded by a whole army.
But what sustains the physician, in the stillness
    of night, in the chamber of pestilence, in the reeking
    hut of the sick beggar—in the cell of the maniac?
A moral courage, *which bids him die*
    rather than desert his charge—
a God, who tells him that
"a faithful shepherd must give his life for the flock!"

Thomas Dent Mütter

WHEN MÜTTER RETURNED TO PHILADELPHIA, HE SAW IT WITH different eyes. By the mid-1850s, the city had stretched its boundaries so far that there were complaints that "there would soon be no rural population left at all." The city's population clocked in at just over half a million, making it the fourth-largest city in the Western world, as well as second-largest in the United States.

London and Paris, from which Mütter had just returned, were much larger, of course (their populations at two and a half million each), and New York City could claim more than 800,000 citizens (provided you included Brooklyn's 266,000). But Philadelphia was firmly in fourth place, the other cities in America not even close to its size. Philadelphia's population had even surpassed such European capitals as Vienna and St. Petersburg and the somewhat similar industrial and commercial cities of Liverpool and Manchester.

When the United States first declared its independence, many of the men of the First Continental Congress thought Philadelphia was "too big and too urban." They could never have imagined the Philadelphia of the mid-nineteenth century, "one of the first of the world's truly big cities . . . an agglomeration of people that made inherited notions of 'a community' obsolete," as the mass of people and crush of industry created a city "too populous and widespread to be truly a community."

Yet Mütter still considered it home. He was heartened by the sight of its coughing smokestacks, its cross-stitch of cobblestone streets, railroad tracks, and telegraph lines, and the large thrashing wheels of the Fairmount Dam and the Fairmount Water Works on the Schuylkill River.

When Mütter finally arrived home, he knew he had no time to waste. He immediately began to set his latest plan into action: to use his remaining time to ensure that all the things he valued in his life would live on after his death—his philosophies, his surgeries, and his collection of unusual specimens.

"Dr. Mütter raised his reputation to the highest pitch during his life," his colleague Pancoast would later say. "It may not, however, be so enduring, or go down so far to posterity, as if the rich fruits of his life's labors had been more fully spread in our journals, or been enshrined in books. This was a distinction too of which he was ambitious. He was desirous of extending his reputation beyond his lifetime along the records of science.

"Fortune had showered so many present favors upon him . . . ," Pancoast said, "he wished for *more*."

WHEN MÜTTER FINALLY RETURNED TO HIS FAMILIAR LECTURE hall at Jefferson Medical College, it was impossible not to see how illness had begun to ravage him: He was very thin and pale now, his hair was changing from premature gray to bright white, and his skin was sallow. But even terminal illness could not dull his bright spirit, and he greeted his students—old and new—in the same energetic and teasingly affectionate manner he always had. When he walked to the lectern to begin what he alone knew would be his final introductory speech, his students could not hide their adoration for him.

"What ardent greeting he received . . . ," a former student would later recall, "after some of his many attacks of painful illness, the warm and often boisterous applause which burst and rang, heedless of his attempts to silence it, indicating a feeling for him not alone of respect and admiration, but of the warmest affection and tenderest sympathy for his suffering."

Mütter attacked his lesson plan with a renewed spirit and vigor, determined to impart all he knew—clearly, completely, and definitively—to this final batch of students. But despite his best efforts to show a brave face, it was evident to his students and peers alike that his condition was not improving.

"During the last course of lectures which he delivered, an anxious, careworn expression evinced that his natural great buoyancy of spirits and extraordinary mental activity were vainly struggling under the crushing burden of disease and suffering," a student forlornly wrote.

Mütter reframed his current tortured state of being as, instead, a gift from God. No longer could he simply show his students the techniques, styles, and approaches he used to help heal the desperate people who sought his care. Now he had to *trust* them to take over the scalpel, the stitching needle, the clean rolls of cloth and lint.

It forced Mütter to be diligent in correcting his students about things that had come so naturally to him: the swift confidence of his accurate, thoughtful cuts; the methodical cleanliness of his surgical kit, operation room, and clothing; the gentle, even temper that he used to comfort and treat every patient who walked through his door.

Before, Mütter had felt it was his role to lead by example—to show his students the heights they should strive to reach, even though their own talents and abilities would likely never match his own.

But now, Mütter realized his task was to create doctors who could replace him.

He had always loved being seen as a singular wunderkind, an unmatched genius whose surgical work was so complex and idiosyncratic that he alone could perform it. But now, that same thought filled him with fear and dread. That his knowledge and methodology would die with him became his greatest fear.

Mütter wanted more than just the surgical techniques he pioneered to live on. He wanted his empathetic philosophies and his humanist approach to be immortal as well.

"[First-century Roman medical writer Aulus Cornelius] Celsus long since urged the possession of certain physical qualities as essential to the surgeon. He must be *young, adroit, ambi-dextrous*—and he adds a moral attribute, which I trust few of you possess—*without pity,*" Mütter explained to his students. "So far as the mere mechanical portion of our art is concerned, the views of Celsus may be considered as partially correct, but fortunately the absence of his 'requisites,' by no means forbids the acquisition of great surgical skill, as a mere operator. . . .

"However, his declaration, that a surgeon would be 'without *pity,*' is most fallacious," he told them firmly, "for surely there is no profession, in the performance of the duties of which such frequent and urgent appeals are made to our sympathy, and he must be more than man—or worse than brute—who can contemplate unmoved, the agony and torture to which his patients are so often subjected.

"No, gentlemen, I would say to you, *cultivate* your *sympathy,* but learn to *control* it. . . . A calm, determined, yet gentle demeanor, is that which you should endeavor to acquire, and beneath it, the deepest and purest sympathy—a sympathy that forces you to spare nothing. . . ."

Mütter began to speak often and ardently about the values and principles he believed were most important to have "*honorable* success."

He implored that each of his students ask themselves, "Am I to live as an influential, well-informed, and man-loving physician, blessing and benefiting those by whom I am surrounded; or shall I endeavor, in the vulgar phrase, to 'enjoy life,' caring nothing for my profession, or estimating it as a trade, make money the basis of all my aspirations, leaving honor and reputation to him who values them?

"If you have never asked yourselves these questions, the time has come when you must do so," he told them. "Your first step must be directed towards either one or the other of these positions. May I not hope that all will select the better path, sterile and thorny though it may prove, and carefully shun the facile and flowery one, that too surely leads to dishonor and despair?"

Again, Mütter felt keenly aware of how he allowed—nay, actively developed—his being a singularly talented genius, blessed by God with gifts one simply could not learn in a classroom. While this vision of him had served for so many years to stoke his ego, he had come to realize its intrinsic harm. How often—too often—good, solid physicians were made to feel humble, discouraged, and hopeless, thinking they had no chance at greatness.

"I cannot admit the opinion of [the French philosopher] Helvétius, that every one is born with equal capacity," he told them, "but I am very sure that nearly every human being possesses nature intellect sufficient, if properly nurtured, and trained, to enable him to become at least a useful member of society, if he does not ultimately reach distinction.

"Starting, then, with this position, it will be my task in the lecture to point out the *mental* and *moral* culture to which each one of you should from this day diligently subject himself," he told his students. "To some, the task will be easy and delightful; to others, a warfare, in which indolence, perverseness, pride, ill-nature, and sensuality will present themselves as foes. But let those who may unfortunately belong to the latter class 'strengthen their hearts' with the truth, that all these natural enemies may, by proper strategy and courage, be certainly overthrown."

If Mütter's students needed an example of what might happen to them if they were not as vigilant as Mütter was in thinking through and then standing up for their own principles, values, and standards, they needed to look no further than the crumbling example of the life and career of Dr. Charles D. Meigs.

CHAPTER TWENTY-THREE

THE VOICES OF THE ILLUSTRIOUS DEAD

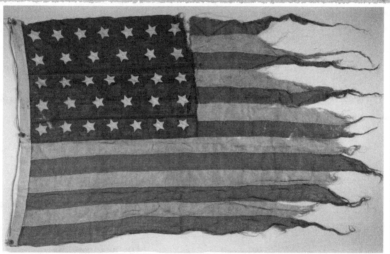

Union Flag Flown over Jefferson Medical College

A PHYSICIAN SHOULD BE
A PATRIOT

I do not mean by this a patriot of the "mob's
decree," but a good old-fashioned patriot.
A man of honest heart, of pure intentions, of firm
and high resolves, of ardent love for his country,
because it is his country;
A man who, if occasion demands, will not hesitate
to shed his last drop of blood in her defense.

Thomas Dent Mütter

CHARLES D. MEIGS, TWENTY YEARS OLDER THAN MÜTTER, WAS still robust and vigorous as he entered his mid-sixties. When the two passed each other in the halls of Jefferson Medical College, Meigs's effortless health served as a startling contrast to the increasingly frail Mütter. But the strength and health of their individual ideas and philosophies could not have been taking more dissimilar paths.

Mütter's ideas—long shunned and mocked by many in the Philadelphia medical community—were slowly being proven correct, and his star was rising even as his health was failing.

The hale and hearty Meigs, however—in almost perfect contrast—was forced to watch as his opinions were disproved, his long-held theories were ridiculed, and his reputation made a staggering, stunning decline.

Meigs's practices and guiding philosophies, which had been seen as so grounded and traditional in the previous decades, now seemed more than just out of fashion—they seemed dangerously out of touch.

And this was true even outside the world of medicine.

LIKE THE REST OF THE COUNTRY, PHILADELPHIA WAS CAUGHT UP in the fear that the nation was going to be "split asunder" by the age's most pressing issue: slavery.

Philadelphia not only allowed slavery when the city was founded in 1682, it was also once one of the country's largest hubs for the slave trade. But attitudes toward slavery gradually changed, and nearly a century later,

in 1780, Pennsylvania became the first state in the Union to pass an abolition act to outlaw slavery in the state.

"When we contemplate our abhorrence of that condition to which the
arms and tyranny of Great Britain were exerted to reduce us," the act began,
"when we look back on the variety of dangers to which we have been exposed, and how miraculously our wants in many instances have been supplied and our deliverances wrought . . . we conceive that it is our duty, and
we rejoice that it is in our power, to extend a portion of that freedom to
others, which hath been extended to us."

The act made very clear the position that Pennsylvania legislators had
taken toward those who believed that white Americans were—and should
remain—superior to all other races.

"It is not for us to enquire why, in the creation of mankind, the inhabitants
of the several parts of the earth were distinguished by a difference in feature or
complexion," the act read. "It is sufficient to know that all are the work of an
Almighty Hand . . . we may reasonably, as well as religiously infer, that He,
who placed them in their various situations, hath extended equally His care
and protection to all, and that it becometh not us to counteract His mercies."

However, even with their "hearts enlarged with kindness and benevo-
lence," the lawmakers believed they wouldn't be able to free all the slaves in
Pennsylvania at once. Hence the law's name and intent: "An Act for the
Gradual Abolition of Slavery." This meant that all children born to a slave
from the date of the act forward would be born *free*, but slaves still could be
purchased or brought into Pennsylvania and continue to be kept as slaves.

However, for the unlucky soul who was still enslaved in Pennsylvania
when the act was passed, it would be left solely up to the discretion of the
slave's owner when—or *if*—the slave would be freed.

Because of the loophole this language caused, there were still slaves in
Philadelphia for decades after the abolition act took effect. Even as late as
the early 1840s, Philadelphia city records show a presence of slaves within
the city limits. It wouldn't be until 1848—nearly seventy years after the act
was passed—that the census showed no slaves living within the city and
Philadelphia's emancipation was finally considered complete.

Despite its Quaker background, Philadelphia was far from welcoming
to free blacks, or anyone considered to be "an outsider." Philadelphians
boasted that their city was "a true American city," citing that it "contained
fewer foreigners than either New York or Boston."

"The city was not showy . . . ," a doctor would later write, "its inhabitants distant and unsocial. . . . The hospitality of a Philadelphia gentleman was proverbial, and often alcoholic."

"Organized gangs of thugs and robbers were numerous and rampant," another doctor recalled, "bearing such refined names as the Rats, the Schuylkill Rangers, the Blood Tubs and the Killers."

Violence in and around the city had grown increasingly common.

The ever-growing population of free blacks—who came to Philadelphia with the hope of making a life for themselves and their families—were a frequent target of that violence.

Much of the anger came from Philadelphia's large working-class and poor populations, who were easily enraged by what they saw as the unfair competition that free blacks presented in the labor market. It was ironic that the racism that emboldened employers to pay free blacks less money than their white counterparts for the same jobs was also the source of so much racist anger volleyed at them by the white workers, who felt they had been robbed by workers who were willing to be paid so much less.

Politicians of the time were not afraid to stoke these feelings of resentment to garner more votes. Philadelphia's mayor was quoted as saying that ninety-nine percent of Philadelphia's own citizens were opposed to abolition, and soon legislation was created to specifically disenfranchise the freed black men and women, stripping them of rights they had been granted since 1780, when the abolition act was first passed.

"There is not perhaps anywhere to be found a city in which prejudice against color is more rampant than in Philadelphia," Frederick Douglass, author, abolitionist, and former slave later wrote. "It has its white schools and its colored schools, its white churches and its colored churches, its white Christianity and its colored Christianity, its white concerts and its colored concerts, its white literary institutions and its colored literary institutions . . . And the line is everywhere tightly drawn between them.

"Colored persons, no matter how well dressed or how well behaved, ladies or gentlemen, rich or poor, are not even permitted to ride on any of the many railways through that Christian city. Halls are rented with the express understanding that no person of color shall be allowed to enter, either to attend the concert or listen to a lecture," he continued. "The whole aspect of city usage at this point is mean, contemptible and barbarous."

But there were many in Philadelphia who committed themselves to the antislavery fight and, furthermore, to the acceptance of the equality of the races. Philadelphia became the founding home of the American

Anti-Slavery Society as well as of the influential abolitionist newspaper the *National Enquirer* (later renamed *The Pennsylvania Freeman*).

Abolitionists had to be creative to circumvent the intolerance of the time. When abolitionists were repeatedly denied rentals at meeting halls around the city because they insisted that both blacks and whites be allowed to attend their meetings, they decided to create a building of their own: Pennsylvania Hall, a large, handsome building they hoped would serve as "a place where freedom of speech could be enjoyed."

Three days after its grand opening, a group of female abolitionists rented the hall for their antislavery convention. In a sign of solidarity with the African American population they were trying to help, blacks and whites entered the hall, arm in arm.

The sight of white women walking arm in arm with black men proved to be too much for the agitated crowd of belligerent onlookers. Within minutes, an uncontrollable mob broke into the hall. They shattered windows, broke chairs and tables, punched and kicked attendees, and eventually burned the entire building to the ground.

But the burning of Pennsylvania Hall would only serve to unify, to rally and strengthen the antislavery cause in Philadelphia. This was important since the city seemed largely in denial about the possibility of an American Civil War.

Despite the growing tension across the country, it was said of Philadelphia that "everything southern was exalted and worshiped." A fact that was likely doubly true for the medical community, where over half the population of both students and doctors were Southern-born . . . including Mütter and Meigs. And as usual, how the two men responded to the threat of a Civil War couldn't be more different.

THOUGH MEIGS WAS RAISED LARGELY IN THE SOUTH, HIS IMMEdiate family embraced his wife's Northern values. His son John would even help found the Union League of Philadelphia, "a patriotic society to support the Union and driven by its founding motto, *Amor Patriae Ducit* ('Love of Country Leads')."

When the gruff Charles D. Meigs surprised his son by asking for the opportunity to speak in favor of abolition in front of his friends at the Union League, the younger Meigs was thrilled and agreed. It turned out to be a terrible mistake.

"All who knew him will remember that the book [that Charles D. Meigs] loved most dearly was a treatise on the races of men by the Count de Gobineau," his grandson Harry I. Meigs remembered. "In these learned volumes my grandfather became wrapped up through and through, and saturated with the ever-flowing stream of their wisdom. . . . My grandfather always put himself among the Aryan or noble race, and he liked to discover in his grandchildren the unmistakable marks of the Aryan outline. . . . The prosperity of our country, and the rapid strides with which it has sprung up to greatness, were by him referred to the weight of Aryan blood in our veins; and his chief source of disgust was the backsliding which he foresaw from the terrible 'commingling of the nations.'"

In his inflammatory speech, the older Meigs argued, before an audience of men and women who were fighting on behalf of the equality of the races, that the great tragedy of slavery was the "half-breed" children who came from white masters raping their black slaves. Not the rape, nor the concept of enslaving another human itself. No, to Meigs, it was the *miscegenation*— the interbreeding of people considered to be of different racial types. It was the horror he felt at the idea that his "godlike race, the archetype of the Grecian demigods and heroes" would procreate with the "nude and barbarous tribes of the African race."

In the free North, he argued, freed blacks knew their place, and white people would never choose to "comingle" with them. But the nature of slavery—the power dynamic in his mind trapped both slave and master— made this "comingling" inevitable.

"Let due honor and reverence be forever rendered, therefore, to those sober, wise, provident philanthropists of Pennsylvania, who erected an impassable wall of separation between the colored and the white races in the Keystone State, by the manumission of all slaves and the prohibition of slavery here forever," Meigs told the audience of his son's abolitionist friends. "It was in 1780 that this wall was builded. . . . It was not alone an anti-slavery wall, but it was an anti-miscegenation wall, and so strong, so thick, and so high is it, that the crime of miscegenation here is not less odious, or less frequent, than *murder itself.*"

The elder Meigs's speech would prove to be so offensive to the gathered crowd of abolitionists that his son John would eventually have to resign his position with the Union League.

MÜTTER, LIKE MEIGS, HAD ALSO BEEN RAISED IN THE SOUTH. Though he had lived in Philadelphia for more than two decades now, he was still close to Colonel Robert Carter, young heir to the Carter family fortune who had agreed to take in the orphaned Mütter as his ward. Mütter himself had grown up in Sabine Hall, the Carters' expansive estate, which was then, and continued to be, the home to dozens of slaves.

But Mütter employed only free men in his own house in Philadelphia, and unlike Meigs, he did not believe there was any biological difference between the races past the superficial. He even included illustrations of people of color in his surgical textbook, and was happy to share what he knew to be the simple truth—that despite all the different skin colors that humans can possess, the bones, organs, muscles, and tissue beneath that skin remain consistent, that once you cut a person open, we all look pretty much the same.

Equally true to Mütter was the feeling that the United States must be kept together if it were to succeed, and that secession of the Southern states—as was often threatened—could never be the answer.

Jefferson Medical College strived to stay apolitical in this charged time, no doubt inspired by the fact that over half its student population came from the South.

The board insisted that its faculty members not speak about politics of the day, calling any debate about slavery or secession "that great maelstrom" that "swallows up time and character, morals, reputation, and money, and which makes no return whatever but disappointment and vexation of spirit."

But Mütter was unable to stop himself from using his position to speak bluntly and passionately to his students.

"Oh, how strange a spectacle has this our 'thrice blessed' country exhibited for the past few months," he told them. "The brother's love supplanted by the fratricide's hate; the pride of greatness smothered beneath the folds of the serpent of discord; the holy spirit of Union nearly put to flight by the demon of anarchy and civil strife!

"And all for what?" he asked. "Simply because our people, forgetting their duty to the 'Constitution and Laws,' have ceased to be true patriots! Will any one believe that the 'magnificent fabric of Union' could for a moment be placed in jeopardy, had we loved it with the true love of a patriot?

"But how fearful responsibility do those assume who dare breathe the word *Disunion*," he said. "*Disunion!*—it makes our blood run cold to hear it even named, and yet men talk about it, predict it, defend it.

"Oh, could these [conspirators] but realize the glory that even now hangs over our land, or, looking into futurity, picture themselves the wondrous and gorgeous destiny that naturally awaits the 'refuge of oppressed,'" he said, clearly announcing his sentiments regarding the still controversial topic of abolition, "possibly their impious hands might be stayed, and the infamy of the traitor transferred to ages yet in the womb of time.

"Go home, then, gentlemen," he implored all the students, but looked directly at Southern ones, "determined to do all in your power to avert so fearful a crime as disunion. Go home, determined to cultivate a spirit of conciliation towards all portions of our land. Go home, determined to be patriots. *Posterity* bids you do this; *the voices of the illustrious dead of every quarter of our land* bid you do this.

"*Go home*," he told them finally, "and let the noble language of the illustrious [American lawyer Daniel] Webster sink deep into your hearts: *I confess that, if I were to witness the breaking up of the Union . . . I should bow myself to the earth in confusion of face—I should wish to hide myself from the observance of mankind, unless I could stand up and declare truly, before God and man, that by the utmost exertion of every faculty with which my creator had endowed me, I had labored to avert catastrophe!*"

But like so many things in Mütter's life, this too was out of his control. And despite the best efforts and fair warnings, so many of the students he lovingly trained in the compassionate art of healing would spend years of their lives on battlefields and in makeshift hospitals, stitching together broken bodies, sawing off shattered limbs, and burying the woeful dead.

As for Meigs, his downfall would not be caused by the comments he made in political forums. No, Meigs's disgrace would come in the form of backlash from one group he never suspected would turn on him: the medical community.

CHAPTER TWENTY-FOUR

LOOK TO GOD FOR PARDON

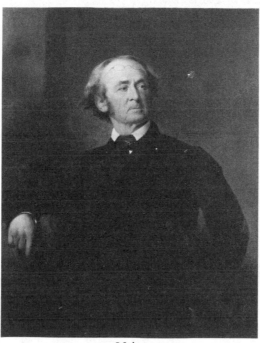

Meigs

INFECTIOUS DISEASE HAD ALWAYS BEEN A PROBLEM FOR Philadelphia—and as its population exploded, the problem only grew worse.

While the city had enjoyed a decline in the mortality rate among its citizens during the years between 1825 and 1850—a triumph considering that similar cities like Boston, Baltimore, and New York City saw increases—their good fortune had begun to run out.

An outbreak of Asiatic cholera killed 1,012 Philadelphians in 1849. An eruption of smallpox took 427 lives in 1852. Yellow fever swept into the city the following year and left 128 corpses in its wake. These numbers were in addition to the deaths caused by illnesses that had become so common in Philadelphia that people thought suffering from them was just an unfortunate, but unavoidable, part of city life.

The frequently recurring disease, typhus, struck the city throughout the 1840s, killing 205 people in 1848 alone. Dysentery terrorized the city every summer, especially the poorest neighborhoods, and would go on to kill more than 1,700 citizens between 1848 and 1851. Meanwhile, malarial fevers spread easily and frequently in the city's low, flat lands between the rivers, and tuberculosis, often called consumption, was also a constant presence.

Ten times as many people died of malaria and tuberculosis in Philadelphia than died of the much more feared cholera, but because the malaria and tuberculosis victims passed away gradually and quietly—they died "romantically," as it was termed—the general public took to dreading cholera more, for it was known for killing its sufferers "with terrifying speed and ugliness."

It was not uncommon for several diseases to have devastating outbreaks at once. In 1852—the same year that smallpox killed more than 400 Philadelphians—433 died of scarlet fever, 558 more of dysentery, and more than 1,200 were claimed by tuberculosis.

Philadelphia civic leaders had finally begun to suspect that there was a connection between sanitation and disease. Starting in 1849, they began thoroughly cleaning streets, waterways, and other public spaces in an effort to discourage the constant scourge of disease. Some politicians and religious leaders still insisted that poverty was "the wages of sin" and spoke out against using public money to clean poor neighborhoods. But the practice spoke highly of the intuitiveness of the day's leaders and would prove a blessing to all the citizens of the city that, for once, its government used sanitary measures—instead of prayer—to fight the constant epidemics.

BUT IF THERE WAS A STUBBORN HOLDOUT IN PHILADELPHIA WHEN it came to not believing in the infectiousness of diseases, it was Charles D. Meigs.

Meigs had become a star in American medicine precisely because of how deeply—and sometimes blindly—he held on to his beliefs, and the incredible lengths to which he would go to fiercely defend them.

Meigs's career had been defined by his passion for what he considered "the right way" to do things and the bold, shamelessly theatrical style—in both lecture and print—with which he espoused these theories. His generation had held that physicians were almost all-knowing gods with whom you should never disagree, and Meigs had qualms about indulging in sentimentalism or speculation to make his point. He thought nothing of belittling his patients, or even his fellow doctors, to ensure his opinions were heard. While it was true that his vision of medicine had begun to be challenged over the course of his career, he had never truly been "one-upped." And because of this, he had always been respected . . . and perhaps a bit feared.

But in the 1850s, the cracks began to show, and the medical community began to look more critically upon the chest-puffing, fact-refuting style of doctors like Meigs.

When the newly formed *American Medical Association* reviewed Meigs's textbook *Observations on Certain of the Diseases of Young Children,* its criticism of the work was clear: "Acknowledging the rare merits which belong to the work as a learned contribution, enriched by the observations of a mind, well-calculated to elicit what is valuable and original in an extensive field of experience, we cannot but speak of it at the same time as presenting *faults too glaring to be overlooked* and of sufficient importance *to merit condemnation.*"

These faults included "an affected obscure style and a fondness for speculations, which, however brilliant and ingenious they may appear, are in many instances *baseless*"; and how Meigs took "the strangest liberties with language, apparently avoiding the simplest and most concise expressions, to extemporize terms more recondite and obscure, framed too without regard to rule or precedent, or indeed to scientific nomenclature, and which are not to be found in any accredited authority." Additionally, "his fondness for what is speculative leads him often to prefer what is novel, ingenious, and peculiarly his own, to that which is more worthy of and sanctioned by common acceptation."

The reviewer continued, remarking that he "notice[d] also a disposition to exclusiveness, exhibited by taking into view some facts in the explanation of a topic *to the disregard of others* which would interfere with the unity of the explanation he would cherish." The reviewer concluded that "[h]owever valuable, suggestive, and instructive these chapters by Professor Meigs may be in the hands of the matured, reflecting, experienced physician, we would hesitate to *expose* the impressible, theorizing mind of the student to their seductions."

To receive such a scathing review from a lauded medical institution must have come as quite a shock to Meigs, whose professional life had always been conducted as if his opinions would never be questioned or proven wrong.

And this was just the beginning.

"MEIGS WAS ALL HIS LIFE A NON-BELIEVER IN THE INFECTIOUS nature of *puerperal fever,*" a fellow doctor later wrote of Meigs, "notwithstanding that for a time numerous facts demonstrative of the incorrectness of his belief almost daily stared him in the face."

Puerperal fever, also known at the time as *childbed fever,* was a tragically common infection among new mothers. In a time before the washing of hands and tools became mandated routine, this highly communicable disease was spread easily and frequently between a doctor and his weakened female patient, whose vulnerable body was still raw, spent, and bleeding from labor.

Within a few days of giving birth, the woman would begin to feel the first symptoms. What first came on as chills and fever would quickly evolve into a "fierce and consuming" infection, which spread with shocking speed and searing pain throughout the woman's entire reproductive system. Many times, the women's bodies could not fight off the infection—severely weakened as they were by pregnancy, breast-feeding, and the aftermath of their long, hard birthing process. It is no wonder the disease earned the harrowing moniker the *destroyer of families*.

But to Meigs, this dreaded pestilence was an absolute mystery—why did it sometimes kill just one of his patients, while other times, he seemed to be in the middle of an epidemic of it, with mortality rates reaching nearly one hundred percent?

The only thing Meigs was absolutely sure about puerperal fever was that his role as doctor had absolutely *nothing* to do with it. And in this way, for the duration of his career, Meigs remained willfully blind to the role he played in sentencing the young mothers in his care to death.

But that was about to change, thanks to a bold and enterprising young doctor named Oliver Wendell Holmes Sr.

EDUCATED IN BOSTON AND PARIS, THE THIRTY-FOUR-YEAR-OLD Holmes was just at the start of his career when he published a controversial paper titled "The Contagiousness of Puerperal Fever."

In it, he convincingly—and seemingly definitively—argued that the deadly infection was most often transmitted to the patient by her own attendants: her doctor, the nurse, or the midwife. He ended the article by advocating the best techniques for preventing the disease's spread: promote a clean and sterile environment for the birth room; remove and/or methodically clean any clothing, bedding, or fabrics that might transmit the disease between patients; and, of course, thoroughly wash the doctor's hands, arms, face, and tools.

The article drew much attention to the young doctor and the case he was making. He was praised for "the clarity and forcefulness" with which he addressed "both the transmission and prevention of this devastating disease."

Strangely, Holmes's boat-rocking realization came to him by chance. As a member of the Boston Society for Medical Improvement, he had noticed an odd coincidence in one of the society's meeting reports. After performing an autopsy on a woman who had died of puerperal fever, a Boston-based physician died of the same infection less than a week later, apparently because of a wound he received while performing the autopsy.

As if that weren't compelling enough evidence, in the interval between being wounded and dying from infection, that same Boston-based physician had served as the obstetrician for several laboring women: Every single one of those women went on to develop puerperal fever.

This inspired Holmes to do further research, and finally write in this paper what he saw as the obvious conclusion, doing so in the plainest language he could: "The disease, known as Puerperal Fever, is so far contagious as to be frequently carried from patient to patient by physicians and nurses."

It was not a new concept. Holmes cited literature that supported his theory, though these articles were mainly published in British journals. However, the specificity of his evidence made his paper uniquely compelling and condemning. To many, Holmes had made the perfect case—an indisputable one.

But, of course, this did not stop the eminent obstetrician Charles D. Meigs—who was just a few years into his appointment as a chair of obstetrics at Jefferson Medical College—from publicly decrying Holmes's conclusion. Meigs's response was particularly horrifying to Holmes, for during the course of his research, he had uncovered a harrowing story that had taken place right in the heart of Philadelphia.

IT HAD BEEN AN OPPRESSIVELY HOT SUMMER IN THE CITY OF Brotherly Love when a particularly vicious outbreak of puerperal fever began to attack the city's women. It got so bad that the medical community demanded an investigation to determine the possible cause of this seemingly unending epidemic. The research revealed that an overwhelming number of Philadelphia's puerperal fever cases could be traced back to one doctor: a man by the name of Rutter.

In one three-month period, *seventy-seven* women whose births were attended by Dr. Rutter contracted the dreaded disease. Fifteen of the women died from it.

After witnessing so many other women under Dr. Rutter's care fall ill and die, several of Rutter's patients decided to seek help when they themselves began to show symptoms. And who better to help them but the city's most renowned obstetrician, Charles D. Meigs?

So Meigs himself was brought in to meet with and consult on several of Dr. Rutter's puerperal fever cases. Though Meigs was fully aware that Dr. Rutter had "a far greater number of such cases than any other practitioner in Philadelphia," the esteemed Meigs waved off any notion that Rutter could be responsible, and instead chalked it up to the fact that Rutter managed such a large practice.

Holmes found Meigs's failure to recognize the true nature of what was happening especially surprising since Meigs had edited a publication on puerperal fever that included the testimonies of four well-known British obstetricians, all of whom wrote about the possible communicable nature of the disease.

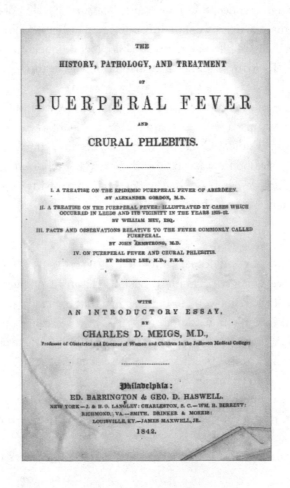

Holmes was outraged that the only conclusion such a lauded professor—the chair of obstetrics at the prestigious Jefferson Medical College no less!—could reach in the face of a "raging epidemic of puerperal fever," isolated largely among the clientele of a single Philadelphia doctor, was *not* that perhaps the disease was clearly contagious (and furthermore was being actively spread by the one person who linked all of these suffering women together), but instead that the "grossly epidemic" proportion of victims in Dr. Rutter's private practice was merely a "coincidence."

Even after Holmes publicly related this story, Meigs refused to accept the contagious nature of puerperal fever and instead disparagingly attacked Holmes for what Meigs perceived as overly "sharp" criticism of his position on the matter.

Holmes followed this rancorous thrust from Meigs by issuing a terse but damning statement: "I take no offense and attempt no retort. No man makes a quarrel with me over the counterpane that covers a mother with her newborn infant at her breast! There is no epithet in the vocabulary of slight or sarcasm that can reach my personal sensibilities in such a controversy."

Meigs and Holmes both refused to budge from their positions.

Holmes believed he had clear facts and science on his side, while Meigs felt that his own extensive career in obstetrics was more than enough evidence to back up his long-held opinion. Frustrating to Holmes was that it didn't seem to be the case that Meigs simply didn't believe puerperal fever could be contagious; rather, it seemed that Meigs was unable or unwilling to understand the concept that diseases could even *be* contagious.

"[I prefer] to attribute these cases [of puerperal fever] to accident, or Providence, of which I can form a conception," Meigs stated, "rather than to a contagion of which I cannot form any clear idea."

The dispute would continue for more than a decade, and even after Holmes made his clear and compelling case, some in the community still sided with Meigs. Among those who did was Hugh Lenox Hodge, professor of obstetrics at the University of Pennsylvania in Philadelphia, who taught in his classroom that the idea of puerperal fever being contagious was pure rubbish, and even went so far as to assure concerned students who wondered if Holmes could be right that they shouldn't worry, because "as physicians, [they] could never be the minister of evil to convey a horrible virus to their parturient patients."

The reason there was still such uncertainty in this debate was because it took place in a "premicrobial era"—that is, a time before the existence of microorganisms was definitively proven, thanks to the invention of the modern microscope and the late-nineteenth-century work of Louis Pasteur (whose experiments helped prove germ theory) and future Nobel Prize–winner Robert Koch (who helped established that microbes can cause disease).

Without the undeniable physical proof later generations of scientists would have, Holmes's article and theory relied almost entirely on deductive logic, looking at the details of the cases to determine that "an unknown contagion existed in the lying-in premises, or was carried to the childbed by an attendant of the mother," and that the presence of an "unseen, transmissible agent" caused the disease.

(When science finally caught up with Holmes, and late-nineteenth-century microbiologists confirmed the theory he had deduced nearly half a century earlier, Holmes was quoted as saying, more than a little proudly, "I took my ground on the existing evidence before a little army of microbes was marched up to support my position.")

But Holmes wasn't alone in his powerful belief in germ theory. At Jefferson Medical College, Mütter and chair of medicine John Kearsley Mitchell were both early proponents of the infectious nature of disease. Mitchell famously lectured that numerous diseases—scarlet fever, consumption, measles, pneumonia, and smallpox, among others—were spread through human contact. Though unable to prove these diseases were related to specific organisms, he would point the finger at "minute spores and fungi."

In addition to his strict insistence on cleanliness before, during, and after operations, Mütter encouraged his students to view diseases as separate entities, produced by separate organisms. When challenged in class about the popular theory that gonorrhea and syphilis were caused by the same pathogen, Mütter quickly corrected the challenger, emphatically stating, "When gonorrhea and syphilis are produced in a patient at the same time, the respective virus of both have been present. One organism *cannot* produce the other disease." At a time when many doctors thought that several diseases were caused by the source (and which of the diseases manifested would be based on a number of different, complicated factors), Mütter's insistence that all diseases—including and especially their causes—must be viewed separately was incredibly forward thinking.

And by 1855—the same year that Mütter would embark on his final year of teaching at Jefferson Medical College, and twelve years after Holmes published his original paper on puerperal fever—it seemed as if the larger medical community was finally also backing Holmes's facts over Meigs's bombast.

In celebration of this clear change of tides, Holmes—now a professor of anatomy and physiology at Harvard University, a post he would hold for thirty-five years—decided to reprint the essay as a stand-alone publication titled *Puerperal Fever, as a Private Pestilence*. Importantly, even though a dozen years had passed, Holmes reprinted the work *without the change of a word or syllable*. The passage of time had not dimmed or diminished his findings at all, and in republishing the work, he hoped to gain a wider audience for its lifesaving message.

However, Holmes had never forgotten Dr. Meigs and his withering remarks and haughty denial of the disease's infectiousness—a truth that Holmes felt the "commonest exercise of reason" should have illuminated.

So, prior to the publication of *Puerperal Fever, as a Private Pestilence*, Holmes penned a fearlessly audacious introduction, in which he called out Meigs by name more than a dozen times. He detailed and deflated Meigs's arguments against his theory, and then warned any medical school students of the dangers of believing any professor whose views were so limited and sophomoric.

"If I am wrong, let me be put down by such rebuke as no rash declaimer has received since there has been a public opinion in the medical profession of America," Holmes boldly declared. "If I am right, let doctrines which lead to professional homicide be no longer taught from the chairs of [Jefferson Medical College and the University of Pennsylvania]. . . .

"Let the men who mould opinions look to it; if there is any voluntary blindness, any interested oversight, any culpable negligence, even, in such a matter, and the fact shall reach the public ear," he concluded, with a statement that would cement Meigs's spectacular fall from power and grace, "the pestilence-carrier of the lying-in chamber must look to *God* for pardon, for *man* will never forgive him."

Meigs never commented on the publication, and would go to the grave without ever admitting that his beliefs on the matter—which he had loudly, persistently espoused for decades—had been utterly and completely wrong.

CHAPTER TWENTY-FIVE

WHILE THERE IS LIFE, THERE IS HOPE

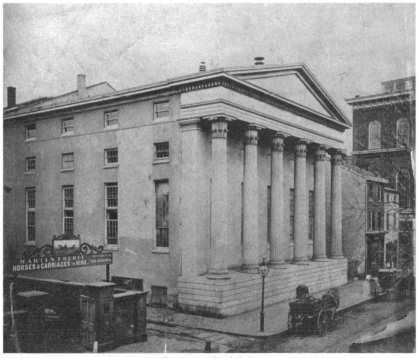

Jefferson Medical College

I̶T WAS EARLY MARCH 1856, AND THE CROCUSES HAD FINALLY begun to push their way through the stone sidewalks of Philadelphia. The petite, persevering flowers exploded across the city's stark landscape like small fireworks in bright whites, yellows, and purples. They served, as they always had, as jubilant reminders that even the cruelest winters will end.

Spring had, at long last, arrived in Philadelphia, but only Thomas Dent Mütter knew it would be the last one he would ever spend as a professor of Jefferson Medical College.

MÜTTER DID NOT WANT TO DISTRACT FROM THE HAPPY FESTIVities associated with a new class of graduates, so he decided to hold off sending his resignation letter until well after the school year was over. Though his friends, peers, and students alike had watched Mütter's condition deteriorate, he knew the news would likely still startle them.

Despite his failing health, Mütter's lectures remained robust and detailed and filled with the same charm that had always defined him. "As zealous as he was efficient," he oversaw the treatment of more than 800 surgical cases at the Jefferson Medical College clinic, and helped perform 267 operations, including amputations of the thigh and leg, amputations of the arm at the shoulder joint, a removal of an upper jaw (an operation that had become more and more common in the harrowing era of phossy jaw), resection of the elbow joint and of the tibia, and numerous plastic surgeries, among others.

Everyone had expressed their hopes that Mütter was simply having a bad year and that his health would be on the mend again soon—perhaps after another trip to Europe? After all, Mütter was forty-five years old—five years *younger* than Meigs had been when Jefferson Medical College had hired them both fifteen years earlier.

Fifteen years, he thought. Mütter had helmed the surgical department of Jefferson Medical College for *fifteen years*. He had taught hundreds upon hundreds of doctors and helped thousands of patients, a significant portion of whom had told him he was their last hope. Through his dedication to innovation and his willingness to experiment, he had been able to introduce and popularize new concepts in medicine and surgery, including numerous forms of plastic surgery and, of course, the now widely accepted ether surgery.

And he tried his best to teach compassion to the eager, ambitious swarms of students. He taught them that the patients who flocked to the clinic for care were not to be defined by their diseases, or their injuries, or their deformities. They were not mysteries to be solved, or cases to add to the docket. They were people, humans. They had names and families, and—maybe if the doctors did their jobs right—they would each have a future too. A good future—one made better by the help these gentlemen should feel privileged to provide.

Taking all of these accomplishments into account, Mütter felt his fifteen years at Jefferson should feel like *enough*. But even recounting all he had done—all the opportunities he felt God had blessed him with—it still seemed hardly sufficient consolation to him for the sacrifice his body was forcing him to make.

As he watched his final class of graduates march into the hall for their commencement ceremony, he tried his best to hide his grief under a trained smile. Among the 215 graduates that year were the sons of two Jefferson Medical College professors: Richard J. Dunglison, the beloved son of Robley Dunglison (who had hand-selected Mütter as chair of surgery so many years ago), and William Henry Pancoast, the only child of Mütter's closest friend and steadfast colleague, Joseph Pancoast.

Mütter had met these young men when they were but children, and had watched them grow for a decade and a half. And now, here they were: doctors.

He looked at the eager faces of the graduating class. Mütter could have no idea what the future held for these man, or for the hundreds more who had also sat on wooden benches in Mütter's lecture hall and learned what it meant to be a physician—a *good* physician—from him.

AMONG THOSE MEN CHANGED FOREVER BY THEIR TIME WITH Mütter was Edward Robinson Squibb.

Squibb, who as a student had been so critical of Mütter, grew more admiring of his old professor in the years since graduation. Watching Mütter work various astounding ether surgeries while struggling with the limitations and complications of working with the earliest incarnations of inhalation anesthesia, Squibb had been inspired to find a way to standardize ether. His vision was to provide doctors and surgeons with stable, constant chemicals for their work, and thereby make ether surgeries safer, more popular, and even more widely accepted . . . and thus also make easier the very difficult job of surgeons like Thomas Dent Mütter.

Squibb would spend over a year developing, creating, and testing a new type of still that would provide a safer, more efficient alternative for distilling ether (which had previously been done over an open flame). After finally building a still that met his high standards, he began months of experimentation with it to determine how to produce the finest and most uniform ether possible, better than anything else on the market.

His journals—which had once been filled with detailed descriptions of meals he ate and the conversations he tolerated with his dim-witted employers—were now filled with charts detailing temperatures, amounts, costs, and specific gravities of solutions. The breakthrough would happen when he struck upon the perfect way to resolve his still's condenser issues and realized that he would be able to wash away most of the impurities that plagued the current market's ether with a combination of potassium carbonate and redistillation.

After years of work—largely in isolation—he had finally done it: He had designed what he considered to be the perfect ether apparatus. It was not only capable of producing "ether of uniform strength by using steam," but also was created in such a way that "nothing short of the grossest carelessness or inattention can interfere with the uniformity of the product."

But Squibb's next move proved to be the most surprising of all.

Instead of rushing to patent either the process or the still—both of which were conceived, created, tested, and perfected by Squibb alone—he gave them to the world for free, publishing an article on his apparatus, including a detailed diagram of his design, in the *American Journal of Pharmacy*. He then began work on making what would become the first truly effective "ether mask" for use in surgery—relieving yet another aspect of ether surgery that vexed surgeons.

It would not be long before Squibb—who made his living as an onshore assistant surgeon for the U.S. Navy—would be encouraged to go into private industry and would found the pharmaceutical company that in his lifetime would be known as E. R. Squibb & Sons (and would develop over the course of 150 years to become the pharmaceutical giant Bristol-Myers Squibb). Their motto was one that Mütter could have stood behind: *"Reliability. Uniformity. Purity. Efficacy."*

Through his company and through his personal work, Squibb would become an advocate for transparency between patient and health-care provider and between doctor and medicine supplier. He was instrumental in launching the movement that produced the first federal Pure Food and Drug Act in 1906, the first of a series of consumer protection laws that, among other things, required drugs to be labeled with their active ingredients and also to maintain recognized purity levels in order to be sold in the United States. This would in turn lead to the creation of the Food and Drug Administration, a national agency dedicated to protecting consumers and regulating the drugs and food they consume.

Squibb never forgot his experiences at Jefferson Medical College. When it was explained to the seventy-seven-year-old Squibb that his hand would have to be amputated due to infection, he immediately set about outlining the exact operation he wanted, planning "the amputation the way he thought his old professors Mütter and Pancoast would have done it . . . with improvements by Squibb." When it came to the surgery itself, he insisted on self-administering his own brand of ether . . . or at least for as long as he remained conscious.

SQUIBB WAS NOT THE ONLY ONE OF MÜTTER'S STUDENTS WHO later went on to transform the world of medicine both locally and worldwide.

Like Squibb, Francis West Lewis decided to spend three years studying medicine at Jefferson Medical College, instead of just the required two. A "marked friendship" grew between Lewis and Mütter, so much so that after his graduation in 1846, Lewis was invited by Mütter to join him during one of his summer trips to Paris and London. Mütter showed the young doctor the innovations and institutions that defined European medicine, and introduced him to doctors and professors who would become Lewis's lifelong friends.

It was during a trip to Europe that Lewis first conceived the idea for what would be his life's legacy. In London, he saw the busy Hospital for Sick Children located on Great Ormond Street. The idea of founding a similar hospital in Philadelphia—one that would focus solely on the treatment of children—was sparked.

Lewis's passion for this idea grew when he returned to the United States, and through his work at the Pennsylvania Hospital, where he saw the appallingly high mortality rate for infants and children treated there. Children were viewed simply as "little adults" and suffered terribly from cross infection, hospital-contracted diarrhea, and even neglect since so many of them were too young to feel comfortable communicating their needs—or were simply unable to—until it was too late.

Finally, in November 1855, Lewis helped open the Children's Hospital of Philadelphia, and what started out modestly as twelve little beds tucked into a small house on Blight Street would develop through rapidly growing stages into a large, well-ordered institution, one of the earliest of its kind in the country—and owing much to "the indefatigable watchfulness and care" of Dr. Lewis.

"Scarcely a day passed, regardless of the weather . . . ," a biographer wrote of Lewis, "that did not find Dr. Lewis at the hospital investigating the minutest detail of its management, planning additions and improvements, and looking after the welfare of his little friends, who upon his appearance in the wards welcomed him with shouts of joy."

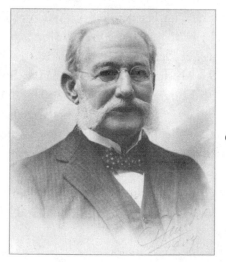

Carlos Finlay

The graduating class of 1855 would include the Cuban-born Carlos Juan Finlay—who was born Juan Carlos Finlay but, like Mütter before him, altered his name slightly after receiving his medical degree, as a form of reinvention. After spending two years studying medicine in Philadelphia, Finlay returned to Cuba with a then-rare microscope in hand, and started a practice in Havana. However, between seeing patients, Finlay made time for research and study—and became obsessed with yellow fever, a disease that plagued both Philadelphia and Havana with equally deadly results. Between 1865 and 1881, Finlay would write and publish ten papers on this devastating disease that no one knew how to prevent.

His breakthrough would finally come in 1881, when he was able to determine that the *Aedes aegypti* mosquito was the agent responsible for transmitting yellow fever. Because of this groundbreaking discovery, yellow fever would be effectively eradicated and Finlay would be responsible for saving countless lives throughout South America, the Caribbean, Africa, and the United States.

In the words of General Leonard Wood, a physician and a military governor of Cuba, "The confirmation of Dr. Finlay's [discovery] is the greatest step forward made in medical science since [the] discovery of vaccination."

LOOKING INTO THE FUTURE, THE ONE THING THAT MÜTTER MAY have been able to predict was that the long-simmering hostilities between the American North and South would finally bubble over into war.

John Brown's ill-fated attack on Harpers Ferry would one day be heralded as the first shot of the American Civil War. Brown was hanged for his crimes on the second day of December 1859, and exactly three weeks later on December 23, 1859—which also happened to be the thirteenth anniversary of Mütter's first ether surgery)—there was a secret exodus of more than two hundred Southern medical students from both Jefferson Medical College and the University of Pennsylvania. The students fled the city under the cover of night, afraid that if they didn't at that moment, they might be trapped in the North if war broke out.

When war did break out, many of Mütter's own students would rush to volunteer, and eventually fight, on both sides of the country's bloodiest war. Some of them would become legends.

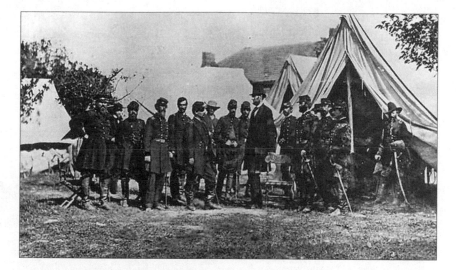

Jonathan Letterman, Army Medical Director (Eighth Figure from Left), Standing between General McClellan (Sixth Figure from Left; Son of Jefferson Medical College Founder George McClellan) and President Lincoln (Sixth Figure from Right) on the Battlefield of Antietam in 1862

Jonathan Letterman, who graduated from Jefferson in 1848, earned the nickname "father of battlefield medicine," thanks to the innovations he developed as a Civil War surgeon. Letterman was named medical director of the Army of the Potomac. The Union Army had entered the war with only ninety-eight medical officers; more than half of the army's medical professionals had resigned to join the South after the start of the war—echoing nearly exactly what happened in Philadelphia that night of December 2, 1859. In an effort to help resolve some of the issues that came up because the Union Army's medical teams were short-handed—supplies that were either almost exhausted or necessarily abandoned; hospital tents that had to be abandoned or were destroyed; medical officers either deficient in numbers or broken down by fatigue—Letterman began drawing up plans and instituting them immediately.

He began introducing a revised concept of the Ambulance Corps— army-issued wagons and trains would be used exclusively for transporting the wounded and, in urgent cases, for transporting medical supplies. Prior to Letterman's ambulance system, there were horrible examples of inefficiency and abuse by personnel tasked to transport the wounded. In one unsettling example, more than three thousand injured soldiers from both sides were left on the battlefield for three days because the civilians respon-sible for moving the wounded had instead picked their pockets, stolen alco-hol from the medical supplies, and left the injured to die.

Letterman also insisted that all surgeons in the Union Army would be tested on their knowledge and be assigned to duty that reflected their skill level. Those who could cut off a limb swiftly and cleanly were sent to the front line; those who could manage the long-term care of patients suffering various unimaginable injuries were kept to work in Northern hospitals.

Last, and perhaps most important, he established field-dressing stations, where wounded soldiers were divided into categories according to the severity of their wounds. Letterman's system of organizing patients into groups of those who would live regardless of their wounds and those who would surely die—known as *triage*—proved to be a revolutionary concept, one still used today.

LETTERMAN WAS HARDLY THE ONLY STUDENT OF MÜTTER'S TO take on a major role in the war. When Robert T. Coleman and John H. Brinton graduated from Jefferson in 1852, after having spent dozens of months studying medicine together in the same room, they could have no idea their futures would see them spending years of their lives aiding two great military men on opposite sides of the Civil War.

Virginia-born Coleman returned to his and Mütter's home state three years after he graduated from Jefferson. When the war broke out, he was appointed surgeon in chief of Thomas Jonathan "Stonewall" Jackson's leg-endary army unit, the Stonewall Brigade. His work would result in Cole-man's being continually promoted until he was the highest-ranking officer in the medical corps of the Confederacy.

Philadelphia-born Brinton—who had been one of Mütter's favorite stu-dents and, like Francis West Lewis, had been invited by his beloved profes-sor on several trips to Europe—would be asked to serve as the personal physician to Ulysses S. Grant. Brinton had been given Mütter's surgical tool kit, which became the tool kit he used to personally treat the wounds of countless soldiers on numerous blood-soaked battlefields, as well as the wounds of their grizzled leader.

Andrew Jackson Foard, whom Mütter watched graduate in 1848, had been the pride of the Jefferson Medical College when he became the U.S. as-sistant surgeon general, a position he held for nine years prior to the Civil War. But once secession began, Foard, a Georgia native, immediately

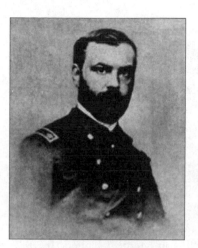

John H. Brinton and his
Certificate of Commission

resigned his prestigious position and enlisted with the Confederacy. He was placed in charge of the medical services of General Braxton Bragg's army and found himself in the middle of some of the most notorious engagements in the war, including the Battle of Shiloh, which killed more than three thousand men and wounded sixteen thousand more in just two days of fighting.

Jefferson Class of 1854 graduate Henry W. Willoughby made history not just for *how* he served, but also *for whom*. Willoughby was proud to be named the assistant surgeon to the 1st Infantry, United States Colored Troops—the first African American troop in U.S. history.

Daniel Leasure, Class of 1846, made a name for himself in the Union Army—not as a doctor, but as a soldier. When he heard of the Confederate Army attack on Fort Sumter, Leasure decided it was his duty as an American to answer President Lincoln's call for seventy-five thousand volunteers to put down the rebellion. Within hours, he had turned over his practice, bid farewell to his wife, and begun to form a regiment. The Union Army would induct him as a colonel and he would go on to lead the immensely popular and storied 100th Pennsylvania Volunteer Infantry, a Scotch-Irish regiment nicknamed the Roundheads who were celebrated for their bravery and for reenlisting—en masse—every year until they had won the war.

Even as a soldier, Leasure still clearly took to heart Mütter's oft-taught philosophy of cleanliness. He became famous for "instruct[ing] his unit in the art of war while keeping a physician's keen eye on sanitation and hygiene."

Because illness and infection were so disproportionately low in Leasure's regiment, his methods were adopted by other commanders. And he earned undying respect from soldiers and doctors alike when, after even the most brutal of battles, Leasure could be found in the hospital tents, assisting the surgeons in their desperate bid to save men's lives.

FOR EVERY MAN WHO TOOK WHAT HE LEARNED FROM MÜTTER and boldly moved into the annals of history, there were even more who earned their degrees and went back home to change the world in smaller but no less important ways.

Robert Sanford Beazley graduated Jefferson Medical College in 1842, and took as his motto "While there is life, there is hope." Having received his medical degree at twenty-five years of age, Beazley enjoyed an incredible sixty-four years of practice, most of which he spent making house calls on horseback. He was said to have "held on to his patients with a grip that seemed to challenge death, making his success in healing almost phenomenal" and he continued to make frequent visits to the sick well into his eighty-ninth year.

John Martyn Harlow left bustling Philadelphia after graduating Jefferson in 1844 and set up a practice in rural Vermont, where the villagers living along the Black River and under the shadow of Ascutney Mountain would "look upon the coming of his carriage, as he flew along the winding and wooded roads, as a harbinger of help to the suffering and of hope to the afflicted in their scattered homes."

Harlow would later have a burst of fame when he was the first doctor to attend Phineas Gage, a railroad worker who survived having a three-and-a-half-foot iron bar driven through his skull because of a workplace explosion. Even though the bar entered through Gage's eye socket and fully exited through the back of his skull, Harlow was able to tend to the man's unusual and extreme injuries with such skill that within three months, Gage was not only walking and talking but was put back to work. When Gage died years later, the family gave the skull and the iron bar to Harlow, who donated both to the Warren Anatomical Museum at Harvard Medical School. When asked to speak at Harvard about the incident, it was a testament to the humble modesty that Mütter taught physicians to have in the face of their more harrowing cases that Harlow ascribed Gage's astonishing recovery not to his own efforts, but rather to the young man's "extraordinary vitality and the unconquerable will."

William S. Forbes graduated from Jefferson Medical College in 1852 to begin a thrilling career in the military. He worked as a surgeon beside the trailblazing nurse Florence Nightingale during Great Britain's Crimean War, served as an army surgeon under Grant during the Siege of Vicksburg, and was named medical director of the 13th Army Corps, before being contracted as a surgeon for the Summit House Hospital in Philadelphia. Once he concluded his military service, Forbes—having never forgotten the experience of watching Pancoast and Mütter working side by side in the Jefferson surgical clinic—began advocating passionately on the importance of dissection and the detailed study of anatomy. In 1866, he presented the Pennsylvania state legislature with his version of a law to provide bodies to medical schools in a fair and legal manner. Although it was dismissively referred to as the Ghastly Act, Forbes's efforts ultimately proved successful, and a board was created to regulate the distribution of bodies to Pennsylvania schools. He returned to his alma mater and became the demonstrator of anatomy at Jefferson, serving in that role for seven years before being appointed professor of anatomy.

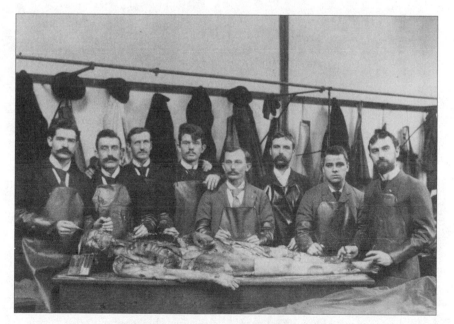

William Pancoast, the Son of Joseph Pancoast,
in the Center of Jefferson Medical College Dissection Room

William Goodell, Class of 1855, knew he wanted to be an obstetrician when he entered the Jefferson Medical College. And while he took ample notes during Meigs's lectures, he followed Mütter's philosophies about creating clean environments for all medical procedures. The son of missionaries, Goodell was elected to be the first physician in charge of the newly established Preston Retreat in Philadelphia ("a lying-in hospital for indigent married women"), and his insistence that the hospital and staff follow Mütter's principles of asepsis and antisepsis was praised for leading to the hospital's astonishing success rate. Of the 2,444 deliveries recorded during Goodell's time there, only six ended in death.

THE RIPPLE EFFECT OF THOMAS MÜTTER'S YEARS OF TEACHING would echo through an entire generation of doctors; and through his students—their work and their influence—Mütter's philosophies and approaches would become an instrumental part of the development of what we now see as the era of modern medicine.

But as Mütter watched his final class of students graduate, he knew none of this. He simply applauded loudly and sincerely as each name was read, and then said his good-byes.

ON MAY 19, MÜTTER FINALLY WROTE THE LETTER HE HAD BEEN dreading and mailed it. It read:

Philadelphia May 19th, 1856

I am compelled by the condition of my health to take the most painful step of my life.

I refer to the resignation of the chair in the Jefferson Medical College with which your board honored me some years since.

In requesting you to lay before the trustees my resignation, I'll aim to refrain from expressing my high appreciation of their uniform kindness to myself and their untiring devotion to the interests of the institution over which they preside.

For sixteen years, trustees and faculty have strived together in harmony and kind feeling towards the accomplishment of one great end and the result proves how richly their efforts have been rewarded.

To leave such trustees and such colleagues occasions me the most poignant regret, and nothing but a firm belief that my life would fall a sacrifice to another winter's work could induce me to tender my resignation.

Please present my warmest regards to each member of the "boards" and that he who "orders all things aright" may continue his protecting influence to us all, shall be the constant prayer of one who is truly and sincerely, your firm friend . . .

Gentlemen, I hereby resign the chair of surgery in the institution over which you preside.

WITH HIGH RESPECT AND
ESTEEM, I REMAIN YOURS,

THOMAS D. MÜTTER

THE JEFFERSON MEDICAL COLLEGE BOARD OF TRUSTEES RECEIVED the letter "with deep regret" and gave "their assent to his request Solely on the ground of his impaired health" and fervently hoped that "a cessation from the arduous professional duties in which he had been engaged may lead to a restoration of his health" so that he might return to his "long career of eminent usefulness."

The board unanimously voted that "as a mark of the high estimation in which the Board of Trustees hold the distinguished service of Professor Mütter during his long connection with the Institution" he be named emeritus professor of surgery, the first time ever that such an honor was bestowed by Jefferson Medical College.

One would think receiving such an honor and leaving on such a high note would be enough for Mütter . . . but there was one more thing he knew he must do before his time on earth came to an end.

CHAPTER TWENTY-SIX

LEAVE NOTHING UNDONE

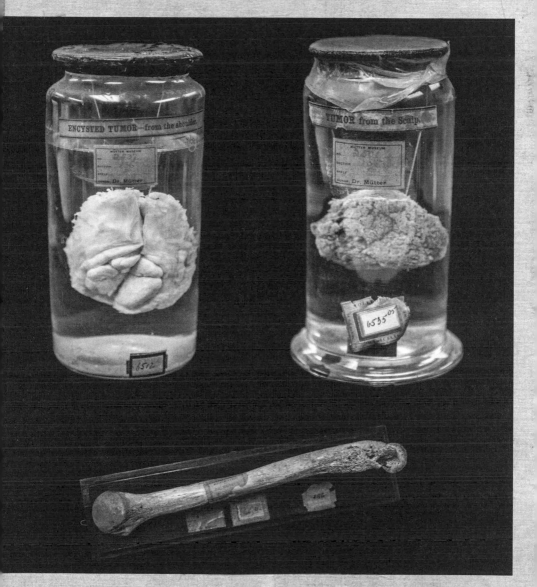

Anatomical Specimens from the Personal Collection
of Dr. Thomas Dent Mütter

Wɪᴛʜ ʜɪs ʀᴇsɪɢɴᴀᴛɪᴏɴ ᴀᴄᴄᴇᴘᴛᴇᴅ, ᴍᴜᴛᴛᴇʀ ʙᴇɢᴀɴ ᴛʜᴇ ᴅɪꜰ-ficult process of leaving the city he loved so much. He gave volumes of books from his personal library to his favorite students, whittling down his enormous collection to one that was "very small, not exceeding seven or eight hundred volumes, and of these many were obsolete." He then gave his unique and impressive collection of surgical tools and tool kits to fellow doctors, so that the tools did not see a day of waste. He donated his piano to the Pennsylvania Hospital for the Insane. He agreed to rent his house, fully furnished, to Samuel D. Gross—the outspoken doctor whom Jefferson Medical College had voted to replace Mütter. He began to write his last will and testament.

But there was still one responsibility he had to fulfill: to find a home for his extensive collection of unusual medical specimens.

Like his idol, Dupuytren, in Paris, Mütter had amassed a large collection of pathological marvels, many extremely unusual. There were "the usual osseous, nervous, vascular, muscular, ligamentotaxis, and other preparations for anatomical demonstration," but his collection also contained a large number of wet preparations (specimens in jars); diseased bones and calculi; an extensive series of paintings and engravings, representing healthy and morbid parts, fractures, dislocations, tumors . . . and the surgical operations that are necessary for their relief; as well as graphic models of medical conditions in wood, plaster, and wax.

Throughout his career, Mütter had always been on the lookout for "fresh acquisitions" and was always sure to tell anyone who asked that his collection was created solely for demonstrations in class, for it was so well curated for "illustrating the various branches taught in the school."

But in truth, to Mütter, it was more than that. Unusual specimens—or medical oddities, as they are sometimes called—were always an attraction to the general public, and it seemed a cruel irony to Mütter that people who suffered so greatly during their life were also stripped of their rightful humanity after their death. One could scarcely imagine a more cruel rejoinder to a life of painful forced isolation than to have one's corpse paraded in a sideshow.

Most of his collection had come from the world of medicine. Mütter had kept and preserved unusual specimens from his own practice. He had solicited strange material from hospitals or fellow doctors whom he knew. And, in the case of the anatomical models, he had sought out expert craftsmen, usually in Europe. But Mütter tried to rescue specimens wherever he found them—taverns, alehouses, sideshows. Sometimes this proved to be an arduous task. The owners would resist, refusing to part with the specimen for any price, no matter how doggedly Mütter used his charms or how wide he opened his wallet. These specimens held too much potential to shock or titillate, which in turn would earn their owners a few extra dollars a year. Mütter always noted that the men never kept the piece for emotional reasons. It was never the case that the specimen couldn't be purchased because it had been plucked from the body of the owner's own family. But Mütter's determination—and the ever-loosening strings of his substantial purse—ensured that more often than not, he obtained the object of his desire.

To Mütter, the marvels he had so carefully gathered deserved more respect than to be scattered to the four winds upon his death. He wanted to find his collection—his entire collection—a worthy home, and vowed that he wouldn't leave the city until it had one.

MÜTTER'S FIRST CHOICE WAS, OF COURSE, JEFFERSON MEDICAL College. He was sure that the board of trustees would welcome the collection. After all, the school's anatomical museum had served as home for many of his more eye-catching pieces during the fifteen years he'd worked there. Mütter offered to donate his collection—which now consisted of about two thousand specimens—to the school if the institution agreed to give it a permanent home.

Jefferson Medical College refused.

The college simply didn't have the space to house such an immense collection, the board explained, nor was it willing to spend the money to build such a space. Mütter was crestfallen, but John Kearsley Mitchell, his longtime friend and fellow faculty member, had an idea. He suggested that Mütter offer his collection to the College of Physicians of Philadelphia.

The College of Physicians was not a school. Rather, it was the nation's oldest professional medical organization, founded in 1787 with a clearly defined objective: "to advance the science of medicine and to thereby lessen human misery."

Mitchell believed that the College of Physicians—which always wanted to be seen as a place for medical professionals and the general public alike to learn about medicine as both a science and an art—might be open to receiving Mütter's impressive collection, and encouraged Mütter to pen a detailed description of what his gift would entail . . . and what the College would be required to provide in exchange for it.

Mütter spent days working on the proposal, and together, Mitchell and he broached the idea with the board of fellows at the College of Physicians of Philadelphia.

Mütter offered to give the organization his complete collection—all two thousand specimens. In addition, he would give them thirty thousand dollars "for the services of a curator, for an honorarium for a yearly lecturer and for enlarging and maintaining the museum."

In exchange for these two gifts, Mütter had only one condition: that the college provide a fireproof building for his collection, which needed to be built within four years.

Much to Mütter's relief, the College of Physicians was interested, but since Mütter's offer required building an entire museum, they told him they would need more time than he allotted. They explained that they had been interested in sometime constructing a new home for the organization—and had started a building fund in 1849—but despite their efforts, they could not secure sufficient funds to begin building even a traditional structure . . . let alone the fireproof one that Mütter demanded.

Mütter was disappointed, but he understood. He offered to postpone his return to Europe until their decision could be made. He spent one last summer in the sweltering heat of Philadelphia, waiting. But once an autumn chill began to enter the air, Mütter—and his "rapidly failing health"— could wait no longer.

He met with the board of the College of Physicians of Philadelphia one last time, and explained to them that, even though he was too ill to stay in the city longer, he didn't want them to think he was abandoning his negotiations with them.

Instead, he provided them a copy of his will, which stated that he would bequeath all his property of every description—"everything which I possess, or to which I may have any claim"—to his "beloved wife, Mary W. Alsop Mütter," with the sole exception of his storied collection of medical specimens, his marvels.

That collection, the will clearly stated, would be given to the College of Physicians of Philadelphia, but only if they carried out "the arrangements entered into, but not completed, at the time of [his] departure for Europe." He expressed his faith and hope that the organization would rally and the museum would be built, but then warned them that if they had not agreed to his terms by the time of his death, the collection—and the money associated with it—would be offered to other medical institutions. Failing that, it would be given in full to his wife, to be handled as she saw fit.

It was the best Mütter could do.

Shortly after that, Mütter handed over the keys to his house to Samuel D. Gross, his successor at Jefferson Medical College, and left.

"It was better to relinquish quickly one's own terms," Gross would remark about the swiftness of the exchange with Mütter. Upon entering the house, it soon became clear to Gross that Mütter's curt brevity was not a sign of rudeness on the part of the departing professor. Rather, when Gross and his wife entered the house, they were moved by Mütter's thoughtfulness, even during this time of his personal suffering.

"On our arrival we were not obliged to go to a hotel, everything being in readiness for our accommodation," Gross wrote, astonished. "In fact, even dinner was awaiting us."

MÜTTER AND HIS WIFE LEFT FOR EUROPE SHORTLY THEREAFTER, deciding that their best option was to go to France, where he could spend the winter in Nice. Despite everything, Mütter held out hope that he might recover—even including a clause in his proposed contract with the College of Physicians of Philadelphia that if his health returned, he would be granted full access to his collection to use in future lectures and classrooms.

When he arrived in Nice, it seemed that if God were to bless him with a place to heal, this would be it. The Mediterranean Sea was a bright, hopeful blue, and sparkled in the region's golden sunlight. His small house was nestled into a vine-covered hillside, where Mary—with whom he had recently celebrated a twentieth wedding anniversary—could pluck olives from the trees if she wanted to. He felt relaxed, finally, his lungs filling with the warm sea air that found its way up the gentle slope of the hill.

But unfortunately for Mütter, the winter of 1856 was one of "unusual severity" in Europe. "His old malady renewed its attacks," it was written by a fellow doctor, "with its customary frequency," and he and Mary made their way back to Paris so that he could convalesce under the care of the best doctors he knew.

But Philadelphia—and the promise of a museum for his collection—was never far from his thoughts. Mütter learned, however, that he was being called insincere in his offer to give his collection to the College of Physicians of Philadelphia—after all, if he were serious about it, why would he have left the country before an agreement could be formally struck? So he wrote an open letter to the College of Physicians, which he would additionally publish in the popular journal *Medical News* to ensure his message was heard.

In the letter, he defended what he considered to be a "grave charge" made against him about his departure from Philadelphia, which he felt was "both unjust and uncalled for." He explained that his ill health had forced him from the country but that, before he left, he gave the organization all the information necessary to form "the basis of a future contract between the College" and himself, and furthermore that these propositions were made "advantageous to both parties" in the hope that it would help accelerate the process. In this way, Mütter wrote, he left Philadelphia feeling that he and the College of Physicians were united in their efforts to see his museum built.

"It will be seen from the foregoing that I have in every way attempted to carry out my promise to the College," he wrote. "I would leave nothing undone to accomplish the chief object of my professional life."

UNDER THE CARE OF HIS PHYSICIAN FRIENDS IN PARIS, MÜTTER was able to extend his life for another year, although it was clear that, while his heart beat and his lungs took in air, the life he lived trapped in his pain-racked body was not an easy one. When asked by concerned friends what they might be able to bring Mütter and Mary to help them, Mütter would quip, "Linen for Mary, Laudanum for me!" referring to the powerful opiate that doctors would prescribe only for patients who were suffering severely.

Mütter spent several seasons in Europe, growing more and more "weary with the endless torture of disease." He realized that his protracted residence abroad brought "no relief to the malad[ies]" plaguing him. Although his friends were keeping him alive, he was no longer living what could be considered a *good* life.

He came to the dark—but true—realization: The "only remedy [to his condition] was to be its own last and fatal attack."

Mütter finally understood how all those patients begging for his help had felt, those who had come to his office door in wretched states and said they were happy and willing to risk their lives on his surgical table if such a risk held the promise of change. He finally knew what it was like to welcome death over continuing to live the life you were forced to live.

Mütter decided that if he was going to die, he did not want to die in Paris. He was an American; he wanted to die and be buried at home, on his native soil. And those close to him sensed a growing impatience about the fate of his collection. He did not want to die without knowing what would happen to it. After saying good-bye to Paris and to his much-loved friends there, Thomas and Mary Mütter set sail for home for the last time.

IN OCTOBER 1858, THOMAS AND MARY RETURNED TO PHILADEL-phia. Mütter, "feeble and dejected, with the graven lines of pain furrowed deeply on his brow," was a shadow of his former self and a shocking sight to his friends and former colleagues.

"Conspicuous from his bright and manly bearing, which frequent and severe suffering had not yet been able to change," Joseph Pancoast would write about his friend's final visit to the school where he had long taught, "his hair blanched prematurely to almost a snowy whiteness, he stood among you, admired and honored, like a tower partly ruined and fallen, yet unspeakably attractive from its lingering charms and former associations."

While in Philadelphia, the gout in Mütter's hands finally subsided enough for him to write a letter in his own handwriting to Colonel Carter, his old guardian, who Mütter was sad to hear had recently lost a child.

"My dear old friend," Mütter wrote. "Ever since my arrival in this country I have been very ill and am still suffering severely. Up to this period, my hands have been nearly useless, hence my delay in writing you. Armistead

[Carter's cousin] had informed me of the death of your darling child. From my whole heart you have my sympathy and were I able to undertake the journey I would go to you at once.

"It appears our heavenly father in his wisdom does by loss and disappointment wean us gradually from this world and its attractions. Does not this community of suffering bring us nearer to each other? My own fate has been to live among strangers and away from those whom I love best in the world."

This letter would be the last Mütter would ever write to Carter—a fact that Mütter seemed oddly prescient of.

"Now that I feel the approach of night," he wrote, "I know that soon I must lie down to sleep until the 'great day' when we shall see [God's] face, and, I trust, rest from our sorrows."

BUT EVEN LOOMING DEATH COULD NOT KEEP MÜTTER FROM HIS determination to ensure that his collection of marvels would find a home. He was relentless in his communications with the College of Physicians of Philadelphia, until finally, in December of 1858, an agreement was struck. An Article of Agreement finalizing the organization's relationship with Mütter and the creation of the Mütter Museum was, at long last, finally formally and legally recognized. Soon after, Mütter fled the freezing Philadelphia winter for the last time.

Three months later, in the warm air and bright sunshine of his native South, Thomas Dent Mütter died at the age of forty-seven.

CHAPTER TWENTY-SEVEN

THE WORLD IS
NO PLACE OF REST

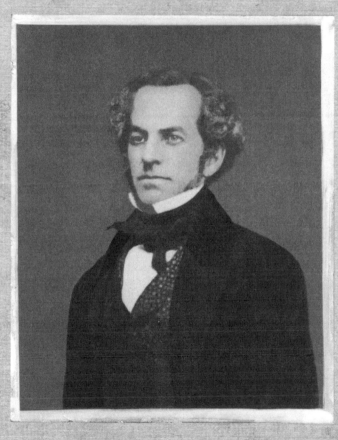

In the weeks and months following his death, tributes to Mütter began to appear in journals and newspapers throughout the country.

"This kind and Christian heart, this generous and accomplished physician has at length found the sad relief which his own art denied him here," read the tribute published in *The North American Medico-Chirurgical Review*. "Among those to whom he gave that ease from suffering in its manifold varieties, which he sought in vain, there will be many to regret his loss."

"The telegraph of the 17th heralded over the western world the mournful intelligence of the death of Dr. Thomas D. Mütter, Emeritus College of Philadelphia, at Charleston, South Carolina, on the 17th day of March, 1859," read the *In Memoriam* that ran in *The Medical and Surgical Reporter*. "A brilliant luminary in the great medical constellation—glorious in its own splendor and deriving reflected beauty from revolving planets—has set in the darkness of an endless night. A lifeboat, which long has floated in gracefulness and usefulness, secured in a peaceful haven, and often shot out in the howling storm rescuing many, *many* a ship-wrecked crew from the perils of a *pestilential* storm, has been cut loose from its moorings, and has drifted far away into the unknown ocean of Eternity."

"The subject of this memoir needs no eulogium from us, before the medical profession, and our humble hands would attempt to wreathe no new laurels for his brow," read the piece in *The Medical and Surgical Reporter*. "The short life of Doctor Mütter illustrated the most remarkable mental abilities and the gentlest qualities of heart. For years, we have viewed him at what seemed the zenith of professional eminence, and yet he continued struggling under the oppression of the severest bodily infirmities, to elevate the science to which he was devoted and to relieve the miseries of others."

Mütter's students, upon hearing the news, shared their memories of their beloved teacher.

"While I recount his manly form and noble bearing, his intellectual face, his kind and genial manner, I convey but a slight conception of that eloquent style and research, wisdom and learning with which his lectures were ever filled—dignity and grace of address—concise and beautiful diction—apt and happy illustrations, which endeared him as a *teacher*," L. Beecher Todd, Jefferson Medical College Class of 1854, wrote; "the skill and neatness, tenderness and sympathy characterizing his operations, which embalmed him forever in the hearts of thousands of the purest citizens and best physicians of our country, who sojourned in Philadelphia to enjoy the wisdom and learning which flowed from his elegant lips. This, as well as many acts of *personal kindness*, justify my affectionate remembrance of him—my teacher, my friend, now no more."

"In every view of him, he was a 'good physician,'" Richard J. Levis, Jefferson Medical College Class of 1848, wrote. "His manner hopefully inspired the desponding; his skill raised many from a lingering couch . . . his great name was ever popularly associated with the relief of suffering, the healing of the sick, joyfully leading away the halt, restoring sight to the blind, or soothing the path of the worn and life-weary to eternal rest."

And with the same breath that his students expressed their undying praise, they also expressed a fearful concern that their late professor might be forgotten.

Todd prayed for an "able hand" to write "the biography of this great and good man" so that it might be "read and remembered, loved, honored and cause the name Thomas Mütter to become a household word of American Surgery."

"Respect for his memory, and the gratitude an obliged pupil feels for a revered preceptor—and which we had hoped in vain that time would have allowed us in some other manner to evince—are the inducements for this feeble offering," wrote Levis. "Other and abler pens will write for him, to coming ages, a deathless name, to be forever blended with the history of American Surgery, and to stand as a synonym for professional excellence and munificence."

"Yet again shall we meet him," Levis would say, "where preceptor and pupil, physician and patient, shall stand in new relations; where disease shall not corrupt, and pain shall not rack; where the palsied hand shall be freed from its fetters, and the darkened eye opened to the light of the life immortal; where the wan and wasted shall be revived; where hopes wreck not, and where sorrows are unknown!"

When it was time to memorialize Thomas Dent Mütter, Jefferson Medical College asked Joseph Pancoast, his longtime friend and surgical brother in arms, to deliver a speech recounting the late professor's life and achievements.

"It is indeed impossible for me even now to revert without pain to the loss of this distinguished friend with whom I was so intimately associated," Pancoast told the gathered crowd of faculty, board, and students, "for, side by side, and step by step, for nearly half an ordinary lifetime, we trod harmoniously together the difficult and somewhat thorny paths of a surgical career.

"Dr. Mütter died early . . . ," he told his audience, "too early, except in cases of men of rare genius, to afford time for the achievement of the highest professional distinction. Yet no one will deny that he had raised himself to the first rank among the members of his profession, and enjoyed confessedly the highest reputation as a practitioner and a teacher of one of the noblest branches of the healing art."

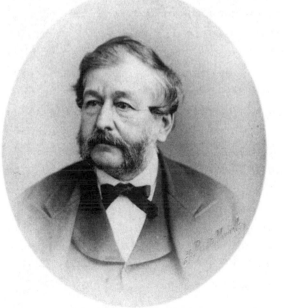

Joseph Pancoast

But like Mütter's former students, Pancoast worried that despite all of Mütter's achievements, his friend's life would be forgotten.

"Dr. Mütter raised his reputation to the highest pitch during his life. It may not, however, be so enduring, or go down so far to posterity," he said, "as if the rich fruits of his life's labors had been more fully spread in our journals, or been enshrined in books. This was a distinction, too, of which he was ambitious. . . . He was desirous of extending his reputation beyond his lifetime along the records of science.

"Often has he talked over such a project with me, and felt, I believe, fully convinced that his future chance of surgical renown might have been safely founded upon achievements in this clinic, which it was his desire to have fully recorded," Pancoast said, referring to the surgical textbook Mütter did not live long enough to write. "Alas! There are many things, as we are apt to discover, to interpose between our wishes and their fulfillment."

Pancoast spoke about the difficulties of the last few years of Mütter's life, how much he suffered, how his attacks of hereditary gout and lung hemorrhages "greatly harassed, distressed, and weakened him" and "forced upon him by slow degrees, and to the great regret of his colleagues," to resign his position and leave Philadelphia.

"The prospect of having to abandon his duties in this place, which had formed so large a part of the happiness of his existence, and was the theatre of so many triumphs," Pancoast said, "he felt as an affliction which seemed to him, as he often expressed it, *like the rending away of his right arm.* . . ."

"For myself especially, who lived so long in his gentle intimacy, his professional merits, great as they were, are not those which swim highest on the seas of thought. It is rather the *sweetness of his character* which I love most to recall; the *kindness of his heart,* which seldom allowed, even towards his enemies, an act of just retaliation to escape him, and I believe his colleagues, in musing over his name, will have their feelings mellowed by a similar sort of retrospection."

Pancoast looked out at the audience. Some of the faces he found in it were people Mütter considered his closest friends and allies; others belonged to colleagues with whom he battled, in private and in public; but most—the new class of students who flooded into Jefferson Medical College that year—knew the man only by name, by reputation, by the legend he left behind. For them, he felt the most pity, to never have met this Mütter, to never have known such a man as he.

"Such, gentlemen, was the surgeon whom the science has lost," he told them with a cracking voice. "Such the professor, full of kindness and knowledge, whom his classes have mourned. Such the friend and colleague, torn from us in the meridian of his existence, whose memory and name we shall ever cherish."

THERE IS NO RECORD OF HOW CHARLES D. MEIGS FELT ABOUT THE death of his longtime adversary. Meigs, at sixty-seven, was still a professor at Jefferson, and celebrating the release of the fourth edition of his textbook *Females and Their Diseases*, when news of Mütter's death broke.

Meigs would turn in his letter of resignation to Jefferson Medical College the following year, having bought thirty-seven acres of land in Delaware County, eighteen miles from the city, where he hoped to spend his retirement. He had built a house on the top of the hill there, as well as a barn and a stable, a tenant house, a springhouse, an icehouse, and a workshop. He was creating an oasis for himself, where he could escape the life he had lived and the vulturous critics who were always trying to tear him down.

He called this new home Hammonasset, after "the Indian name of a small river in Connecticut [where] his forefathers had settled." And looked forward to a time when all he had to do was read and write poetry, paint and eat and drink, and enjoy the company of his numerous children and grandchildren as they played in the fresh country air and the "luxuriant growth of noble woods" that covered over half the property.

"Men ought to retire from public appointments, whilst they were still somewhat fresh in health," he told his son. "If they retained such positions to a late period of life, they sometimes lost the power of judging of their own fitness for duty."

But Meigs's resignation was not accepted. The war had begun, and no suitable replacement could be found. Meigs agreed to give one more course of lectures, which he accordingly did, "though against his will or wishes."

"I am now old and well stricken in years," Meigs angrily wrote in his diary, "and yet I labor diligently in my calling! How long!"

Finally, on February 25, 1861, six days after his sixty-ninth birthday, Charles D. Meigs gave his last lecture at Jefferson Medical College.

"This afternoon I delivered my last lecture at the Jefferson Medical

College, and shall never more appear in public as a teacher . . . ," he wrote in his diary. "I am surprised that this *finale* of my public life causes in me not the slightest excitement; I am simply glad to get out of it."

After resigning, Meigs dropped out of public life nearly altogether, for he was "entirely weary of all medical responsibilities" and had "lost . . . taste for medical literature, and rarely looked into a medical book." He was happy to disengage from the community he felt had turned against him and his beliefs, and leave behind this new world of medicine he increasingly found too confusing to understand.

But retirement for Meigs would not be the idyllic vision of which he had long dreamed. The Civil War, which some had predicted would be over within a matter of weeks, had been raging for months. Isolated in the country, Meigs made an agreement with the conductor of a train that passed his land daily. If any battle of disastrous end should be known to the city, the conductor would give two whistles with his engine, but for a successful contest, "he should whistle twice as often."

Meigs had every reason to be interested in the war. His family was fighting in it—including his firstborn son, Montgomery C. Meigs, who was quartermaster general for the Union—and it wouldn't be long before someone in his family would die in it.

John R. Meigs—firstborn son of Meigs's own firstborn son, who was born the same year that Mutter and Meigs joined the Jefferson Medical College faculty—was Meigs's "favorite and pride among all his descendants in the third generation. . . . High actions and noble exploits were looked for at the hands of this grandson."

But Meigs's dreams for his grandson—who had left his schooling at West Point, so eager was he to fight—were dashed when a bullet exploded inside the twenty-year-old soldier's body as he was fighting "in one of the most luckless engagements of our war." He was killed instantly.

The death of his favorite grandchild in such a brutal manner shook Meigs to his foundation, though it was said that his "mind rose faithful still, and strong, above the dreadful sorrow." However, fate was not through with Meigs yet.

"The Angel of Death had not gone back to his abode among the spirits, but was fluttering about still," another grandson would later write, "waiting only to come again and afflict yet more grievously the gray, vulnerable state of my grandfather."

Just seven months after his beloved grandson's death—just when "the keenness of [Meigs's] grief had begun to lose his edge"—Meigs was devastated when Mary, his wife of just over fifty years, died as well. Her death broke him.

"She was not my grandfather's better half; she was his whole earthly existence," a grandson later wrote, "without whom he desired not to live. The world, that had long been embittered to him, became irksome to him now, and he would gladly have left it."

But much to his own disappointment, death did not come for Meigs. His lungs, heart, and mind remained in good working order, even as the rest of his body—and his life—began to fall apart. Months passed as Meigs wandered about Hammonasset, alone, "slowly pining away in grief both of soul and body." When he wasn't mourning the loss of Mary, he began to suffer "untold distresses with a bodily infirmity that took away his peace." He refused to let any doctor—even his friends—see him.

Meigs's children finally demanded that their now elderly father return to the city, where he could be looked after more dutifully by the large family of children and grandchildren who were his only legacy now that his standing within the medical community had been irrevocably shattered. Meigs refused, but his family gave him no choice.

With that, Meigs left the house he had built for himself and his wife, and unhappily returned to Philadelphia, "whose hot red bricks and monotonous lanes he had long ago learned to hate," haunted by the memories of his old patients, "the distressed women and dying children that he had known as [the city's] inmates."

"Cooped up in a second-story room, he pined for the peace and quietude of his pleasant home at Hammonasset," one grandson recalled, "and each year he frightened his friends and neighbors by threatening to leave the ugly town, and find a little happiness in the fields alone."

Meigs openly wished for death, telling his children and grandchildren that he would welcome it as a blessing—"a quiet night and an end of [my] toils."

"There was only a little left of his mortal self; his flesh and bones were all out of joint," according to a grandson, "and he pined for dissolution."

But death still would not come to Meigs.

"All of him thought his life was now near its end," a grandson wrote, "but the soul was laughing . . . proud of its own strength."

It would take four long years "full of misery and rent with shame" before Meigs would finally die, alone in his sleep, at the age of seventy-seven.

THOMAS DENT MÜTTER'S WIFE, MARY ALSOP MÜTTER, WAS WITH her husband when he died, and rode with his body back to Connecticut, where her family took in the grieving widow and offered her a plot of land in the family cemetery in Middletown. Mary decided to build a small mausoleum to house her husband's body.

The small, dark gray building would bear Mütter's name—umlaut and all—in a sea of stones marked with *Alsop*. Mary made sure the mausoleum was built large enough to fit five tombs in it.

Thomas, her beloved husband, filled one. Mary's tomb remained empty until her death eighteen years later, in 1877. She never remarried. The other three tombs would remain empty, built to honor the family she never knew. The names of Mütter's father, mother, and baby brother were now etched in stone alongside Thomas's and Mary's, and in this way, Mütter's family—who died apart from one another and whose bodies had been buried in distant and disparate cemeteries—could be joined together, finally and for all time.

But Mary's mausoleum in Connecticut would not be the memorial to Mütter that would be most remembered.

IN 1861, TWO YEARS AFTER MÜTTER'S UNTIMELY DEATH, THE College of Physicians of Philadelphia finally began construction on what would become the Mütter Museum. The three-story stone building, constructed on the corner of Thirteenth and Locust Streets, took two years to complete and was, per its namesake's demand, fireproof.

In 1863, the Mütter Museum opened, billing itself as the permanent "repository for specimens, models, historical instruments and many other unusual medical memorabilia and incunabula" that Mütter had collected from all over the world.

The largesse Mütter gave to the organization along with his collection would be spent not just for lumber, carpentry, bricklaying, painting, and plumbing, but also for the acquisition of new cases and jars needed to accommodate the more than two thousand specimens. The salary for the museum's curator came from Mütter's trust, which also paid for an annual lectureship so the community could hear and learn about the latest innovations happening in medicine. And even more important to Mütter, any student of medicine or current doctor could attend the Mütter lecture series, or visit the collection and attend a lecture, "without charge or fee."

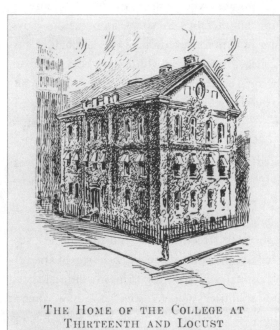

THE HOME OF THE COLLEGE AT
THIRTEENTH AND LOCUST
STREETS, 1863–1909.

The Mütter Museum,
1863

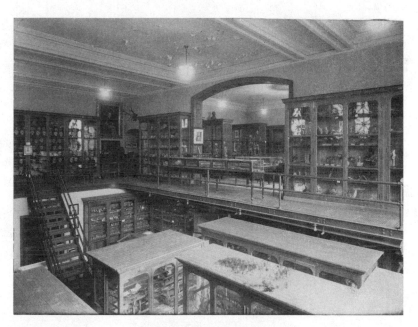

Early Interior of the Mütter Museum

Around this time, John H. Brinton, who was perhaps Mütter's most devoted protégé, was following his mentor's footsteps in numerous ways. After Samuel Gross's retirement, Brinton would take over as chair of surgery at Jefferson Medical College, the position Mütter had held for fifteen years. Brinton would also become chairman of the committee on the Mütter Museum, and—inspired by Mütter's example and Brinton's own experience as a Civil War surgeon—would found the Army Medical Museum, to preserve unusual medical specimens collected by doctors at war.

In 1880, Brinton was asked to give a speech at the Tenth Annual Meeting of the Jefferson Medical College Alumni Association to share his memories of the famous Faculty of '41.

Brinton recounted for the crowd, to peals of laughter, the exploits of those early days: the sharpshooting street urchins who hit Mütter's students with snowballs as he led the class on yet another field trip in an overstuffed omnibus; the school hospital, which during Brinton's time had been "[a] stove-maker's room and [a] bottler's upper stories," and how when it was his turn to staff the clinic, he would use the small stove there to cook himself a "savory oyster" and "a steaming midnight cup of coffee served by

John H. Brinton

the order of a crafty Faculty to ensure the wakefulness of the [exhausted] watcher"; the story of Meigs and the etherized sheep that refused to die.

He spoke about each faculty member individually, but he saved his memories of Mütter for last. Brinton remarked on how Mütter was "beloved, nay almost worshiped by his class," before he praised him as a teacher (where "his great charm lay in his enthusiasm and in his power of imparting something of his own spirit to hearers"), as a surgeon (showing "powers and capabilities which shone so conspicuously"), and as the originator of the Mütter Museum, which Brinton believed made good on "the anticipations and cherished hopes of its founder."

"Time in his flight brings many changes, levels many landmarks, wipes out many names," Brinton said in the conclusion of his speech. "Yet I feel sure that through the mist of fleeting years, which is fast settling down between us and those of whom I have spoken, their figures will not wane but rather stand out with an increasing grandeur. For in good truth this Faculty of 1841 were men of mark. Some were great men . . . all were great professors . . . and we owe them much."

"THIS WORLD IS NO PLACE OF REST," THOMAS DENT MÜTTER taught his students. "It is no place of rest, I repeat, but for effort. Steady, continuous undeviating effort."

One hundred and fifty years after his death, Thomas Dent Mütter's legacy does not rest. It lives on in the surgical techniques he created and which are still being used today; in the innovations and institutions created by the young men who learned from him what it means to be a good physician; and in his namesake museum, now located on Twenty-Second near Market in Center City Philadelphia, which has only grown in size and popularity since its original 1863 opening.

There—for the modest price of admission—you can stand in front of a giant's skeleton. Or marvel at a colon the size of a cow, extracted from a man known only as the Human Balloon. Or, of course, peer into the face of *Madame Dimanche*, that French widow who one day began to grow a horn from her forehead, and whose wax model had so bewitched Mütter, he had carried it with him across an ocean.

There, you will also find a woman dubbed *the Soap Lady*, her body having turned into a waxy soaplike substance after her death, freezing her

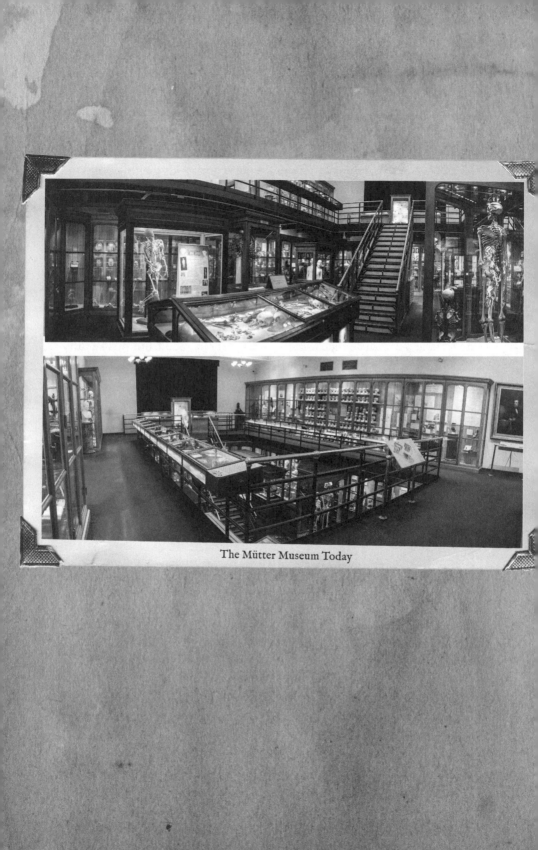

The Mütter Museum Today

small face in what looks like a perpetual scream. There are skulls collected from around the world, with details of their death carefully transcribed in ink on the surfaces of their bones—such as *Julius Farkas, age 28. Protestant, soldier. Suicide by gunshot wound of the heart, because of weariness of life* or *Girolamo Zini, age 20, Rope-walker. Died of a broken neck.* There, you can read from books bound in human skin, a doctor's final gift to a grieving family: the story of a man's health covered in leather made of his own flesh.

Over the past century and a half, the museum's collection has grown to include tumors cut from presidents, the jarred brains of madmen and geniuses, deformed skeletons displayed in delicate glass cases, Civil War surgical tools still caked in dried blood, and even the death cast of Chang and Eng Bunker, the famous sideshow act, a pair of conjoined brothers who inspired the term *Siamese twins.* The Mütter Museum was asked to do Chang and Eng's autopsy—an endeavor successfully led by none other than Joseph Pancoast's son, William Henry Pancoast.

All of this and more can be found under one roof, and all of it is watched over by the dashing portrait of one man: Thomas Dent Mütter.

"Thus, in dying," his old friend Pancoast would say of the museum, "has he left a precious heritage to the profession."

What started as a public home for his ambitious private collection has now evolved into one of the most popular science museums in the United States, where tens of thousands of people flock every year to be intrigued, awed, and provoked by its fantastic collection of artifacts. And like Mütter himself, the museum challenges its visitors to see past their own shock and initial revulsion and instead find the humanity of the people whose remains are on display.

"While these bodies may be ugly," the late Mütter Museum curator Gretchen Worden once wrote, "there is a terrifying beauty in the spirits of those forced to endure these afflictions."

And every week, fresh groups of scientists and doctors come to the museum and its library to study its holdings, unlock its clues, and perhaps even help its long-dead founder to finish his timeless mission: *to alleviate human suffering.* It was a goal Mütter believed was possible, and one toward which he believed all people should strive, regardless of background, birth, skill set, or innate talent.

"Place no dependence on your own genius, even if you possess it. If you have great talents, industry will improve them; if you have but moderate

talents, industry will supply their deficiency—nothing is denied to well directed labor; nothing is obtained without it," he taught his students, and
believed it applied to everyone, including and especially himself. "This
world is no place of rest. . . . Our work should never be done, and it is the
daydream of ignorance to look forward to that as a happy time, when we
shall wish for nothing more, and have nothing more to accomplish."

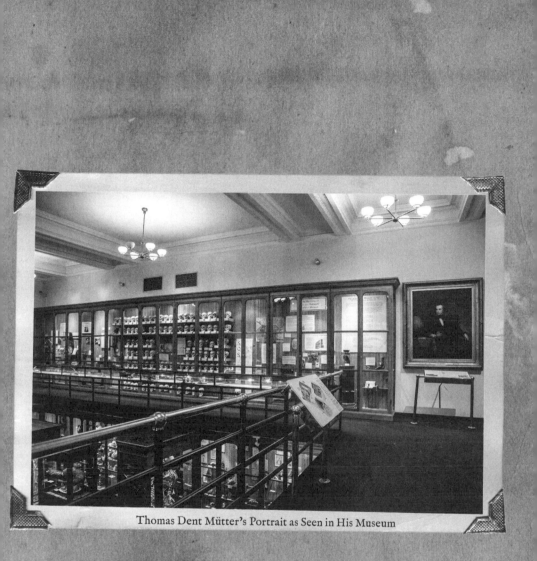

Thomas Dent Mütter's Portrait as Seen in His Museum

ACKNOWLEDGMENTS

THIS BOOK WOULD NOT HAVE BEEN POSSIBLE IF NOT FOR THE EX-traordinary force that was Gretchen Worden (1947–2004). Her relentless efforts to open the museum up to the greater public during her long tenure as the director of the Mütter Museum allowed hundreds of thousands of people to experience the strange wonder of its collection, including a school-age me growing up in Northeast Philadelphia. Gretchen would later offer me—a lowly undergrad with a hunch—full access to the muse-um's archives and library to begin my research into Mütter's astonishing life and times, which a decade and a half later has resulted in this book. Gretchen's joyful light, sharp wit, and determined passion were a constant source of inspiration and comfort, and the sadness I feel that she didn't live to see this book is gratefully tempered by the fact that her influence can be found throughout it . . . and throughout me as well.

In the course of writing this book, I have been extremely lucky to work with generous institutions that have allowed me access to their collections, as well as with the charming and brilliant champions of knowledge who call those institutions home. These heroes not only gifted me with their time, wisdom, and insight but also laughed at my terrible jokes and, on more than one occasion, sneaked me slices of cake from their office parties. To these saints of research, I salute thee:

Robert Hicks, Anna Dhody, Annie Brogan, and Evi Numen at the Mütter Museum at the College of Physicians of Philadelphia;

F. Michael Angelo at the Thomas Jefferson University, Archives & Spe-cial Collections, Philadelphia;

Nicole Joniec and Sarah Weatherwax at the Library Company of Phila-delphia;

Jamison Davis at the Virginia Historical Society;

Michael Frost at Yale University's Sterling Memorial Library;

Benjamin Bromley, Anne T. Johnson, and Gerald Gaidmore at the Special Collections Research Center at the College of William and Mary Swem Library.

And lastly, special thanks are owed to the late Virginia historian Richard W. Slatten D.D.S. (1925–1990), who, in 1983, wrote a small paper on the life of Thomas Dent Mütter, mining heavily the resources at the Virginia Historical Society. Though the work was never published, Slatten thoughtfully sent a copy to the Mütter Museum. It was an immensely helpful document to use as reference, especially in terms of seeing Mütter's story from the Southern perspective.

I am also greatly indebted to several arts organizations and institutions which helped support and fund the creation of this book. I express sincere thanks and gratitude to:

The University of Pennsylvania/Kelly Writers House for gifting me the 2010–2011 ArtsEdge Writer-in-Residency;

The Mütter Museum at the College of Physicians of Philadelphia's Francis C. Wood Institute for awarding me their 2010 Wood Institute Fellowship;

The National Endowment for the Arts for awarding me a 2011 Fellowship in Literature;

The Berkshire Taconic Community Foundation for awarding me their 2013 Writer-in-Residency at the Amy Clampitt House in Lenox, Massachusetts;

And the Alfred P. Sloan Foundation, the Hamptons International Film Festival, and the Greater Philadelphia Film Office/Philadelphia Film Festival, all of which supported my earliest efforts to capture Mütter's story.

In order to pursue my dream of writing this book, I had to leave behind three important families in New York City: my fantastic coworkers at the Artists Rights Society; my fellow rabble-rousers at the Bowery Poetry Club; and the inspiring poets whom I am lucky enough to call friends within the New York City poetry community, especially at the NYC-Urbana Poetry Slam. I want to take this moment to thank them for all of their glorious and buoying support.

It took several vagabond years to research and write this book, and I am grateful to the following people who opened their homes to me during stretches of this project:

In Philadelphia: Stephanie, Joe, Bernadette, and Claire Napoleon; Kevin, Katie, Cian, Lucas, and Declan Aptowicz; Ed, Jeannie, Violet, and Oliver Garcia-Wong; and F. Omar Telan;

In New Jersey: my parents, Maureen and Bruce Aptowicz;

In New York City: Susan Rice; Caitlin, Leo, Camilo, and Ramiro Trasande; Jeff, Jan, and Sarah Kay; and Taylor Mali and Rachel Kahan;

In Boston: David Pantalone;

In Chicago: Shanny Jean Maney and Roy Magnuson;

In Albany: Daniel, Maisie, Miriam, and Beatrice Nester;

In Vermont: Wess Mongo Jolley and Ivan Goguen;

In Austin: Ernie Cline and Libby Willett-Cline; Derrick Brown and Jessica Blakeley; and Anis and Alexis Davis Mojgani.

I also thank each of the following friends and colleagues who read and offered valuable suggestions to parts or all of the manuscript: Aaron Myers, Seth Myers, Anne Horowitz, Amy David, Susan Rice, Derrick Brown, and especially Alexis Davis Mojgani, Sarah Kay, and Ernie Cline.

Enormous thanks are owed to my literary agent, the dazzlingly fantastic Yfat Reiss Gendell, whose belief in this project and in me as its writer was absolutely instrumental in pushing it to where it is today. Thanks as well to Erica Walker, Cecilia Campbell-Westlind, and the rest of the Foundry Literary and Media family.

A special debt of gratitude is also owed to my editor, the sly, insightful Charlie Conrad, as well as his whip-smart assistant, Leslie Hansen, who have made me feel fortunate at every step of this project to have been able to work with them.

And grateful thanks goes to the incredible photographer and artist Dan Winters for gracing this project with its stunning cover, and this grateful author with her amazing author portraits.

Finally, I offer my most humble and grateful thanks to the following people who played an important part in this project every step of the journey:

Jeffrey Shappy Seasholtz, who sacrificed much to help me see this dream come true and for whose enduring friendship I will remain forever grateful;

Kevin Aptowicz and Katie Eyer, whose devoted, boundless support of me and this project was a necessary and guiding force;

Stephanie Dobbins Napoleon, whose friendship, care, and brilliance have sustained me for so many years, but especially during the writing of this book;

My mother, Maureen O'Keefe Aptowicz, from whom I inherited my love of reading and writing, and whose belief in me and my writing has always been deeply felt and immensely appreciated;

Ernie Cline, whose generous and unwavering support of me over the last fifteen years can be seen clearly in the DNA of my entire writing career, but especially in this project.

And lastly and always, Gretchen Worden, who made this all possible in so many ways.

NOTES AND SOURCES

DESPITE HIS FLAMBOYANT PERSONALITY AND OUTGOING NATURE, Mütter was rather an elusive character to research. Neither he nor his wife kept a diary, and the majority of their correspondence has been lost to history. However, I am grateful to have been able to capture his incredible story using a wide variety of source material.

The bulk of the research for this book was conducted at the Archives and Special Collections at the Scott Memorial Library of Thomas Jefferson University and at the Historical Medical Library of the College of Physicians of Philadelphia/Mütter Museum. I am grateful to both of these institutions for the access they provided me to speeches, lectures, journals, correspondence, meeting minutes, and out-of-print textbooks and memoirs, which make up much of the backbone of this book.

A few publications were absolutely invaluable to me during every stage of this book, particularly *Philadelphia: A 300-Year History* (Editor: Russell F. Weigley, WW Norton & Company, 1982) and *American Surgery: An Illustrated History* by Ira M. Rutkow, MD (Lippincott Williams & Wilkins, 1998), whose exhaustive attention to detail was matched only by the charm of their writing. Paris in the nineteenth century was so amazing, strange, and beautiful, you could write a whole book on it—and somebody did! I highly recommend David McCullough's *The Greater Journey*, which was an extremely helpful reference for me during those chapters set in Paris. The *Autobiography of Samuel D. Gross, M.D.* by Samuel Gross (George Barrie, 1887) was also a fantastic and consistently used resource. Although Gross wasn't always the most reliable of narrators, his tendency to be as effusive in his praise as he was hilariously damning in his criticism helped me in my understanding of the full spectrum of Mütter's world. And lastly, I would also like to highlight the work of late Virginia historian Richard W. Slatten, whose unpublished paper on the life of Thomas Dent Mütter was incredibly helpful from the earliest stages of this project.

Any text between quotation marks comes from a letter, memoir, speech, lecture, article, or other written document. Additionally, numerous adjectives and descriptive phrases (which are not found in quotes but are recognized in the endnotes) were mined from period sources.

The speech excerpts found throughout the book are all collected from the same speech: Mütter's March 8, 1851, "Charge to the Graduates of Jefferson Medical College of Philadelphia," which he gave just three days before his fortieth birthday, at the height of his career. It should be noted that the excerpts are often edited down for length and are not presented in Mütter's original order, as my hope was that the placement of these excerpts would help to contrast or complement Mütter's core philosophies with the action of the story.

Descriptions of people, places, and objects were often based on images I found in my research, some of which are included in this book. Descriptions of diseases and medical conditions (such as pregnancy)—including symptoms, stages, and statistics—were pulled both from publications of the time and contemporary reports created by the Centers for Disease Control and Prevention (CDC).

All descriptions of Mütter's surgeries were taken from his published works, and the lithographic images of patients are from his own textbook. The descriptions of specimens from Mütter's personal collection were pulled from numerous inventory lists provided by the Mütter Museum. The wax model of Madame Dimanche, featured in the first chapter of this book, is one of the Mütter Museum's most popular specimens and part of Mütter's original donation. While there is no receipt of its purchase, the rareness of the specimen (the Mütter Museum model is the only one currently known to still exist) and the timing of Madame Dimanche's surgery helped me to conclude that it was likely purchased on Mütter's earliest trip to Paris.

As per other images in the book, please note that special care was taken to acquire images of people and places as close as possible to the time period described in the chapter in which the image appears, but it was not always possible. With this in mind, please note that the portrait of George McClellan was taken in the 1840s, the photograph of "The Pit" was taken in the 1890s, and the image of Mütter performing his first ether surgery was created for and published in *JMC Clinic*, a student yearbook, in 1929.

Additionally, I feel I should mention that the "Muscle Man" image that opens Chapter Seven was a teaching illustration used to show the placement and function of the muscles within the body; the American flag shown at the beginning of Chapter Twenty-Three flew over Jefferson Medical College for all four years of the Civil War; and, though it is impossible to know from seeing the image in its black-and-white form within the book, I am delighted to share that Mütter's Surgical Admission Ticket, which serves as one of the opening images for Chapter Fifteen, was printed—in typical Mütter style and in contrast to the beige-and-gray admission tickets of the day—on bright *pink* paper.

As with all nonfiction projects, it was not unusual to come across conflicting information and/or bald spots within the research. I mined the extensive research seen in these endnotes to draw the best possible conclusions when those circumstances arose, and I would love to quote Erik Larson speaking about his own research for *The Devil in the White City* (an enormous inspiration for this book): "The citations that follow constitute a map. Anyone retracing my steps ought to reach the same conclusions as I."

—PROLOGUE—

endless torture of pain and disease: R. J. Levis, M.D., "Memoir of Thomas Dent Mütter," *The Medical and Surgical Reporter,* whole series no. 129, new series II, no.6 (May 7, 1859): 113–118 (Philadelphia: Crissy & Markley, 1859)

Levis had been Mütter's student at: "Part I: Jefferson Medical College 1846 to 1855 (pages 55–88)" in Frederick B. Wagner Jr., MD, and J. Woodrow Savacool, MD (eds.), *Thomas Jefferson University—A Chronological History and Alumni Directory, 1824–1990,* 1992, http://jdc.jefferson.edu/wagner1/16

1859, the year Levis would be named lead: Ibid.

His ingenuity, his early excellence: Levis, "Memoir of Thomas Dent Mütter"

the poor and humble: Ibid.

Mütter's office was thronged with patients: Ibid.

gather around him with a confidence and infatuation . . . I shall be whole: Ibid.

An expert and efficient surgeon . . . requisite appliance: Ibid.

constant physical struggles that made Mütter's too-short life blaze so brightly: Ibid.

by the failings of his own body: Ibid.

trips across the Atlantic, where he was greeted . . . medical men of London and Paris: Ibid.

spared no labor or expense in securing the most . . . private surgical cabinets of his time: Ibid.

"The subject of this memoir needs no eulogium from us . . . relieve the miseries of others": Ibid.

"His life, until his retirement, was one of incessant labor. . . . the close of a useful life": Ibid.

"What an epitome of this life it is to know that . . . hushed in the endless silence of the tomb": Ibid.

"other and abler pens write for him, to coming ages . . . the history of American Surgery": Ibid.

"The Medical Man Must Obtain a Thorough Medical Education . . . human wit": Thomas D. Mütter, *Charge to the Graduates of Jefferson Medical College of Philadelphia*, delivered March 8, 1851 (Philadelphia: T. K. and P. G. Collins, Printers, 1851)

—CHAPTER ONE—

high cheekbones, full upturned lips, glittering deep-set eyes: All physical descriptions of Madame Dimanche are based on the wax model from Mütter's original collection, on display at the Mütter Museum and as seen in Gretchen Worden, *The Mütter Museum of the College of Physicians of Philadelphia* (New York: Blast Books, 2002).

twenty years old when he graduated from . . . storied medical college: Richard W. Slatten, "Thomas Dent Mütter, Surgeon and Teacher" (Unpublished biographical sketch, 1983)

the absolute pink of neatness: *Autobiography of Samuel D. Gross, M.D., with Sketches of His Contemporaries* (in 2 vols.) (Philadelphia: George Barrie, 1887)

secured just enough money to get him to his destination . . . wits to get him back home: Slatten, "Thomas Dent Mütter"

"am afraid that I shall not be able to obtain an order . . . furtherance of my plan": Correspondence, Carter Family Papers, 1667–1862, Special Collections, Earl Gregg Swem Library, College of William & Mary, Mss. 39.1 C24

the *Kensington* . . . had sold after all, to the Imperial Russian Navy: Slatten, "Thomas Dent Mütter"

(later to be renamed the *Prince of Warsaw* by Tsar Nicholas himself): Ibid.

colorfully dressed women sweeping the streets . . . on Sundays, absolutely everyone did: Descriptions of Paris are based on descriptions found in August K. Gardner's *Old Wine in New Bottles, or, Spare Hours of a Student in Paris* (New York: C. S. Francis, 1848)

"principal error is rather too much fondness . . . proper for a boy his age": Correspondence, Carter Family Papers

"experience be acquired by the attentive student . . . field for observation . . .": Gardner, *Old Wine*

the most frightful instances of venereal ravages: B. H. Benjamin, "The Hospitals and Surgeons of Paris," *The New World*, October 28, 1843

publicly whipped: Ibid.

the lowest classes of society . . . already in a hopeless or dying condition: Ibid.

(called *sages-femmes*): Ibid.

one in every fifty women who entered Hôpital de la Maternité did: Ibid.

vast majority of the children there had arrived via *le tour*: Ibid.

Every night, a dozen or so infants were received in precisely this way: Ibid.

adopt children from the Hôpital des Enfants-Trouvés . . . fallen out of fashion: Ibid.

sixteen thousand children were considered wards . . . would live to adulthood: Ibid.

There were hospitals for lunatic women... married couples who wished to die together: Ibid.

École Pratique d'Anatomie... dogs kept tied up in the back: David McCullough, *The Greater Journey: Americans in Paris* (New York: Simon & Schuster, 2011)

using marvelous speed to incise the face and rip out the bones with a huge forceps: Samuel X. Radbill, "Joseph Pancoast (1805–1882): Jefferson Anatomist and Surgeon, and His World," *Transactions & Studies of the College of Physicians of Philadelphia*, ser. 5, vol. 8, no. 4 (1986): 233–246

the spectacle of it, how the partially conscious... fainted in their seats: Ibid.

the hospital system maintained its very own wine... extensive collection: Benjamin, "Hospitals and Surgeons of Paris"

"natural consequence of this state of things... obtain distinction and worldly prosperity": Ibid.

"had not Monsieur Dupuytren been compelled from poverty... Baron Dupuytren": Ibid.

"the bandit of the river bank": J. Chalmers Da Costa, M.D., "The French School of Surgery in the Reign of Louis Philippe," *Annals of Medical History* Vol. IV, Spring, Summer, Autumn, and Winter 1922

"that man with the face of an ape and the heart of a crouching dog": Ibid.

dazzled his classes with his graceful and brilliant: Ibid.

"his operations were the poetry of surgery": Ibid.

an *interne* at the hospital to which Dupuytren was attached: Levis, "Memoir of Thomas Dent Mütter"

"quick, active, appropriative mind... readily imbued... distinguished [Parisian] teachers": Ibid.

Thomas Dent Mütter—with a perfectly European umlaut over the *u*: Slatten, "Thomas Dent Mütter"

—CHAPTER TWO—

"The Physician Should Be an Ambitious Man... it gives life and heat to all around": Mütter, *Charge to the Graduates*, 1851

the entire government shut down:, Russell F. Weigley (ed.), *Philadelphia: A 300-Year History* (New York: W. W. Norton, 1982)

all but abandoned by friends and family: Ibid.

the Pennsylvania Hospital and Almshouse refused to receive yellow fever victims: Ibid.

die alone in the streets: Ibid.

"depository [for] victims of the plague who had nowhere to go and nobody to care for them": Ibid.

"heroic bleeding and purging": Ibid.

more than one-tenth of the city's entire population was dead: Ibid.

Philadelphia publishing house Carey, Lea & Blanchard... of medical books: Ibid.

inform the public of the progress and hopeful treatment of this terrible disease: Ibid.

"heroic role of the medical profession in battling the infection": Ibid.

silver pitchers of recognition: Ibid.

she became pregnant with Thomas in the summer of 1810: Slatten, "Thomas Dent Mütter"

she was fifteen and he was twenty-five: Ibid.

Lucinda had been born into the established Gillies family... prestigious families in the South: Ibid.

(five Armistead brothers would fight in the War of 1812 . . . future U.S. national anthem): Ibid.

(whose family would include not only governors . . . future leader of the Confederate Army): Ibid.

(whose patriarch, Robert Carter, was so powerful . . . farmland, and more than one thousand slaves): Ibid.

women were frequently married in their late teens: Michael R. Haines, "Long Term Marriage Patterns in the United States from Colonial Times to the Present" (NBER Historical Paper No. 80, Issued March 1996), http://www.nber.org/papers/h0080.pdf

father endeared himself to his new countrymen . . . in the Revolutionary War: Joseph Pancoast, *A Discourse Commemorative of the Late Professor T. D. Mutter, M.D., LL.D.*, Introductory Lecture to Anatomy Course at Jefferson Medical College, Delivered October 14, 1859 (Published by the Jefferson Medical College, 1859)

John ran a healthy business as a factor and commission agent: Slatten, "Thomas Dent Mütter"

these men not only aided farmers in selling their crops . . . purchase of slaves for a client: Clement Eaton, *A History of the Old South* (Prospect Heights, IL: Waveland Press, 1975), 230.

Lucinda named him Thomas, after her husband's late father: Slatten, "Thomas Dent Mütter"

She named him James, after her own late father, a beloved doctor: Ibid.

luck began to run out: Ibid.

buried her small body in Baltimore's St. Paul's Church: Helen W. Ridgeley, "The Ancient Churchyards of Baltimore," *The Grafton Magazine of History and Genealogy* 1, no. 4: 8–23 (New York: Grafton Press, 1908)

thirty-three, a widower, and a single father to Thomas, who was only three: Slatten, "Thomas Dent Mütter"

bought a large house in Henrico County, Virginia . . . He called it Woodberry: Ibid.

couldn't shake a rattling cough: Ibid.

placing him in the care of Tom's grandmother, Frances Gillies, his late wife's widowed mother: Ibid.

Four months into this journey, on a winter's passage of the Alps, John Mutter died: Ibid.

a martyr for many years to gout: Pancoast, *A Discourse Commemorative*

Frances Gillies . . . passed away too: Slatten, "Thomas Dent Mütter"

he didn't even need a license—a practice that Philadelphia . . . of the nineteenth century: "Part I: Jefferson Medical College 1835 to 1845 (pages 27–54)" in Frederick B. Wagner Jr., MD, and J. Woodrow Savacool, MD (eds.), *Thomas Jefferson University— A Chronological History and Alumni Directory, 1824–1990*, 1992, http://jdc.jefferson .edu/wagner1/15

Almost every act a doctor performed—invasive examinations . . . sun or lamplight: J. Chalmers Da Costa, M.D., "Then and Now: Oration Delivered at the Celebration of the Fiftieth Anniversary of the Founding of the Philadelphia County Medical Society, January 14, 1899," in Joseph M. Spellissy, M.D., ed., *Proceedings of the Philadelphia County Medical Society, Vol. XX, Session of 1899*

infectiousness of diseases, were still under heavy dispute: Ibid.

Tetanus was widely thought to be a reflex irritation: Ibid.

Appendicitis was called peritonitis, and its victims were simply left to die: Ibid.

"The grim spectre of sepsis" was ever present: Ibid.

It was absolutely expected that wounds would eventually fester with pus: Ibid.

"yellow ooze" was seen as a good "laudable pus": Richard Gordon, *Great Medical Disasters* (London: Hutchinson, 1983)

"ichorous pus" (a thin pus teeming with shredded tissue) . . . of cadaverous putrefaction": Ibid.

Medicine was not standardized, so accidental poisoning was common: Da Costa, "Then and Now"

drugs were often bulky and nauseating: Ibid.

doses of purgatives were given by even the most conservative men: Ibid.

To treat a fever with a cold bath would have been "regarded as murder": Ibid.

There was no anesthesia—neither general nor local: Ibid.

If you came to a doctor with a compound fracture, you had . . . chance of survival: Ibid.

Surgery on brains and lungs was attempted only in accident cases: Ibid.

"a pauper in the almshouse more comfortable . . . than a king": Ibid.

In the early 1800s, there was not a single female physician in Philadelphia: Ibid.

"very generally ignorant, often dirty and sometimes drunk": Ibid.

***The Boston Medical and Surgical Journal* ran a letter . . . better things are expected:** *The College and Clinical Record* 1, no. 5 (May 1880): 78 (JMC)

"Individual discoveries are glorious and worthy . . . fame and wealth apply them": Da Costa, "Then and Now"

"Our fathers did wonders with the resources they could . . . science lives and advances": Ibid.

—CHAPTER THREE—

The Willing Mansion . . . his first office for the practice of surgery: Slatten, "Thomas Dent Mütter"

to become distinguished would require not only earning . . . professional colleagues: Ibid.

showcasing the fantastic techniques he'd learned in Paris: Levis, "Memoir of Thomas Dent Mütter"

"Adopting, with all the enthusiasm of his nature . . . more endurable": Pancoast, *A Discourse Commemorative*

he tried his best "to be agreeable, to be useful, and to be noticed": Slatten, "Thomas Dent Mütter"

"cut[ting] quite a swathe": Ibid.

in a low carriage behind a big gray horse, driven by a servant in livery: Ibid.

"Youthful looking, neat and elegant in his attire . . . fashionable thoroughfares": Pancoast, *A Discourse Commemorative*

"immaculately dressed young man riding about . . . an intrusion": Slatten, "Thomas Dent Mütter"

"one Frenchman [is] equal to a dozen Americans": Howard A. Kelly, M.D., LL.D., F. A.C.S. Hon. F.R.C.S., and Walter L. Burrage, A.M., M.D., *American Medical Biographies* (Baltimore: The Norman, Remington Company, 1920)

The oft-repeated stories of the surgical exploits . . . *drawing a long bow*: *Autobiography of Samuel D. Gross*

"Mütter's early disappointment professionally was . . . to be helpful as well as to be noticed": Slatten, "Thomas Dent Mütter"

His life and future were now entirely dependent on . . . all but strangers to the boy: Ibid.

keen intelligence and an unfailingly amiable disposition: Ibid.

Sabine Hall, the Carter family's sprawling estate: Frances Archer Christian and Susanne Williams Massie, eds., *Homes and Gardens in Old Virginia* (Richmond, VA: Garrett and Massie, 1932) two trunks of clothing, a small toy hobby horse . . . a drawing of his mother in ink: List of Items with which Thomas Mutter arrived, courtesy of Carter Papers, Special Collections, Earl Gregg Swem Library, College of William & Mary

The enormous brick and stone building featured four large white cypress columns: Christian and Massie, *Homes and Gardens in Old Virginia*

six meticulously curated gardens extending over five opulent terraces . . . fields: Ibid.

enormous front parlor flanked by a hand-carved staircase. . . . Colonel Carter himself: Ibid.

a broad classical pediment was added to the roof . . . carpentry to finish: William M. S. Rasmussen, "Sabine Hall: A Classical Villa in Virginia," *Journal of the Society of Architectural Historians* 39, no. 4 (Dec. 1980): 286–296 (Published by University of California Press on behalf of the Society of Architectural Historians)

entire redbrick exterior be painted white and . . . the roof and chimneys be lowered: Ibid.

"gay and splendid city": Ibid.

its streets "as beautiful as any in the world.": Ibid.

First Bank of the United States had a similar oversize portico . . . very similar to: Ibid.

"I felt for our friend Mr. Mutter the most sincere . . . Estate as possible": Carter Papers

"I certainly feel much delicacy and reluctance by assuming . . . unremitted condemnation": Ibid.

forced to sell both Woodberry . . . debts that no one knew John Mutter had: Slatten, "Thomas Dent Mütter"

the court system to release the funds to him: Ibid.

"The charge Mr. Bradley makes for the child's clothes . . . the present submit": Carter Papers

Charles Goddard . . . The established rapport between tutor and pupil: Slatten, "Thomas Dent Mütter"

relieving the Carter household of some of the disciplinary duties: Ibid.

However, when Thomas turned twelve, Carter decided . . . boarding schools: Ibid.

$140 a year, Thomas learned English, French, and Latin . . . boarded with his own teacher: Ibid.

"Early in the spring he had a slight attack . . . considerably grown": Carter Papers

"His general health has been better than it was . . . attacked by bilious colic": Ibid.

"I wrote to Aunt to send me two pairs of shoes . . . as I am in want of them": Ibid.

"As the warm weather is coming very fast . . . at Fredericksburg and are spoilt in the making.": Ibid.

"I am in great want of shirts as I have but two . . . nor nice enough to wear in town": Ibid.

The bill shows that Thomas—who was just sixteen . . . and even several dozen cigars: Clothing Bill as found in the Carter Papers

distinguished in scholarship, industry, and behavior . . . chapel without an excuse: Carter Papers

praised for his natural gifts as a captivating presenter . . . its range and amplitude: Slatten, "Thomas Dent Mütter"

borrowing enough money to make it to his desired destination . . . the funds to get back home: Ibid.

spend a semester at Yale, a college . . . in the northern city of New Haven, Connecticut: Ibid.

sent home when none of the Connecticut doctors could stop him from coughing up blood: Ibid.

outstanding bills with a tailor and a shoemaker, which . . . contacted to pay: Ibid.

spend time in Fredericksburg and Alexandria, places . . . without Colonel Carter's permission: Ibid.

the grandson of their long-dead friend, Dr. James Gillies: Ibid.

too ill to return to college anytime soon, they advised, and this . . . for the rest of his life: Ibid.

Thomas took the news with fortitude and equanimity: Ibid.

what he wanted to do with his life: to study medicine: Ibid.

"My dear Sir, Owing to your short stay in the District . . . Thomas D. Mutter": Carter Papers

the guardian grew more and more impressed with the actions of his young ward: Slatten, "Thomas Dent Mütter"

officially "come of age," Colonel Carter felt . . . Thomas to stand on his own: Ibid.

success would have to depend on his own efforts alone: Levis, "Memoir of Thomas Dent Mütter"

found himself in feeble health: Slatten, "Thomas Dent Mütter"

make an extended visit to one of Virginia's famed health spas: Ibid.

to develop a sizable practice among the spa's clientele: Ibid.

collect material for what he hoped would be . . . article on "watering spas" . . . properties: Ibid.

excellent prospects of success: Levis, "Memoir of Thomas Dent Mütter"

English or American physician actively working: Ibid.

had formed such associations and acquired such favorable . . . residence in Paris: Ibid.

proficient in both French and German: Ibid.

anticipate receiving the patronage of the English, American, and German tourist: Ibid.

Jackson was an assistant to one of the medical college's best-known professors: Ibid.

(the subject of Mütter's doctoral thesis was "Chronic Inflammation of the Testis"): Ibid.

"If at the end of that time the prospect should then seem . . . permanent residence in Paris": Ibid.

an assistant to the popular, and increasingly sickly, Dr. Thomas Harris. . . . Medical Institute: Ibid.

—CHAPTER FOUR—

"The Physician Should Possess Self-Respect. . . . disgraceful herd": Mütter, *Charge to the Graduates*, 1851

the first and only medical school in the thirteen American colonies in the fall of 1765: "Penn in the 18th Century: School of Medicine Historical Development, 1765–1800," University of Pennsylvania Archives; http://www.archives.upenn.edu/histy/features/1700s/medsch.html

all serious American aspirants toward the medical profession were compelled . . . their education: James F. Gayley, M.D, *A History of the Jefferson Medical College of Philadelphia* (Philadelphia: Joseph M. Wilson, 1858)

"anatomical lectures" and "the theory and practice of physik": "Penn in the 18th Century"; http://www.archives.upenn.edu/histy/features/1700s/medsch.html

a student had to: attend at least one course of lectures . . . (the art of healing, or medicine): Ibid.

attend at least one course of clinical lectures: Ibid.

study for one year under the doctors working at the Pennsylvania Hospital: Ibid.

be examined privately by medical trustees and professors: Ibid.

be examined publicly: Ibid.

at least twenty-four years of age: Ibid.

was regarded as "something extra among the people": Gayley, *History of the Jefferson*

"some of the eccentricities of genius": Ibid.

first male public figure who ventured to carry a silk umbrella . . . (then "a scouted effeminacy"): Ibid.

first doctor to send his patients to an apothecary . . . herbs, tinctures, and salves himself: Ibid.

In his first public address about his vision for the school . . . institutions of a similar nature: Ibid.

By 1825, Philadelphia's population had exploded . . . medical students: Slatten, "Thomas Dent Mütter"

medical school population of closer to 500 . . . classrooms and lecture halls: Ibid.

Every physician had private students who apprenticed . . . other schools opened: Ibid.

nor could they be assured that the doctor under whom . . . or even correct: Gayley, *History of the Jefferson*

accusations of favoritism in filling its department chairs and teaching positions: Ibid.

criticism of the faculty's recent duplicitous practice . . . fees for teaching their classes: Edward Louis Bauer, M.D., *Doctors: Made in America* (Philadelphia: J. B. Lippincott, 1963)

"for Philadelphia to retain her position as the medical Athens of America": Gayley, *History of the Jefferson*

Several physicians in the city were popular enough . . . connected to their offices: Bauer, *Doctors*

the University of Pennsylvania would use its political power to thwart: Ibid.

would ostracize any doctor who didn't share its belief . . . medical school in Philadelphia: Ibid.

Several efforts to establish a second medical . . . unsuccessful: Gayley, *History of the Jefferson*

in 1824, when the irascible Dr. George McClellan's . . . Medical College: Slatten, "Thomas Dent Mütter"

"duly-qualified alumni [who] may give . . . institutions of a similar nature": Gayley, *History of the Jefferson*

saved a man's life before he even entered the . . . skin to make flaps for the stump: Bauer, *Doctors*

speaker with "a resounding voice that bespoke authority." . . . practitioners, and laymen: Ibid.

one of those Philadelphia doctors who needed their own lecture hall: Ibid.

"Some of his best friends . . . inconsiderate and imprudent": W. Darrach, M.D., *Memoir of George McClellan, M.D.* (King & Baird, Printers; Philadelphia, 1847).

an excellent judge of character: Bauer, *Doctors*

known to heckle other surgeons while they . . . surgical lectures: Slatten, "Thomas Dent Mütter"

simply the "*sans ceremonie* and *en avant* spirit" of his "sleepless genius": Darrach, *Memoir of George McClellan, M.D.*

"In public, he was inconsiderate" . . . "alone, he was the grave, profound Philosopher": Ibid.

attempts to obtain a charter for a second school failed: Bauer, *Doctors*

coordinated with Jefferson College in Canonsburg . . . department of that college in Philadelphia: Slatten, "Thomas Dent Mütter"

prominent place as a literary institution: Gayley, *History of the Jefferson*

"a respectable contingent of educated intellect to our country . . . other seminaries of learning": Ibid.

which prided itself "in extending the benign influences . . . and an elevating morality": Ibid.

rented the Tivoli Theater on the south side of Prune Street: Ibid.

the merits of the new school: Ibid.

The first class numbered an impressive 107, with 20 graduating at the end: Ibid.

which they had considered to be only "an experiment": Ibid.

instituted from year one: that all students must... in the care of patients: Bauer, *Doctors*

important factor in the training of medical students: Ibid.

by having them observe... treated patients: "George McClellan, MD," Thomas Jefferson University online historical profiles; http://www.jefferson.edu/university/jmc/departments/surgery/history/mcclellan.html

an idea that had never been tried before: Ibid.

to be McClellan's most important contribution to medical education: Bauer, *Doctors*

reshaping the way medicine would be taught throughout the world: "George McClellan, MD"; http://www.jefferson.edu/university/jmc/departments/surgery/history/mcclellan.html

—CHAPTER FIVE—

"The Physician Must Also Be a Thinking, Observing... the road yourself": Mütter, *Charge to the Graduates*, 1851

well devised, amply demonstrated, and outstandingly delivered: Slatten, "Thomas Dent Mütter"

natural energy and enthusiasm, combined with his... complicated subjects: Pancoast, *A Discourse Commemorative*

those around him would say his ability seemed "almost intuitive": Ibid.

"At his first essay from this perch... he seems to have taken a falcon flight": Ibid.

"In orators, this early perfection is not often seen": Ibid.

"great generals, who learn to fight by fighting, and whose only real school is war": Ibid.

Two long-simmering crises were coming to a head... course of American medicine: Slatten, "Thomas Dent Mütter"

The first crisis grew out of a challenge to the old private... lectures to as many students: Ibid.

he would undergo an examination for an MD degree: Ibid.

Lecturers worked in isolation: Ibid.

"purely private enterprise[s] whose standards derived... the individuals involved": Ibid.

to standardize medical teaching by bringing it more... of the admininstration: Ibid.

detractors called "rather unwholesome tactics": Ibid.

The university was accused of conspiring to monopolize... university's favor: Ibid.

that no man could look for success as a private teacher... with the university: Ibid.

"period of accommodation" between the university and its... public confrontations: Ibid.

"It is said that one should not speak ill of the dead.... the lecture-room": *Autobiography of Samuel D. Gross*

Gibson had rightfully earned his reputation as an "impressive lecturer": Ibid.

never failed to command the attention of his classes with "clearness, accuracy and earnestness": Ibid.

Gibson... often indulged in offensive language against... their mutual disdain: Ibid.

Gibson openly accused McClellan of falsehood for... this subject between the rival schools: Ibid.

to bear witness to Gibson's performing the surgery . . . in front of Gibson's own class: Ibid.

"who had come to see the fun": Ibid.

the operation was over, Gibson turned . . . "a *tumor* . . . *not the gland itself*": Ibid.

"my distinguished friend has extirpated the parotid gland . . . doesn't know it": Ibid.

The remark caused "convulsions of laughter" in the large assembly: Ibid.

period second to none in America's medical history. . . . "rivalry marked with jealousy and unfairness": Slatten, "Thomas Dent Mütter"

Medical lore and literature would record abundant evidence . . . especially that of treatment: Ibid.

It still possessed two great schools, and its doctors were still revered . . . any serious career: Da Costa, "Then and Now"

gaining rivals in places like New York, Baltimore, and Chicago: Ibid.

"one of the best of good fellows": Pancoast, *A Discourse Commemorative*

"He possessed spontaneously, as it were, the art . . . to do what he could to please others": Ibid.

habit of sending Mütter to make house calls: Slatten, "Thomas Dent Mütter"

Mütter began to develop a healthy private practice: Ibid.

defiantly occupied "the difficult domain of reparative and reconstructive surgery": Ibid.

"strangers from various parts of this wide domain . . . sufferings demanded": Pancoast, *A Discourse Commemorative*

"He succeeded with patients for the same reason as with students . . . and liked": Ibid.

distinguished Philadelphia doctors—Randolph, Norris, and Anderson: Robert Liston, *Lectures on the Operations of Surgery and on Diseases and Accidents Requiring Operations, with Numerous Additions by Thomas D. Mütter, M.D.* (Philadelphia: Lea & Blanchard, 1846), 193–203

match the color of his expensive suit to the carriage in which he was riding: *Autobiography of Samuel D. Gross*

Nathaniel Dickey . . . intelligent, funny, and in perfectly good health: Liston, *Lectures on the Operations of Surgery*

against the chest of a seated Dr. Norris, and his arms held down . . . a tight white sheet: Ibid.

Mütter had already explained the surgery to Nathaniel in detail: Ibid.

thrice daily massage Nathaniel's face: Ibid.

inviting dangerous infection to nest in his already beleaguered mouth: Ibid.

a knife, a hook, a pair of long forceps, needles . . . leeches, opiates, and a sharp lancet: Ibid.

to obstruct the entrance of light into the mouth as little as possible: Ibid.

the insertion of a sharp hook into the roof of Nathaniel's mouth . . . muscle and skin back: Ibid.

the silk thread straining at the incision sites: Ibid.

—CHAPTER SIX—

"The Physician Should Also Be a Gentleman . . . should be made": Mütter, *Charge to the Graduates*, 1851

"See this unobvious, apparently vile lump of animal texture?" . . . this subject sufficiently?: Charles D. Meigs, M.D., *Woman: Her Diseases and Remedies: A Series of Letters to His Class* (Philadelphia: Lea & Blanchard, 1851)

"Women possess a peculiar trait—it is modesty." . . . one of their most charming attributes: Ibid.

"But scan her position in civilization, and it is easy to perceive . . . and it is true to say so": Ibid.

"The great administrative faculties are not hers" . . . idea of a Hamlet, or a Macbeth? *No*": Ibid.

"Such is not woman's province, nature, power, nor mission. . . . of worship and service": Ibid.

"She has a head too small for intellect" . . . "but it is just big enough for love": Ibid.

nursed all the children herself, and was so faithful . . . during infancy and childhood: J. Forsyth Meigs, M.D., *Memoir of Charles D. Meigs, M.D.* (Philadelphia: Lindsay & Blakiston, 1876)

by the prejudices and false modesties: Bauer, *Doctors*

many religious leaders: Ibid.

an obstetrician could examine the abdomen of a pregnant woman only through blankets?: Ibid.

frightened patient told Meigs she'd "rather die": Meigs, *Memoir*

"*Ce que femme veut, Dieu le veut aussi!*": Ibid.

—CHAPTER SEVEN—

on January 1, 1841, the city was frozen solid: Weigley, *Philadelphia*

"It will, perhaps, long be remembered by the present . . . continued until the 15th of May": Ibid.

warmly called him Mac: Frederick B. Wagner Jr. and J. Woodrow Savacool, eds., *Jefferson Medical College: Legend and Lore* (Philadelphia: William T. Cooke, 1996)

lacked two important requisites of great surgeons and . . . judgment and patience: Ibid.

frequency with which he jumped to conclusions: Ibid.

years of the Jefferson Medical College were plagued with financial problems: Ibid.

harassment by the University of Pennsylvania: Ibid.

John Revere (the son of patriot Paul Revere): Ibid.

Granville Sharp Pattison (whose nickname was the Turbulent Scot): Ibid.

William Barton . . . his legendary "Navy vocabulary": Ibid.

"[Dr. Barton]'s favorite epithet, almost constantly applied . . . I shall not mention it": Ibid.

"spirit of independent thinking": Ibid.

"a parcel of politicians" and a "blackguard Board of Trustees": Ibid.

that Jefferson was "rotten and going to the dogs": Ibid.

failed to reckon with the power and stability of the board of trustees: Ibid.

to vacate all the chairs and to elect new professors: Ibid.

McClellan's connection with the school he had fought so hard . . . unceremonious end: Ibid.

Dunglison had earned his nickname, the Great Peacemaker: Ibid.

Dunglison had come up with his list . . . ultimate vote on April 2: Jefferson Medical College Minutes, No. 1 (April 19, 1838, to November 26, 1873), Archive of Jefferson Medical College of Philadelphia

the dawn of a new era at Jefferson Medical College: Ibid.

For some chairs . . . the board unanimously agreed . . . there was serious competition: Ibid.

"Meigs possessed all the requisites for success upon the stage . . . to keep awake": *Autobiography of Samuel D. Gross*

(Meigs described the labia of virgins as being plump . . . except with fat persons"): Charles D. Meigs, M.D., *The Philadelphia Practice of Midwifery* (Philadelphia: James Kay, Jun. & Brother, 1838)

(Meigs strongly recommended bleeding the woman . . . leeches directly onto her genitals): Ibid.

The British-born Dunglison made his name in the 1820s and 1830s . . . and James Madison: John H. Brinton, M.D., "Alumni Address: The Faculty of 1841," delivered before the Alumni Association of the Jefferson Medical College of Philadelphia at its Tenth Anniversary, March 11, 1880, *The College and Clinical Record* I, no. 3 (March 15, 1880)

chair of Jefferson's Institutes of Medicine and Medical Jurisprudence. . . . for him: Ibid.

It would be a position he would hold for over a third of a century: Ibid.

"still a fine-looking old lady, dressed in the old style, wearing a turban": Ibid.

"This, it need not be said, was a great disappointment . . . best boy that ever was": Ibid.

Aglae, passed away in 1835. Bache, "faithful to her memory," never remarried: George B. Wood, M.D., *Biographical Memoir of Franklin Bache, M.D.: Prepared at the Request of the College of Physicians of Philadelphia, and Read Before the College, May 3d and June 7th, 1865* (Philadelphia: J. B. Lippincott, 1865)

Bache had a full head of hair, thick bushy eyebrows . . . calm sweetness: Bauer, *Doctors*

Meigs was thin, with sallow visage, and a large balding head: Ibid.

considered themselves austere, honest, and forthright: Ibid.

not easily lend themselves to any compromise that might lie between right and wrong: Ibid.

"If I were to describe Franklin Bache, I would speak of him . . . intermediate shades": Brinton, "Alumni Address: The Faculty of 1841"

"If it should be deemed unfair . . . opposite their record": Meigs, *Memoir*

"If as a lecturer [Bache] was dull . . . he was earnest and faithful . . . examination": *Autobiography of Samuel D. Gross*

Mutter's gifts as a lecturer had been amply demonstrated . . . now firmly established: Slatten, "Thomas Dent Mütter"

prominent in both arenas: L. Riordan, biography, April 1970, from Jefferson Medical College Library (Vertical File)

"a very fine needle, turned near the point into a sort of hook . . . inch behind the cornea": *"Joseph Pancoast"* in William B. Atkinson, MD, ed., *Physicians and Surgeons of the United States* (Philadelphia: Charles Robson, 1878)

The invention of the plough and groove, or plastic suture . . . the flaps, come together: Ibid.

"good-looking substitute" for a destroyed eyebrow ("made by . . . cut for it up to the brow)": Ibid.

And a surgical technique (involving "an abdominal tourniquet . . . excessive blood loss: Ibid.

of decided convictions, professional, moral, and political . . . an upright citizen: *Autobiography of Samuel D. Gross*

to help free medicine from an inherited body of superstition: Slatten, "Thomas Dent Mütter"

As a professor, Pancoast was respected by his peers: *Autobiography of Samuel D. Gross*

"He possessed all the attributes of a great operator . . . and his eye never winced": Ibid.

Dr. Jacob Randolph, the son-in-law of Philip Syng Physick: J. Chalmers Da Costa, MD, LLD: "Osteitis Deformans (Paget's Disease of the Bones)," The Mütter Lecture for 1920, *Transactions of the College of Physicians*, ser. 3, vol. 42 (1920): 455–458 (Philadelphia: College of Physicians, 1920)

But Randolph was utterly unsupportive of splitting the chair of surgery ... weakened position: Jefferson Medical College Minutes

And they voted to give that chair ... Thomas Dent Mütter: Ibid.

Schuylkill River overflowed, flooding into the city ... on each side: Weigley, *Philadelphia*

—CHAPTER EIGHT—

"The Physician Must Be an Industrious Man ... prevents us from determining": Mütter, *Charge to the Graduates*, 1851

"JEFFERSON MEDICAL COLLEGE. Session Of 1841–42. ... *Dean of the Faculty*": *The Boston Medical and Surgical Journal* XXV, ed. V. C. Smith, M.D. (Boston: D. Clapp Jr. Proprietor and Publisher, 1842)

The *New* Jefferson Medical College: Frederick P. Henry, A. M., M.D., ed., *Standard History of the Medical Profession of Philadelphia* (Chicago: Goodspeed Brothers, 1897)

strength of Jefferson had always lain in the personal power ... scholarly Dunglison hoped: Ibid.

evenly split between old and new, Northerners and Southerners: Ibid.

the Ely Building, the main lecture hall of the college ... ever-growing population of students: Julie S. Berkowitz, *Adorn the Halls: History of the Art Collection at Thomas Jefferson University* (Philadelphia: Thomas Jefferson University, 1999)

two "capacious" lecture rooms ... two additional large halls in the rear of the building: Ibid.

The first hall would be ... used exclusively for dissecting: Ibid.

The second hall would be used as an "anatomical museum" ... used in their lectures: Ibid.

models of human faces or body parts made of wood ... as seen in both paint and pen: Ibid.

Over the years, Mütter had amassed an ambitious collection ... extraordinary material: "Catalogue of the Specimens Belonging to the College of Physicians" (Curator's Report for 1862, presented January 7, 1863)

intestines pulled from cholera victims ... a wax cast of a hermaphrodite: Ibid.

"He surrounded himself richly with materials of illustrations ... and [inspire] wonder": Pancoast, *A Discourse Commemorative*

For six long hours each day ... overcrowded lecture rooms: John Kearsley Mitchell, *Charge to the Graduates of Jefferson Medical College of Philadelphia*, delivered March 9, 1850 (Philadelphia: C. Sherman, 1850)

"task to the utmost [his] powers of memory and analysis": Ibid.

"trim [their] lamps for a toilsome study": Ibid.

"Many a time, in the midnight rambles of my medical duty ... instincts of his nature": Ibid.

The students hailed from all over the newly formed country ... and South Carolina: Wagner and Savacool, eds., *Jefferson Medical College: Legend and Lore*

small in stature and delicately framed, with a clear blue eye ... thick black hair: Brinton, "Alumni Address: The Faculty of 1841"

a wonderfully musical voice, which, even in its lowest notes: Ibid.

His gestures were relaxed and comfortable, and his speech was smart and sharply prepared: Ibid.

the great charm of his enthusiasm: Ibid.

Mütter was the first professor to introduce this informal style ... the United States: Thomas Jefferson Department of Surgery (Undated)

"I can well remember him . . . exertion invariably brought him": Brinton, "Alumni Address: The Faculty of 1841"

diagrams, models, and specimens collected from around the world: Ibid.

"so as to impress yet not confuse": Ibid.

"kindness and enthusiastic devotion . . . and ornate developments": Levis, "Memoir of Thomas Dent Mütter"

—CHAPTER NINE—

The clinic . . . was a prominent feature in the weekly curriculum: Henry, *Standard History of the Medical Profession*

referred to as the right arm of the college: Ibid.

"Brilliant as Dr. Mütter was in his didactic teachings . . . he surpassed himself in the clinical arena": Brinton, "Alumni Address: The Faculty of 1841"

"considerable emphasis" on the care and attention he paid to patients: Slatten, "Thomas Dent Mütter"

"accustomed to manipulation," by massaging each hand and . . . prior to the operation: Ibid.

"If his orders are not immediately obeyed . . . describe his disease": McCullough, *The Greater Journey*

patients underwent operations . . . sent immediately home in a carriage: Slatten, "Thomas Dent Mütter"

John Kearsley Mitchell . . . shared a Scottish ancestry: Brinton, "Alumni Address: The Faculty of 1841"

a handsome man, tall and portly, with a gentle, polished bearing: Bauer, *Doctors*

He wore his brown hair severely combed from left to right . . . about this ring": Ibid.

bound to Calcutta and Canton: Brinton, "Alumni Address: The Faculty of 1841"

Philadelphia as a practitioner: Ibid.

"In sickness and trouble, they turned to him . . . and none the wiser": Henry, *Standard History of the Medical Profession*

among the first advocates of the germ theory of disease: Ibid.

to find a building with grounds close to the college . . . at minimal cost: Brinton, "Alumni Address: The Faculty of 1841"

that the Jefferson Medical College board move forward with the plan as soon as possible: Henry, *Standard History of the Medical Profession*

But the petition was summarily rejected: Ibid.

could not hide his frustration with the decision: Brinton, "Alumni Address: The Faculty of 1841"

"Mütter, he of the musical voice and charming personality . . . the gods fight in vain . . .": Ibid.

"But that didn't diminish his love of Jefferson . . . the potential . . . entering a great era" Ibid.

"This disorderly transportation . . . and boyish sharp-shooting": Henry, *Standard History of the Medical Profession*

even formal portraits of him often show his tie and clothing askew: Berkowitz, *Adorn the Halls*

"He made anatomy so plain, that the dullest pupil . . . not fail to be enlightened": *Autobiography of Samuel D. Gross*

"Pancoast, the dexterous, the dramatic . . . quick as a flashing sunbeam": *The Papers and Speeches of J. Chalmers Da Costa* (Philadelphia: W. B. Saunders, 1931)

"You have but just now listened . . . the honor to address to you": Joseph Pancoast, M. D., *Introductory Lecture to the Course of Anatomy, Delivered in Jefferson Medical College,* October 19, 1849 (Philadelphia: C. Sherman, Printer, 1849)

"work in seemingly perfect harmony": Thomas Jefferson Department of Surgery (Undated)

"Mütter and Pancoast, Pancoast and Mütter . . . each striving . . . Medical College": Brinton, "Alumni Address: The Faculty of 1841"

instruction should be denounced and "sneered at": John H. Gibbon, M.D., "Thomas Dent Mütter, Professor of Surgery, Jefferson Medical College, 1841–1856," *Annals of Medical History* 25 (1925): 237–241

They accused it of being imperfect, insufficient: Ibid.

mislead rather than instruct: Ibid.

not the best surgeon, nor the best teacher: Ibid.

"his personal attractions, features, voice and bearing": Ibid.

accused him of "playing for popularity" in his lectures: Ibid.

"In no period in our medical history was rivalry so marked . . . we have in America": Slatten, "Thomas Dent Mütter"

"a Varginny student": Meigs, *Memoir*

this appointment gave him the first opportunity of showing fully what was in him : Ibid.

was horrified by some of the brutal scenes that were commonplace in slave states: Ibid.

threw himself into being a Jefferson Medical College professor with the greatest ardor: Ibid.

"He took great pleasure in his lectures during the first years . . . routine work among the sick: Ibid.

"Being thoroughly versed in all his subjects, and having . . . what latent powers he had": Ibid.

shouldn't "bother too much" when it came to patients' comfort: Bauer, *Doctors*

avoid "fussing about," . . . when their female patients were in labor: Ibid.

"read and write in another room until the delivery [is] ready.": Ibid.

antisepsis **was not a term or concept used at the time, Mütter . . . "clean" in his technique:** Thomas Jefferson Department of Surgery (Undated)

worked under "as near an aseptic technique as was possible at the time": Bauer, *Doctors*

Mütter spoke out against this "filthy abomination": Thomas D. Mütter, M.D., *On Recent Improvements in Surgery: An Introductory Lecture to the Course on the Principles and Practice of Surgery in Jefferson Medical College of Philadelphia,* Delivered November 3, 1842 (Published by the Class) (Philadelphia: Merrihew & Thompson, Printers, 1842)

"mild, clean, and simple warm water dressing": Ibid.

"doctors were not gentlemen" because "all gentlemen were clean men": Richard W. Wertz and Dorothy C. Wertz, *Lying-In: A History of Childbirth in America* (New Haven, CT: Yale University Press, 1989)

"heroic role of the medical profession in battling the infection": Weigley, *Philadelphia*

so unrecognized that the appearance of pus in an infected . . . "a successful surgical outcome": Ibid.

"the most illustrious faculties in the history of American medical education.": *Jefferson Medical College: Legend and Lore* by Wagner, Frederick B., Jr. and J. Woodrow Savacool (eds.) (Philadelphia: William T. Cooke Publishing Company, 1996)

a period of remarkable prosperity and growth: Henry, *Standard History of the Medical Profession*

period of the true rise and healthy growth of the school: Ibid.

"the golden age of the second great School of Medicine in Philadelphia": Ibid.

such decadent meals as oyster pies made with . . . paid for a half a week's work: Weigley, *Philadelphia*

"The mere acquisition of great wealth did not guarantee admission . . . it is in Philadelphia": Ibid.

brown coat with high stiff white collar, black bengaline cravat . . . pleated jabot: Berkowitz, *Adorn the Halls*

—CHAPTER TEN—

"The Physician Should Have a Reverence for His Art. . . . almost necessarily attended": Mütter, *Charge to the Graduates*, 1851

"Philadelphia, Nov 10, 1842. To Professor Mutter. . . . most grateful remembrances": Mütter, *On Recent Improvements in Surgery*

"We have the honor to subscribe ourselves, Your most obedient servants": Ibid.

"No one who attended his lectures . . . by no means inconsiderable": Pancoast, *A Discourse Commemorative*

"Philadelphia, Nov 12, 1842. Gentlemen—Your note requesting . . . yours, Thos. D. Mütter": Mütter, *On Recent Improvements in Surgery*

"a retrospective view of surgery for the last few years": Ibid.

His first, *The Salt Sulphur Springs, Monroe County, Va.*, had been a disaster: Slatten, "Thomas Dent Mütter"

That first publication was inspired by Mütter's 1834 visit to the Virginia spa: Ibid.

agreeable temperature and dry atmosphere: Ibid.

the waters themselves did *not* have any curative properties: Ibid.

and especially did not cure cases of consumption (now called tuberculosis): Ibid.

regarded as heresy by defenders of the springs: Ibid.

the therapeutic merits of such springs: Ibid.

well patronized, they were massively profitable: Ibid.

so the proprietors had a vested interest in maintaining the illusion that mineral springs: Ibid.

earned him the displeasure of one specific spring owner by the name of William Burke: Ibid.

less than enthusiastic about Mütter's comments on the efficacy of springs. . . . with scorn: Ibid.

Since Mütter had [chosen] to introduce . . . *Diseases to Which They Are Applicable*: Ibid.

"It is well known" . . . "that an excess of oxygen in the air . . . and other internal remedies": Ibid.

"ignored the fact that many owner-proprietors bottled . . . those unable to come to springs": Ibid.

"One need look no further for confirmation . . . that of azote [i.e., nitrogen] great": Ibid.

the "overwhelming evidence" Burke provided: Ibid.

"I have said to many, as I would say to you . . . well-wisher, Thos. D. Mutter": Ibid.

Whether Burke ever realized Mütter's sneaky double entendre . . . book on the subject: Ibid.

"The renown of an art, the noblest of all . . . alleviation of human suffering": Mütter, *On Recent Improvements in Surgery*

"This has been called the *age of progression* . . . dictates of our predecessors: Ibid.

"A contrary disposition, indeed, seems to prevail . . . crowded into the science": Ibid.

"But it is a surprising as well as humiliating reflection . . . disgraceful to all concerned: Ibid.

"And why does this obscurity arise? . . . of which they are to be constructed": Ibid.

"the numerous operations to be discussed . . . hastily condemned": Ibid.

"patient and unprejudiced investigation, aided by experience and reason . . . in their true light": Ibid.

("a new field of investigation . . . hitherto the most obscure"): Ibid.

("I fear much remains to be done ere we arrive at its true origin and proper treatment"): Ibid.

"most ingenious operation in certain varieties . . . rectum distended with feces": Ibid.

"No operation of modern times is more deserving . . . under similar circumstances": Ibid.

"It is the boast of modern surgeons . . . cured by constitutional treatment alone": Ibid.

"incurable deformity, permanent maiming . . . was the inevitable fate": Ibid.

"Allow not then the temptings of the demon . . . no comfort, no satisfaction": Ibid.

"The dark clouds of ignorance, and error . . . these great men are before us": Ibid.

"It must have been obvious to you that American . . . our country to the other": Ibid.

"most daring courage, intrepid coolness . . . and practical experience": Ibid.

"Shall [this progress] be permitted to subside? . . . let pass this golden era?": Ibid.

"Will you not rather 'gird up your loins' . . . also boast of her medical sciences": Ibid.

"There are many among you who are discouraged . . . reap an abundant reward": Ibid.

"Dwell not then upon what has been done . . . but what remains to do": Ibid.

—CHAPTER ELEVEN—

One neighborhood . . . earned the nickname the Infected District: Weigley, *Philadelphia*

"4,000–5,000 people": Ibid.

"incapable of reporting their full horrors to his readers": Ibid.

shops to charge a penny for a meal . . . scraps begged at the back doors of the wealthy: Ibid.

a common custom for one enterprising individual . . . bargain price of two cents a head: Ibid.

police were known as watchmen because . . . "watch-boxes" to protect themselves: Da Costa, "Then and Now"

"were very respectable" while others "were the reverse": Ibid.

"The more humble and gentle the name . . . would fight *anything* at *any time*": Ibid.

"When there was a fire, hand engines . . . joy to the heart of a Comanche or Pawnee'": Ibid.

"Great disorders and riotous demonstrations . . . the Delaware by a rival company": Ibid.

In the Infected District, rum was commonly sold for a penny a glass: Weigley, *Philadelphia*

"Rum is at the root of the trouble": Ibid.

the county supported nineteen temperance societies . . . seven thousand members: Ibid.

Total-abstinence societies . . . topped them with more than ten thousand members: Ibid.

"He that is down needs fear no fall": Ibid.

The population of the city exploded . . . 250,000 by 1842: Ibid.

There were mills for spinning cotton . . . and chandeliers: Ibid.

The factories of Philadelphia produced . . . the nation's steel: Ibid.

the city's twelve sugar refineries . . . supplier of commercial sugar: Ibid.

Unskilled factory operatives, coal heavers . . . six days a week: Ibid.

factories recognized only the Fourth of July . . . sick time were, of course, nonexistent: Ibid.

Of those 300 employees, 225 were boys, "some not yet eight years of age": Ibid.
The area's matchstick factories . . . paying a wage of $2.50 a week: Ibid.

—CHAPTER TWELVE—

"The Physician Must Be a Charitable Man. . . . the physician should chiefly cultivate":
    Mütter, *Charge to the Graduates*, 1851
earliest moment a woman could be certain she was pregnant . . . the quickening: An-
    thony Joseph, "The 'Pennsylvania Model': The Judicial Criminalization of Abortion
    in Pennsylvania, 1838–1850," *American Journal of Legal History* 49 (2007): 284–320
Nineteenth-century philosophers and theologians . . . as the absolute truth: Ibid.
It was a common and widely accepted belief . . . when those first movements were felt:
    Ibid.
Therefore, the quickening was not just the unborn . . . child received its *rational soul*:
    Ibid.
womb "seemed capable of producing growths . . . mere 'moles' or 'false conceptions'":
    Ibid.
"Not everything which comes from the birth parts of a woman is a human being": Ibid.
pregnancy was a nine- to ten-month process: Ibid.
the quickening became the main determining . . . the moral responsibility to that life:
    Ibid.
abortifacient drugs and surgical abortions . . . along the Eastern Seaboard: Ibid.
where advertisements for abortion services ran in the local papers: Ibid.
Abortions were so popular and common that one woman in New York City: Ibid.
offering abortions commercially in the late 1830s. . . . included pills and surgery: Ibid.
opened additional storefronts in Boston and Philadelphia: Ibid.
Physicians were moving toward the view . . . than at the quickening: Ibid.
medical testimony in nineteenth-century criminal cases had a growing influence: Ibid.
"mute testimony to medicine gone wrong": Ibid.
She swallowed magnesia, and tansy, and pennyroyal: Ibid.
She was bled: *The Medical Examiner: A Monthly Record of Medical Science* II (1839) (Phila-
    delphia: Lindsay & Blakiston, 1839)
She consumed cups of tea made from powdered roots: Ibid.
the promise that it would "make her regular": Ibid.
which she said was "sharp to the taste": Ibid.
she couldn't, as they said at the time, "get to rights": Joseph, "The 'Pennsylvania Model'"
a self-described "botanical physician": Ibid.
gave Eliza a new round of tinctures . . . black-powder tea, ergot, savin oil: Ibid.
"shined and looked like a knitting needle": *The Medical Examiner* (1839)
replacing the hot bricks at her feet to keep her warm: Ibid.
"I found her with a livid face . . . her extremities cold and she was pulseless": Ibid.
There was no saving her: Joseph, "The 'Pennsylvania Model'"
Rush convinced Chauncey to move her to his house: Ibid.
the next day, either in transit or soon after arriving at Chauncey's house: Ibid.
Meigs found his first patients among the poor and destitute: Meigs, *Memoir*
the position of his wife's family in society: Ibid.
did not, and indeed they could not be expected . . . that of their family obstetrician:
    Ibid.
fit to be trusted: Ibid.
higher and increasingly more impressive social rank: Ibid.

difficult cases of childbirth . . . "greatly disturbed and tried his strength and nerves": Ibid.

In one of the cases, he made a wrong diagnosis . . . survived, relatively unharmed: Ibid.

"so disgusted" with himself for the error: Ibid.

"the painful responsibility which belongs to that branch": Ibid.

For two straight years, he worked purely as . . . gynecological cases to his friends: Ibid.

his expenses increasing: Ibid.

"began to fancy that the wolf was approaching his door": Ibid.

For the sake of his family and his finances, Meigs returned to obstetrics: Ibid.

"endowed with a clear perceptive power . . . doctrines of a good medical school": Charles D. Meigs, M.D., *Females and Their Diseases: A Series of Letters to His Class* (Philadelphia: Lea & Blanchard, 1848)

his business and reputation only increased: Meigs, *Memoir*

Chauncey, who at first denied that Eliza was even pregnant when he began treating her: Joseph, "The 'Pennsylvania Model'"

that it was a simple case of inflammation: Ibid.

excess food and drink as well as exposure to a damp draft in Sowers's room: Ibid.

"period of religious ecstasy": Ibid.

placid smile: Ibid.

"blissful immortality in the world to come": Ibid.

"the milk flowed freely": *The Medical Examiner* (1839)

"to spare the feeling of the family": Joseph, "The 'Pennsylvania Model'"

"resulting from a laceration of the uterus caused by an instrumental abortion": Ibid.

Chauncey was arrested and indicted for the murder of Eliza Sowers: Ibid.

Chauncey had four distinct charges: Ibid.

murder by simple assault, and murder by means of poison: Ibid.

murder by means of assault and abortion, and murder by means of mere abortion: Ibid.

released on bail on the grounds "that it was . . . a murder case at all?": Ibid.

"The death of the mother following criminal abortion . . . responsible for all its results": Ibid.

"necessarily attended with great danger . . . they are practiced" . . . injure the woman: Ibid.

termed abortion the "destruction of . . . the fruit of [the woman's] womb": Ibid.

harm to the mother *as well as* the death of the unborn: Ibid.

the trial became a citywide obsession . . . week before a crowded courtroom: Ibid.

one of the three physicians who examined Eliza Sowers's body: Ibid.

he did not clearly understand how conception took place: Ibid.

"very great nonsense on the part of the lawyers": Ibid.

chastise any woman . . . who approached . . . "know their own duty as well as their physicians?": Ibid.

"I love my profession as a ministry . . . nature of man so clearly and so plainly?": Bauer, *Doctors*

the courts of Pennsylvania issued some of the strictest laws . . . a woman found herself in: Joseph, "The 'Pennsylvania Model'"

—CHAPTER THIRTEEN—

"The Physician Must Be a Man of Strict Integrity and Virtue. . . . ye comforted me'": Mütter, *Charge to the Graduates*, 1851

"It is now generally admitted that 'plastic surgery' originated in India": Mütter, *On Recent Improvements in Surgery*

Indian criminals earned "peculiar punishments" . . . sliced off, ears, lips, limbs: Ibid.

a black market for doctors who claimed to be able to replace missing body parts: Ibid.

"And what the knife of the executioner called forth . . . in Europe and America": Ibid.

fame depended on his having practiced the art . . . by grafting: "Gaspar Taliacotius (1546–1599)" in Alexander Chalmers, ed., *The General Biographical Dictionary* / T / Vol. 29 (1812): 114

from the skins of other people: Mütter, *On Recent Improvements in Surgery*

the skin from the arm of a porter onto the noseless face of his patient: Ibid.

"All went well for the space of thirteen months . . . original owner of the nose had died!": Ibid.

"The sympathy between the nose and its parent . . . cut from [the skin of] the same porter": Ibid.

this ridicule: Ibid.

"no attempt to perform these operations . . . the latter end of the last century": Ibid.

"an art nearly lost, yet of the greatest value to mankind": Ibid.

"Even now *plastic surgery* must be considered . . . fully established": Ibid.

"I received a burn when five years old . . . medical aid was not called . . .": Thomas Dent Mütter, *Cases of Deformity from Burns, Successfully Treated by Plastic Operations* (Merrihew & Thompson, Philadelphia, 1843)

"Dr. Burns, a neighboring physician, hearing of my circumstances . . . which was never done": Ibid.

chronic hypertrophy: Ibid.

"When I was eleven years of age, an attempt . . . did not experience any relief": Ibid.

The clavicle on her right side was also . . . inch and a half of the top of her sternum: Ibid.

"My condition has been most humiliating and made my life a burden": Ibid.

"Death is preferable to a life of such misery as mine": Ibid.

fully explained: Ibid.

any of the usual operations for such deformities: Ibid.

entirely different: Ibid.

"Although [the surgery would be] severe . . . promised partial, if not entire relief": Ibid.

placed her in "preparatory treatment": Ibid.

—CHAPTER FOURTEEN—

two doctors whom Mütter had asked to assist him and four medical students: Mütter, *Cases of Deformity*

the "sound" unscarred skin, outside of the most heavily scarred . . . skin on its opposite side: Ibid.

"the most vital part of the neck": Ibid.

"a most shocking wound six inches in length by five and a half in width": Ibid.

"for I knew very well, that if permitted to heal . . . be made worse than before": Ibid.

carrying the scalpel downward and outward over the deltoid muscle: Ibid.

six and a half inches in length, by six in width: Ibid.

leave the flap attached: Ibid.

the upper part of her neck: Ibid.

He placed the skin in the gap: Ibid.

Once he saw that the edges of the wounds: Ibid.

to support the sutures: Ibid.

that no other dressing at this stage was advisable: Ibid.

Mütter realized that scars, by nature, contract . . . need to heal in a stretched position: Ibid.

"The fortitude with which this truly severe operation was borne . . . period of its duration": Ibid.

"Rest and quietude were enjoined": Ibid.

eating or drinking of any kind had been strictly prohibited by Mütter: Ibid.

other than a slightly raised pulse and . . . she seemed perfectly well: Ibid.

"A little nervous, but no fever; no swelling . . . another day without sustenance": Ibid.

"an enema to be administered at once . . . barley water to be taken every hour or two": Ibid.

The treatment, thankfully, worked: Ibid.

"The wound united along the edges . . . pus at the most dependent part of the flap": Ibid.

evacuated the pus through a small opening in its vicinity . . . dressed the shoulder: Ibid.

"a little mutton broth" followed by an enema of salt and water: Ibid.

noticed a "troublesome circumstance" where "a band . . . wider than a small wire": Ibid.

straighten her lower teeth—including the removal of one . . . the lower jaw: Ibid.

move about and "enjoy the full benefit of the operation": Ibid.

"The whole appearance of the patient is so . . . scarcely recognize her as the same individual": Ibid.

"It will be sufficient to state that no unfavourable symptom made its appearance": Ibid.

"The comfort and satisfaction I feel . . . a blessing that cannot be described!": Ibid.

"For nearly eight years she had been unable . . . nearly in contact with the sternum": Ibid.

"this case was even more unfavourable": Ibid.

"determined to perform the operation which had proved so successful": Ibid.

"speaking, swallowing, or motions of the neck of any kind": Ibid.

a nine-year-old boy who had "a deformity of the mouth and throat": Ibid.

His mouth was kept permanently open . . . throat from chin to sternum: Ibid.

"The operation . . . was performed before the medical . . . hopeless, was effected": Ibid.

"Two years and more have elapsed since the first . . . cases are also doing well": Ibid.

"[Mütter] felt it a glorious thing to be able to . . . higher grounds": Elizabeth S. Harris and Raymond F. Morgan, "Thomas Dent Mutter, MD: Early Reparative Surgeon," *Annals of Plastic Surgery* 33, no. 3 (September 1994)

—CHAPTER FIFTEEN—

The Physician Should Be a Self-Relying Man. . . . profession of which he is a member": Mütter, *Charge to the Graduates*, 1851

ever-growing prestige of the college: "Part I: Jefferson Medical College 1835 to 1845" http://jdc.jefferson.edu/wagner1/15

stature as an American institution: Ibid.

Paris's Hôtel-Dieu's need for leeches was so great . . . part of the hospital staff: McCullough, *The Greater Journey*

John Kearsley Mitchell recommended that his students . . . suffering from typhoid: Lawrence G. Blochman, *Dr. Squibb: The Life and Times of a Rugged Idealist* (New York: Simon & Schuster, 1958)

leeches directly into a woman's uterus, using a sleek wooden speculum: Charles D. Meigs, M.D., *Obstetrics: The Science and the Art* (Philadelphia: Blanchard & Lea, 1856)

rent floors above the two stores next to the college . . . fifteen patients: "Part I: Jefferson Medical College 1835 to 1845" http://jdc.jefferson.edu/wagner1/15

serve as the college's only hospital for another thirty years: Ibid.

Students eagerly volunteered to provide nursing care: Ibid.

meals brought from a nearby restaurant: Ibid.

"Mütter's fancy was full and free, and in its brilliant play . . . might deem *excessive*": Pancoast, *A Discourse Commemorative*

"These advantages were not coveted by him, however, for personal . . . his support": Ibid.

family had always been valued above wealth: Weigley, *Philadelphia*

Mütter had met and married Mary Alsop . . . the elite Connecticut Alsops: Slatten, "Thomas Dent Mütter"

the upper class would accept some members of the . . . considered to be virtue: Weigley, *Philadelphia*

upper social stratum in Philadelphia and were generally seen as "vulgar": Ibid.

"The lines of demarcation in [Philadelphia] 'society' . . . the exclusives and the excluded": Ibid.

"How am I able to communicate a just notion . . . delicate beauty of their ladies": Ibid.

He was born on the island of St. George's: Meigs, *Memoir*

a little frontier town, whose population numbered "only two hundred and seventy souls": Ibid.

in this semi-wild, sparsely inhabited country: Ibid.

was still occupied by Native Americans . . . and Chickasaw: Ibid.

short distance from Hiwassee . . . Colonel Return J. Meigs . . . lived: Ibid.

all through the Revolutionary War: Ibid.

a sword for gallant conduct: Ibid.

"erect as a tree": Ibid.

the White Chief: Ibid.

It was in this land "of law and lawlessness . . . downright barbarism" . . . formative years: Ibid.

"Here was a spot, a climate—forest and stream, hill and dale . . . broad and deep": Ibid.

"a truly savage life": Ibid.

"He had made the acquaintance of a certain Jim Vann . . . *pony in the country*": Ibid.

"a most violent and brutal fellow": Ibid.

at first flatly "and with high indignation" refused even to listen to such a project: Ibid.

"never ceased to beg and entreat and knock, until finally . . . she yielded": Ibid.

Meigs would live "in the Nation" for over a month. He was twelve years old: Ibid.

Vann's savagery and wildness: Ibid.

"As I grew older, I came to think that some of his stories . . . been quite within the truth": Ibid.

"Poor Vann has *ceased from troubling* . . . his death was a public blessing": Ibid.

extensive literary work: J. Whitridge Williams, M.D., "A Sketch of the History of Obstetrics in the United States up to 1860," *American Gynecology*, Volume 3 (American Gynecology Publishing Co., 1903), 38–42, 266–294, 340–366

translation in 1831 of Velpeau's *Traité* . . . flowed in rapid succession from his hand: Ibid.

He prepared many of his books within a few months: Ibid.

composed one of his bestselling textbooks . . . between two teaching sessions: Ibid.

"a meager book": Ibid.

"the task would be useless": Ibid.

"very misty": Ibid.

"a haze of words": Ibid.

that the placenta was entirely fetal in origin . . . between it and the uterine wall: Ibid.

the muscular structure of the womb: Ibid.

physician who, upon introducing his hand to remove . . . relaxed by copious bloodletting": Ibid.

was an cloquent advocate of the use of the lancet: Ibid.

overcome the rigidity of the birth canal, and as his cure of eclampsia: Ibid.

vividly impress into the minds . . . views he wanted to promote: Ibid.

not only to positively *deny* the contagious nature . . . opposed with him: Ibid.

Squibb was a local boy, born on the Fourth of July of 1819: Blochman, *Dr. Squibb*

"ineffectual invalid for the rest of his days": Ibid.

working as an apprentice for a Philadelphia pharmacist . . . house of J. H. Sprague: Ibid.

"unqualified favorites": Ibid.

"Dr. Bache, with his patriarchal white beard and distinguished lineage": Ibid.

"with his clear, playing, logical and unforgettable . . . contrasts strongly with some of the rest": Ibid.

"the clean-shaven, dramatic, Bermuda born": Ibid.

"the originality of idea, and erratic, familiar manner . . . not fit well elsewhere": Ibid.

"He and Bache are wildly different as good and bad" . . . "And yet both are capital teachers": Ibid.

"a striking figure as he stood before his class . . . his high forehead": Ibid.

his skill and knowledge: Ibid.

humor in his lectures: Ibid.

doleful expression: Ibid.

attempted to examine her . . . *"Ah, mon pauvre docteur, c'est tout gâté pour jamais!"*: Ibid.

with an admiring but not uncritical eye: Ibid.

"small, blue-eyed Mütter with his dark curly hair graying prematurely, and his finely chiseled features": Ibid.

clear, musical voice: Ibid.

"round faced Pancoast, bald except for a monastic fringe . . . sandy handlebar mustache": Ibid.

wiping his bloody fingers on his pocket handkerchief and . . . "on whatever was handy": Ibid.

openly discussed his differences with them: Ibid.

in the amphitheater for their lectures: Ibid.

Bache invited Squibb to his "medical-club meeting": Ibid.

strictly professional conversation was prohibited by rule: Ibid.

"keep down the rebellion in [their] stomachs": Ibid.

"beyond any real medical help" *The British and Foreign Medical Review* 18 (July–October 1844): 525–526 (London: John Churchill, 1844)

"There are few, if any, deformities consequent on accident . . . transatlantic surgery": Ibid.

the fastest knife in the West End: Gordon, *Great Medical Disasters*

"Time me, gentlemen, time me!": Ibid.

removal of a forty-five-pound scrotal tumor in four minutes: Ibid.

prior to the operation, the poor patient . . . carry his scrotum around in a wheelbarrow: Ibid.

sawed off the patient's testicles: Ibid.

"a distinguished surgical spectator": Ibid.

"dropped dead from fright": Ibid.

"the only operation in history with a 300 percent mortality [rate]": Ibid.

"surgeons operated in blood-stiffened frock coats": Ibid.

"the stiffer the coat, the prouder the busy surgeon": Ibid.

"There was no object in being clean . . . manicure his nails before chopping off a head": Ibid.

his suggestions for hygiene improvement to reduce obstetric . . . from puerperal fever: Ibid.

"outraged obstetricians, particularly in Philadelphia": Ibid.

"abrupt, abrasive, argumentative" . . . "charitable to the poor and tender to the sick": Ibid.

"He relished operating successfully in the reeking tenements . . . and made a fortune": Ibid.

incisions, hemorrhage, and the dressing and union of wounds: Liston, *Lectures on the Operations of Surgery*

It covered injuries of the scalp, the cranium, and the brain, including the most effective trephining techniques: Ibid.

"In presenting to the profession in this country . . . veterans of our art": Ibid.

"It will be observed that this volume contains all the lectures . . . hands of every surgeon": Ibid.

"The additional matter furnished by the editor . . . publication of the lectures be continued": Ibid.

That year, Jefferson Medical College could not only claim . . . in the entire United States: "Part I: Jefferson Medical College 1846 to 1855"; http://jdc.jefferson.edu/wagner1/16

The college celebrated by renovating its main lecture hall: Ibid.

The upper and lower lecture rooms were enlarged to seat 600 students: Ibid.

the upper lecture hall—known as the pit: Ibid.

This "miniature hospital" would represent a precursor . . . built nearly thirty years later: Ibid.

six Corinthian columns that graced the facade: Ibid.

the form of a Grecian temple: Ibid.

"In every respect, the comfort and advantage of the students . . . successful teaching": "Annual Announcement of Jefferson Medical College of Philadelphia: Session of 1847–48" (1847), *Jefferson Medical College Catalogs*, Paper 62; http://jdc.jefferson.edu/jmc_catalogs/62

"[We] expected . . . to be back yesterday . . . remain some time longer": Ibid.

"the irreparable loss our Nation has sustained . . . Andrew Jackson": Jefferson Medical College Minutes

crepe on the left arm for sixty straight days: Ibid.

the building itself was shrouded in black mourning bunting for six months: Ibid.

"Mütter has no children and makes a good income by his profession": "The Diaries of Sidney George Fisher, 1844–1849," *The Pennsylvania Magazine of History and Biography* 86, no. 1 (Jan. 1962): 49–90

"At so large a dinner conversation is never general . . . chiefly owes his success": Ibid.

—CHAPTER SIXTEEN—

If a person inhales the right quantity . . . no pain during medical or surgical procedures: Ira M. Rutkow, M.D., *American Surgery: An Illustrated History* (Philadelphia: Lippincott-Raven, 1998)

continuously screamed out in wretched pain whenever Wells . . . rotten tooth: Ibid.

They called Wells a swindler: Ibid.
said his discovery was a humbug: Ibid.
his career never recovered: Ibid.
"incident of history gone awry": Ibid.
common side effects of inhaling nitrous oxide gas: Ibid.
agitated behavior: Ibid.
a medical breakthrough was showcased . . . even knew it: Ibid.
"laughing gas parties" or "ether frolics": Ibid.
"exhilarating features": Ibid.
The sudden loss of equilibrium and inhibition . . . roaring crowds: Ibid.
sulphuric ether and nitrous oxide: Ibid.
"It is the greatest discovery ever made! . . . prick of a pin!": Ibid.
John Collins Warren, the influential professor . . . Massachusetts General Hospital:
    Ibid.
Charles Thomas Jackson, "one of the most eccentric . . . surgical anesthesia": Ibid.
Jackson, a graduate of Harvard Medical School, began inhaling nitrous in 1841:
    Ibid.
by 1844, he had persuaded several local dentists . . . patients' toothaches: Ibid.
it was Jackson who suggested in September 1846 . . . than nitrous oxide: Ibid.
John Collins Warren if he might share this latest innovation with his class: Bauer,
    Doctors
October 16, 1846, in the same surgical amphitheater as Wells's fiasco: Ibid.
"anonymous" liquid on a patient: Ibid.
the dawn of a new era in surgery: Ibid.
"Gentlemen, this is no humbug": Ibid.

—CHAPTER SEVENTEEN—

"The Physician Must Be a Determined, . . . most successful": Mütter, *Charge to the
    Graduates*, 1851
"unqualified triumph": Ibid.
which he called Letheon, after Lethe . . . mythology's river of forgetfulness: Ibid.
who already imagined that Letheon contained sulphuric ether: Ibid.
challenged Morton to use his "preparation" . . . full amputation at the thigh: Ibid.
"It was the custom to bring the patient . . . before the advent of anesthesia": Ibid.
the patient "unconscious and insensitive to pain": Ibid.
detailed public announcement . . . Boston Society for Medical Improvement: Ibid.
Medical and Surgical Journal a week later: Ibid.
Bigelow's actions represent the first formal announcement . . . medical profession:
    Ibid.
considerable controversy: Ibid.
the first *use* of ether anesthesia: Ibid.
Dr. Crawford W. Long . . . anesthesia for minor procedures as early as 1842: Ibid.
unlike Morton and Wells, Long did not share the news . . . Morton's demonstrations:
    Ibid.
Two days before Christmas in 1846 . . . pit of Jefferson Medical College: Thomas Jef-
    ferson Department of Surgery (Undated)
"appeared often at operations to be painfully sympathetic . . . the patient": Levis,
    "Memoir of Thomas Dent Mütter"
the first surgeon in Philadelphia to administer anesthesia: Berkowitz, *Adorn the Halls*

—CHAPTER EIGHTEEN—

Much to Mütter's shock, the medical community's . . . in Philadelphia: Berkowitz, *Adorn the Halls*

"We are persuaded that the surgeons of Philadelphia . . . younger brethren": Rutkow, *American Surgery*

there was a great number of deaths: Ibid.

"The last special wonder has already arrived at the natural . . . of its predecessor novelties": Ibid.

These agents have been employed to relieve pain in all sorts . . . to be regarded as an evil: Ibid.

The board of Philadelphia's Pennsylvania Hospital . . . surgical anesthesia for seven years: Ibid.

"I acknowledge that I am an enthusiastic admirer . . . and so plainly?": Meigs, *Memoir*

"He taught in his lectures not only the absolute duty of the student . . . that of the preacher": Ibid.

"He always held that there was in the practice of medicine . . . desire to escape from": Ibid.

"great pains to demonstrate the dangers of ether inhalation": Brinton, "Alumni Address: The Faculty of 1841"

how easily a life might be destroyed by this . . . than by etherizing a sheep to death: Ibid.

in order to afford his students, as he alleged, "a practical illustration of its dangers: Ibid.

"Prejudice was an element deeply rooted in his character": *Autobiography of Samuel D. Gross*

"His opposition to [anesthesia] was founded, not upon personal . . . its evil effects": Ibid.

"Certainly, my dear friend," was the invariable answer: Ibid.

"Then, by God, I hope you will kill your patient!" was the invariable rejoinder: Ibid.

"You will find it hard when you die to pass the gates of St. Peter . . . the altar of science": Ibid.

hearty laugh: Ibid.

brought a sheep into the amphitheater to be "heroically etherized" to death: Brinton, "Alumni Address: The Faculty of 1841"

Ellerslie Wallace . . . Meigs's dutiful assistant, poured the freshly prepared ether from a demijohn: Ibid.

"My long and extensive practice of midwifery has rendered . . . daughters of Eve: Meigs, *Obstetrics*

"Perhaps, I am cruel in taking so dispassionate a view" . . . however rarely: Ibid.

"So I ask you? Should I exhibit a remedy for pain . . . the risk of *killing* one woman?: Ibid.

"My *God*, . . . if that were to happen, I ask that you clothe me in . . . should any of us?": Ibid.

"conversational, not at all rhetorical. . . . of anybody else": *Autobiography of Samuel D. Gross*

in the lecture room Meigs was the best actor he had ever seen: Ibid.

"possessed all the requisites for success upon the stage . . . strong perception of the ludicrous": Ibid.

once-dead sheep: Brinton, "Alumni Address: The Faculty of 1841"

—CHAPTER NINETEEN—

"The Physician Should Be a Discreet Man. . . . from troubles": Mütter, *Charge to the Graduates*, 1851

by having his students rush into church and falsely claim there was an emergency: Unattributed Mütter note in a biography found in Thomas Jefferson University Archive in the Alumni Address re: the Faculty of '41 File

"The operation was an extensive one . . . Pancoast assisted . . . have good effect": Blochman, *Dr. Squibb*

"the most bungling demonstration I ever saw": Ibid.

shrieking patient's "blood and tears detracted from the artistic effect": Ibid.

"The patient was not easily etherized": Ibid.

"but was finally brought under the full effect . . . and replied he did not know it was done": Ibid.

no groaning or noise during the operation . . . when the anesthetic effect would diminish: Ibid.

operation to be "very well and prettily and quickly done": Ibid.

"Some notable bleeding from the end of the bone but probably not serious": Ibid.

"A large audience and only one case of fainting": Ibid.

operation as a grand performance—"Barnum by Dr. Mütter": Ibid.

"zealous and enduring attention": "Annual Announcement of Jefferson" (1847); http://jdc.jefferson.edu/jmc_catalogs/62

"ample opportunities . . . for pursuits in practical anatomy": Ibid.

"the student has much more leisure than during the session": Ibid.

a thorough renovation of the building: Ibid.

"So satisfied are the faculty of the value to the students . . . the business of instruction": Ibid.

796 patients: Ibid.

the much larger Pennsylvania Hospital, with its full staff . . . patients in its *twelve-month* period: Ibid.

"The Clinic enables the professors to exhibit to the class . . . operated on before the class": Ibid.

Of the 796 patients . . . 409 people—came to be treated in Mütter's surgical ward: Ibid.

176 of the 796 patients were under the age of ten: Ibid.

82 of those were under the age of three: Ibid.

399 males and 397 females: Ibid.

diseases of the mouth, the stomach, and the intestines: Ibid.

They treated chronic enlargement of the spleen, herpes . . . and impetigo: Ibid.

lupus, cholera, epilepsy, and gonorrhea: Ibid.

"idiocy" or "insanity" or "hypochondria": Ibid.

fingers that had been crushed between train cars . . . by gunpowder, and broken bones: Ibid.

"conical stumps": Ibid.

"Multitudes of surgical patients, as attested by the register . . . employed in vain": Pancoast, *A Discourse Commemorative*

surgeries because of "spontaneous contraction of hands and feet . . . a diseased sternum": "Annual Announcement of Jefferson" (1847); http://jdc.jefferson.edu/jmc_catalogs/62

elephantiasis: *The Journal of Edward Robinson Squibb, M.D.* (private printing, George E. Crosby Co., 1930) took up a collection for the man: Ibid.

"He loved . . . to match himself with the most difficult cases . . . energy of the strife": Pancoast, *A Discourse Commemorative*

"His office was thronged with patients from every part of the Union . . . to consult him": Levis, "Memoir of Thomas Dent Mütter"

"At the clinic of the College, on his entrance . . . *but touch his garment, I shall be whole*": Ibid.

"At no time had the ample resources of Philadelphia . . . more triumphantly exhibited": "Annual Announcement of Jefferson" (1847), http://jdc.jefferson.edu/jmc_catalogs/62

"In no hospital which I have visited, abroad or at home . . . application of instruments": Pancoast, *A Discourse Commemorative*

did not largely decrease the percentage of deaths that resulted from operations: Rutkow, *American Surgery*

still died at the same rate as surgical patients who endured operations without anesthesia: Ibid.

John Collins Warren wrote a second monograph . . . to educate the public on the subject: Ibid.

"The introduction of chloroform produced an excitement . . . within little more than a year": Ibid.

Removing this element from the act of surgery seemed strange and unnatural to some: Ibid.

American Journal of the Medical Sciences, army surgeon John B. Porter: Ibid.

"the blood is poisoned, the nervous influence and muscular . . . adhesion is prevented": Ibid.

A System of Operative Surgery: Based upon the Practice of Surgeons in the United States: Ibid

"In the majority of cases, the creation of pain by any operation . . . by every operator": Ibid.

did not yet employ antiseptic or aseptic measures: Ibid.

patients died of common postoperative problems . . . wound sepsis, and shock: Ibid.

by writing a series of articles: Ibid.

"the supposed dangers of anesthetic agents" (later released as an authoritative monograph): Ibid.

"I think anesthesia is of the devil," Dr. William Atkinson . . . God intended them to endure!": Ibid.

—CHAPTER TWENTY—

"a singularly handsome man": Da Costa, "Osteitis Deformans"

slender, and graceful: Ibid.

with a clear sweet voice of remarkable strength and carrying power: Ibid.

"a style of dress not altogether proper for a boy his age": Carter family papers.

scrupulously neat: Da Costa, "Osteitis Deformans"

"in fact, almost a dandy": Ibid.

"a delightful conversationalist and an admirable raconteur": Ibid.

his lungs had begun to shudder and ache in his chest: Slatten, "Thomas Dent Mütter"

"inconceivably sensitive to pain": James B. McCaw, M.D., and George A. Otis, M.D. eds., *Virginia Medical Journal*, Vol. XIII (Richmond: Ritchie and Dunnavant, 1859)

No matter what treatment he sought or to what preventive care he devoted himself, nothing helped: Ibid.

("Few can boast of [being ambidextrous] . . . and often, many who can have in fact *only two left hands*," a fellow doctor once quipped): Thomas Dent Mütter, *Introductory Lecture to a Course on the Principles and Practice of Surgery*, Delivered in Jefferson Medical College, November 1, 1847 (Philadelphia: Merrihew and Thompson, 1847)

The famed clinic of Jefferson College was only becoming more popular: Levis, "Memoir of Thomas Dent Mütter"

His office was flooded with the ill and injured, the desperate . . . needed to consult with him: Ibid.

"some of the greatest achievements of American surgery": Ibid.

"In the every-day surgical operations Mütter was . . . in the Surgical Clinic": Brinton, "Alumni Address: The Faculty of 1841"

his advice and aid in consultation: Levis, "Memoir of Thomas Dent Mütter"

"his feeble physical abilities enabled him to": Ibid.

member of Philadelphia's Protestant Episcopal Church: Ibid.

ward for incurables: Ibid.

"The consolations of religion supported him through his long sufferings . . . and hopefulness": Ibid.

American Medical Association was founded in Philadelphia in 1847: Da Costa, "Then and Now"

the following year, the Philadelphia County Medical Society: Ibid.

a forum where all "respectable physicians" could meet, debate, and exchange experiences: Ibid.

bind the profession together: Rules of gentlemanly conduct . . . and to the greater public: Ibid.

respectable school, was of good moral and professional standing . . . active practitioner: Ibid.

who "prescribes a remedy without knowing its composition": Ibid.

These societies were not only successful: Ibid.

Children's Hospital of Philadelphia . . . Northern Home for Friendless Children: John H. Packard, M.D., ed., *The Philadelphia Medical Register and Directory* (Philadelphia: Collins, 1868)

"long violently opposed to [the idea of] the female doctor": Da Costa, "Then and Now"

a group of Quakers . . . Female Medical College of Pennsylvania within the city limits in 1850: Ibid.

Woman's Medical College of Pennsylvania . . . Pennsylvania Medical . . . *against* women practitioners: Ibid.

"cannot stand the strain of practice": Ibid.

"their physiological necessities forbid the attempt": Ibid.

"if married they will neglect home duties": Ibid.

"not consent to only attend women": Ibid.

"nerves are too delicate for the work": Ibid.

expelling any of its members who dared to teach at a . . . with women physicians: Ibid.

physician at the Pennsylvania Hospital was so appalled . . . teach even one single woman: Ibid.

the first female doctor was elected into the same . . . role in the profession entirely: Ibid.

"Woman, as usual, finally had her way. . . . And yet the earth did not rock . . . stars did not fall": Ibid.

"*Anesthesia* . . . I need not, on this occasion, enter upon the history . . . *offspring of the New World*": *The Medical Examiner: A Monthly Record of Medical Science* LXXXV (January 1852)

"In England, Scotland and Ireland, and on every portion . . . in the practice of surgery": Ibid.

"You will be anxious, I doubt not, to learn the estimation . . . advocates and inventors . . .": Ibid.

"These operations were for many years considered almost . . . of an established operation": Ibid.

what they considered to be "the exploitation of the manual art of surgery": Rutkow, *American Surgery*

"seemingly boundless enthusiasm for questionably appropriate surgical intervention": Ibid.

the jargon of American medicine: *conservative surgery* and *radical surgery*: Ibid.

The words took on different meanings at different times: Ibid.

sharp philosophic difference: Ibid.

Earlier surgeons would define *conservative surgery* . . . often life-endangering injury: Ibid.

Conservative surgery therefore was defined as any surgery "devised . . . who would hold still": Ibid.

"The more bloody, and even the more uniformly fatal . . . cutting performed by others": Ibid.

"And they too become partakers in the popular idolatry . . . surgery into human butchery": Ibid.

"To answer this question in a satisfactory manner . . . it is necessary . . . pace in different cases.": Thomas Dent Mütter, M.D., *Introductory for 1844–5, on the Present Position of Some of the Most Important of the Modern Operations of Surgery* (Philadelphia; Merrihew & Thompson, 1844)

"a welcome messenger": Ibid.

"a martyr to unspeakable sufferings, and a loathsome object to her friends": Ibid.

"It is true, that some of the French, who adopt the view . . . becomes involved, or *none at all*": Ibid.

"It is urged by some, that we are justified . . . and that she must die in a few months: Ibid.

"But, gentlemen . . . whenever I have done so, it has been with . . . voluntarily subjected": Ibid.

"the knife promises nothing": Ibid.

"it will serve to satisfy the patient in part, and prevent . . . utterly abandoned by the surgeon": Ibid.

John Watson, an influential New York City surgeon . . . "Surgery . . . better for your patients": *The Medical Examiner* (1852)

The early years of the 1850s were a transformative time in Philadelphia: Weigley, *Philadelphia*

"The old axiom, *mens sana in corpore sano* . . . have been imparted to his frame": Mütter, *Introductory Lecture,* 1847

"Without health . . . the professional life of a man is . . . of suffering and disappointment": Ibid.

professional visits to Europe: Levis, "Memoir of Thomas Dent Mütter"

"numerous eminent friends": Ibid.

"was greeted warmly by the most eminent medical men . . . their operations and consultations": Ibid.

"favored by him with letters of introduction to distinguished medical men": Ibid.

"found them passports at once to the society and attentions of the recipients": Ibid.

his presence seemed "at once known among the numerous . . . pleasure seekers in Paris": Ibid.

throngs of people who both sought his company socially as well as . . . consulted by him professionally: Ibid.

among his most "distinguished and attentive friends": Ibid.

severe attacks of his "frequently recurring malady": Ibid.

"You ought to conceive, therefore, of the tenor of a medical life . . . gravity of your concerns" Charles D. Meigs, *Charge to the Graduates of Jefferson Medical College*, Delivered March 6, 1852 (Philadelphia: T. K. and P. G. Collins, Printers, 1852)

"You must go, in and out, before the people, daily . . . touches neither extreme in anything": Ibid.

"Therefore, we charge you: be good men, and learned men . . . of the public welfare in short": Ibid.

"only means of securing relaxation and escaping the incessant calls for his services at home": Levis, "Memoir of Thomas Dent Mütter"

"his only hope for healing the same painful infirmities which always oppressed him": Ibid.

—CHAPTER TWENTY-ONE—

"The Physician Should Be an Honest Man. . . . 'I dressed him, but God healed him'": Mütter, *Charge to the Graduates*, 1851

There had been considerable improvement in ocean travel: Slatten, "Thomas Dent Mütter"

the Collins Line, which in 1850 began offering . . . the British Isles and the United States: Ibid.

ships were the biggest and fastest steamers afloat: Ibid.

A solo trip cost Mütter a thousand dollars, and that number . . . for both himself and his wife: Ibid.

his body still felt weakened and "at the point of breaking down completely": Pancoast, *A Discourse Commemorative*

"a full and systematic work on surgery": Ibid.

gathering and arranging material for his new book: Ibid.

"Merely to have breathed a concentrated scientific atmosphere . . . excellence is *defied*": John Harley Warner, *Against the Spirit of System: The French Impulse in Nineteenth-Century American Medicine* (Princeton, NJ: Princeton University Press, 1998)

"Be *honest* at the *bedside* . . . of great danger . . . 'bourne from which no traveler returns'": Mütter, *Charge to the Graduates*, 1851

"If the physician fails under these circumstances . . . agent by which an immortal soul is lost": Ibid.

Skeletons, wax castings, deformed or defective organs . . . drawings, prints, and instruments: From the Musée Dupuytren website, translated from French by Google: http://translate.google.com/translate?hl=en&sl=fr&u=http://www.upmc.fr/fr/culture/patrimoine/patrimoine_scientifique/musee_dupuytren.html&prev=/search%3Fq%3DMus%25C3%25A9e%2BDupuytren%26biw%3D1126%26bih%3D617

He had authored some of the country's earliest articles on plastic surgery: Rutkow, *American Surgery*

"very explicit descriptions, including drawings": Levis, "Memoir of Thomas Dent Mütter"

"an accurate idea of what was involved from the surgeon's point of view": Ibid.

surgical textbook. . . (he would surely be forced to abandon when his health hopelessly failed): Ibid.

—CHAPTER TWENTY-TWO—

"The Physician Must Possess Moral Courage. . . . 'shepherd must give his life for the flock!'": Mütter, *Charge to the Graduates*, 1851

"there would soon be no rural population left at all": Weigley, *Philadelphia*

the fourth-largest city in the Western world, as well as second-largest in the United States: Ibid.

London and Paris . . . were much larger . . . (provided you included Brooklyn's 266,000): Ibid.

Philadelphia's population had even surpassed such European capitals . . . and Manchester: Ibid.

"too big and too urban": Ibid.

the Philadelphia of the mid-nineteenth century, "one of . . . to be truly a community": Ibid.

the large thrashing wheels of the Fairmount Dam and the Fairmount Water Works: Ibid.

"Dr. Mutter raised his reputation to the highest pitch . . . the records of science": Pancoast, *A Discourse Commemorative*

"Fortune had showered so many present favors upon him . . . he wished for *more*": Ibid.

"What ardent greeting he received . . . after some . . . tenderest sympathy for his suffering": Levis, "Memoir of Thomas Dent Mütter"

it was evident to his students and peers alike that his condition was not improving: Ibid.

"During the last course of lectures which he delivered . . . burden of disease and suffering": Ibid.

"Celsus long since urged the possession of certain physical qualities . . . mere operator . . . : Mütter, *Introductory Lecture*, 1847

"However, his declaration, that a surgeon would be 'without *pity*' . . . so often subjected: Ibid.

"No, gentlemen, I would say to you, *cultivate* your *sympathy* . . . to spare nothing . . .": Ibid.

"*honorable* success.": Mütter, *Charge to the Graduates*, 1851

"Am I to live as an influential, well-informed, and man-loving physician . . . who values them?": Ibid.

"If you have never asked yourselves these questions, the time . . . to dishonor and despair?": Ibid.

"I cannot admit the opinion of [the French philosopher] Helvétius, that . . . reach distinction": Ibid.

"Starting, then, with this position, it will be my task in the lecture . . . be certainly overthrown": Ibid.

—CHAPTER TWENTY-THREE—

"A Physician Should Be a Patriot. . . . to shed his last drop of blood in her defense": Mütter, *Charge to the Graduates*, 1851

to be "split asunder": Da Costa, "Then and Now"

Philadelphia not only allowed slavery when the city was founded . . . hubs for the slave trade: Weigley, *Philadelphia*

"When we contemplate our abhorrence of that condition . . . been extended to us": "An Act for the Gradual Abolition of Slavery," Commonwealth of Pennsylvanias Legislative Reference Bureau, http://www.palrb.us/statutesatlarge/17001799/1780/0/act/0881.pdf

"It is not for us to enquire why, in the creation of mankind . . . to counteract His mercies": Ibid.

It wouldn't be until 1848—nearly seventy years after the act . . . slaves living within the city: Weigley, *Philadelphia*

"a true American city" . . . "contained fewer foreigners than either New York or Boston": Da Costa, "Then and Now"

"The city was not showy . . . gentleman was proverbial, and often alcoholic": Ibid.

"Organized gangs of thugs and robbers were numerous . . . Blood Tubs and the Killers": Ibid.

Philadelphia's mayor was quoted as saying . . . opposed to abolition: Weigley, *Philadelphia*

soon legislation was created to specifically disenfranchise the freed . . . act was first passed: Ibid.

"There is not perhaps anywhere to be found a city in which prejudice . . . between them": Ibid.

"Colored persons, no matter how well dressed . . . mean, contemptible and barbarous": Ibid.

Philadelphia became the founding home of the American Anti-Slavery Society: Ibid.

the founding home of the influential abolitionist newspaper the . . . *Pennsylvania Freeman*: Ibid.

"a place where freedom of speech could be enjoyed": Ibid.

In a sign of solidarity with the African American population . . . entered the hall, arm in arm: Ibid.

They shattered windows, broke chairs and tables, punched . . . entire building to the ground: Ibid.

strengthen the antislavery cause: Ibid.

"everything southern was exalted and worshiped": Ibid.

"a patriotic society to support the Union and driven by . . . ('Love of Country Leads')": The Union League of Philadelphia, website: http://www.unionleague.org/about.php

"All who knew him will remember that the book . . . terrible 'commingling of the nations'": Meigs, *Memoir*

"godlike race, the archetype of the Grecian demigods and heroes": Charles D. Meigs, M.D., *Address Delivered before the Union League of Philadelphia, October 31, 1864* (Philadelphia: Collins, Printer, 1864)

"nude and barbarous tribes of the African race": Ibid.

"Let due honor and reverence be forever rendered . . . less frequent, than *murder itself*": Ibid.

"that great maelstrom": Mütter, *Charge to the Graduates*, 1851

"swallows up time and character, morals, reputation . . . and vexation of spirit": Ibid.

"Oh, how strange a spectacle has this our 'thrice blessed' country . . . anarchy and civil strife!": Ibid.

"And all for what? . . . Simply because our people, forgetting . . . the true love of a patriot?": Ibid.

"But how fearful responsibility do those assume who dare breathe . . . predict it, defend it": Ibid.

"Oh, could these [conspirators] but realize the glory that even now . . . in the womb of time": Ibid.

"Go home, then, gentlemen . . . determined to do all in your power . . . bid you do this": Ibid.

"*Go home* . . . and let the noble language of the illustrious . . . *labored to avert catastrophe!*": Ibid.

—CHAPTER TWENTY-FOUR—

Asiatic cholera killed 1,012 . . . in 1849: Weigley, *Philadelphia*

smallpox took 427 lives in 1852: Ibid.

Yellow fever swept into the city the following year and left 128 corpses: Ibid.

typhus . . . killing 205 people in 1848 alone: Ibid.

Dysentery . . . more than 1,700 citizens between 1848 and 1851 : Ibid.

malarial fevers spread easily and frequently in the city's low, flat lands between the rivers: Ibid.

Ten times as many people died of malaria and tuberculosis . . . more feared cholera: Ibid.

gradually and quietly—they died "romantically," as it was termed: Ibid.

"with terrifying speed and ugliness": Ibid.

In 1852—the same year that smallpox killed more than 400 Philadelphians . . . tuberculosis: Ibid.

Starting in 1849, they began thoroughly cleaning streets, waterways . . . scourge of disease: Ibid.

poverty was "the wages of sin": Ibid.

sanitary measures—instead of prayer—to fight the constant epidemics: Ibid.

"indulging in sentimentalism or speculation": Richard Harrison Shryock, *The Development of Modern Medicine: An Interpretation of the Social and Scientific Factors Involved* (Philadelphia: University of Pennsylvania Press, 1936)

"Acknowledging the rare merits which belong to the work . . . *to merit condemnation*": *Transactions of the American Medical Association*, Vol. IV (Philadelphia: T. K. and P. G. Collins, 1851)

"an affected obscure style and a fondness for speculations . . . in any accredited authority": Ibid.

"his fondness for what is speculative leads him often to prefer . . . by common acceptation": Ibid.

"notice[d] also a disposition to exclusiveness, exhibited by taking . . . he would cherish": Ibid.

"[h]owever valuable, suggestive, and instructive these chapters . . . to their seductions": Ibid.

"Meigs was all his life a non-believer in the infectious nature . . . him in the face": *Autobiography of Samuel D. Gross*

"fierce and consuming": "Oliver Wendell Holmes" in *Stanford University School of Medicine and the Predecessor Schools: An Historical Perspective*, Chapter 5.2, http://elane.stanford.edu/wilson/html/chap5/chap5-sect2.html

the *destroyer of families*: Ibid.

dreaded pestilence: Ibid.

published a controversial paper titled "The Contagiousness of Puerperal Fever": Ibid.

argued that the deadly infection was most often transmitted . . . by her own attendants: Ibid.

He ended the article by advocating the best techniques for preventing the disease's spread: Ibid.

"the clarity and forcefulness" with which he addressed "both the . . . this devastating disease": Ibid.

apparently because of a wound he received while performing the autopsy: Ibid.

the interval between being wounded and dying: Ibid.

Every single one of those women went on to develop puerperal fever: Ibid.

"The disease, known as Puerperal Fever, is so far contagious as . . . by physicians and nurses": Ibid.

Holmes cited literature that supported his theory, though . . . published in British journals: Ibid.

Charles Meigs . . . publicly decrying Holmes's conclusion: Ibid.

particularly horrifying to Holmes, for during the course . . . right in the heart of Philadelphia: Ibid.

seventy-seven women whose births were attended by Dr. Rutter . . . women died from it: Ibid.

"a far greater number of such cases than any other practitioner in Philadelphia": Ibid.

Meigs waved off any notion that Rutter could be responsible . . . such a large practice: Ibid.

Meigs had edited a publication on puerperal fever . . . communicable nature of the disease: Ibid.

in the face of a "raging epidemic of puerperal fever": Ibid.

"grossly epidemic" proportion of victims in Dr. Rutter's private practice . . . a "coincidence": Ibid.

Meigs refused to accept the contagious nature of puerperal fever . . . on the matter: Ibid.

"I take no offense and attempt no retort. No man makes a quarrel . . . in such a controversy": Ibid.

"[I prefer] to attribute these cases [of puerperal fever] to accident . . . form any clear idea": Ibid.

"as physicians, [they] could never be the minister of evil . . . virus to their parturient patients": Ibid.

"an unknown contagion existed in the lying-in premises . . . an attendant of the mother": Ibid.

the presence of an "unseen, transmissible agent" caused the disease: Ibid.

"I took my ground on the existing evidence before a little army . . . to support my position": Ibid.

early proponents of the infectious nature of disease: Frederick B. Wagner Jr., M.D., ed., *Thomas Jefferson University: Tradition and Heritage*, 1989, http://jdc.jefferson.edu /cgi/viewcontent.cgi?article=1007&context=wagner2

diseases—scarlet fever, consumption, measles, pneumonia . . . through human contact: Ibid.

these diseases were related to specific organisms: Ibid.

"minute spores and fungi": Ibid.

gonorrhea and syphilis were caused by the same pathogen: Ibid.

"When gonorrhea and syphilis are produced in a patient . . . *cannot* produce the other disease": Ibid.

professor of anatomy and physiology at Harvard University . . . hold for thirty-five years: "Oliver Wendell Holmes", http://elane.stanford.edu/wilson/html/chap5 /chap5-sect2.html

reprint the essay as a stand-alone publication titled *Puerperal Fever, as a Private Pestilence*: Ibid.

reprinted the work *without the change of a word or syllable*: Ibid.

a truth that Holmes felt "the commonest exercise of reason" should have illuminated: Ibid.

He detailed and deflated Meigs's arguments against his theory . . . of believing any professor: Ibid.

"If I am wrong, let me be put down by such rebuke as no rash declaimer . . . Pennsylvania . . . : Ibid.

"Let the men who mould opinions look to it; if there is any . . . never forgive him": Ibid.

<h2 style="text-align:center">—CHAPTER TWENTY-FIVE—</h2>

startle them: Levis, "Memoir of Thomas Dent Mütter"

"As zealous as he was efficient": "Annual Announcement of Jefferson Medical College of Philadelphia: Session of 1856–1857," (1856): 31–32 (From the Jefferson Medical Archive)

he oversaw the treatment of more than 800 surgical cases . . . plastic surgeries, among others: Ibid.

hardly sufficient consolation to him for the sacrifice: Pancoast, *A Discourse Commemorative*

Among the 215 graduates that year were the sons of two . . . colleague, Joseph Pancoast: "Part I: Jefferson Medical College 1855 to 1865 (pages 89–124)" in Frederick B. Wagner Jr., MD, and J. Woodrow Savacool, MD, eds., *Thomas Jefferson University— A Chronological History and Alumni Directory, 1824–1990*, 1992, Paper 17, http://jdc .jefferson.edu/wagner1/17

Squibb would spend over a year developing, creating, and testing . . . for distilling ether: Ibid.

were now filled with charts detailing temperatures, amounts, costs, and . . . of solutions: Ibid.

to wash away most of the impurities that plagued the current market's . . . and redistillation: Ibid.

"ether of uniform strength by using steam": Ibid.

"nothing short of the grossest carelessness or inattention . . . uniformity of the product": Ibid.

he gave them to the world for free, publishing an article . . . *American Journal of Pharmacy*: Ibid.

first truly effective "ether mask" for use in surgery . . . ether surgery that vexed surgeons: Ibid.

"the amputation the way he thought his old professors . . . with improvements by Squibb": Ibid.

he insisted on self-administering his own brand of ether . . . as long as he remained conscious: Ibid.

"marked friendship": *Transactions of the College of Physicians of Philadelphia, ser. 3, vol. 25* (1903), ed. William Zentmayer (Philadelphia: College of Physicians of Philadelphia, 1903)

Lewis was invited by Mütter to join him during one of his summer trips to Paris and London: Ibid.

Mütter showed the young doctor the innovations and institutions . . . Lewis's lifelong friends: Ibid.

In London, he saw the busy Hospital for Sick Children . . . Great Ormond Street: Ibid.

Lewis's passion for this idea grew when he returned to the United States: Ibid.

Pennsylvania Hospital, where he saw the appallingly high mortality rate . . . treated there: Ibid.

cross infection, hospital-contracted diarrhea, and even neglect: History of the Children's Hospital of Philadelphia (From the official CHOP website): http://giving.chop.edu /site/PageNavigator/Gift_of_Childhood/About/childrens_hospital_history.html

in November 1855, Lewis helped open the Children's Hospital of Philadelphia: *Transactions of the College of Physicians of Philadelphia (*1903)

owing much to "the indefatigable watchfulness and care" of Dr. Lewis: Ibid.

"Scarcely a day passed, regardless of the weather . . . welcomed him with shouts of joy": Ibid.

altered his name slightly after receiving his medical degree: "10 Notable Jefferson Alumni," Exhibition of Thomas Jefferson University Archives online: http://jeffline .tju.edu/SML/archives/exhibits/notable_alumni/index.html

Between 1865 and 1881, Finlay would write and publish ten papers on this devastating disease: Ibid.

His breakthrough would finally come in 1881, when he was able . . . transmitting yellow fever: Ibid.

countless lives throughout South America, the Caribbean, Africa, and the United States: Ibid.

In the words of General Leonard Wood . . . "The confirmation . . . discovery of vaccination": Ibid.

exodus of more than two hundred Southern medical students . . . the North if war broke out: "Part I: Jefferson Medical College 1855 to 1865" http://jdc.jefferson.edu /wagner1/17

"father of battlefield medicine": L'éinelle C. Frederick, "Jonathan Letterman," Pennsylvania Center for the Book: Biography Project, Spring 2010; http://www.pabook.li braries.psu.edu/palitmap/bios/Letterman__Jonathan.html

medical director of the Army of the Potomac: Ibid.

The Union Army had entered the war with only ninety-eight medical officers . . . of the war: Ibid.

supplies that were either almost exhausted or necessarily abandoned . . . by fatigue: Ibid.

Ambulance Corps—army-issued wagons and trains . . . for transporting medical supplies: Ibid.

more than three thousand injured soldiers . . . were left on the battlefield for three days: Ibid.

picked their pockets, stolen alcohol from the medical supplies, and left the injured to die: Ibid.

surgeons in the Union Army would be tested on their knowledge . . . reflected their skill level: Ibid.

he established field-dressing stations, where . . . according to the severity of their wounds: Ibid.

Letterman's system of organizing patients into groups of those . . . would surely die: Ibid.

appointed surgeon in chief of Thomas Jonathan "Stonewall" Jackson's . . . Stonewall Brigade: Kelly and Burrage, *American Medical Biographies*

highest-ranking officer in the medical corps of the Confederacy: Ibid.

became the U.S. assistant surgeon general, a position he held . . . Bragg's army: "Part I: Jefferson Medical College 1846 to 1855," http://jdc.jefferson.edu/wagner1/16

named the assistant surgeon to the 1st Infantry, United States Colored Troops . . . U.S. history: Granville P. Conn, M. M. D., *History of the New Hampshire Surgeons in the War of Rebellion* (Concord, NH: Ira C. Evans, Printers,1906)

President Lincoln's call for seventy-five thousand volunteers . . . to form a regiment: Joseph Leasure (a lateral descendant of Col. Daniel Leasure), "Exploits of Dr. Leasure and Roundheads," 100th Pennsylvania, Veteran Volunteer Infantry Regiment, aka "The Roundheads" website; www.100thpcnn.com/drleasure.htm

Scotch-Irish regiment nicknamed the Roundheads who were celebrated . . . had won the war: Ibid.

"instruct[ing] his unit in the art of war while keeping . . . keen eye on sanitation and hygiene": Ibid.

his methods were adopted by other commanders: Ibid.

Leasure could be found in the hospital tents, assisting the surgeons: Ibid.

"While there is life, there is hope": Lyon Gardiner Tyler, L.L.D., *Encyclopedia of Virginia Biography, Vol. V* (New York: Lewis Historical Publishing, 1915)

"held on to his patients with a grip that seemed to challenge death . . . almost phenomenal": Ibid.

continued to make frequent visits to the sick well into his eighty-ninth year: Ibid.

"look upon the coming of his carriage, as he flew along . . . in their scattered homes": Samuel Atkins Eliot, A.M., D.D., ed., *Biographical History of Massachusetts, Vol. 1* (Boston: Massachusetts Biographical Society, 1911)

such skill that within three months, Gage was not only walking and talking . . . back to work: Ibid.

When Gage died years later, the family gave the skull and . . . Harvard Medical School: Ibid.

"extraordinary vitality and the unconquerable will": Ibid.

worked as a surgeon beside the trailblazing nurse Florence Nightingale: "10 Notable Jefferson Alumni", http://jeffline.tju.edu/SML/archives/exhibits/notable_alumni/index.html

surgeon under Grant during the Siege of Vicksburg . . . medical director of the 13th Army Corps: Ibid.

surgeon for the Summit House Hospital in Philadelphia: Ibid.

presented the Pennsylvania state legislature with his version . . . fair and legal manner: Ibid.

Ghastly Act: Ibid.

a board was created to regulate the distribution of bodies to Pennsylvania schools: Ibid.

the demonstrator of anatomy at Jefferson, serving in that role . . . professor of anatomy: Ibid.

elected to be the first physician in charge of the newly established . . . ("married women"): "Part I: Jefferson Medical College 1846 to 1855" http://jdc.jefferson.edu/wagner1/16

Mütter's principles of asepsis and antisepsis: Ibid.

Of the 2,444 deliveries recorded during Goodell's time there, only six ended in death: Ibid.

"Philadelphia May 19th, 1856. I am compelled by the condition . . . Yours, Thomas D. Mütter": Jefferson Medical College Minutes

Jefferson . . . board of trustees received the letter . . . "long career of eminent usefulness": Ibid.

board unanimously voted that "as a mark of the high estimation . . . Institution" . . . College: Ibid.

—CHAPTER TWENTY-SIX—

donated his piano to the Pennsylvania Hospital for the Insane: Pennsylvania Hospital, Department for Mental and Nervous Diseases, *Physician in Chief and Administrator's Report . . .* , Vols. 16–20 (1856) "the usual osseous, nervous, vascular, muscular, ligamentotaxis ... demonstration": "Annual Announcement of Jefferson" (1847), http://jdc.jefferson.edu/jmc_catalogs/62

a large number of wet preparations (specimens in jars); diseased ... wood, plaster, and wax: Ibid.

demonstrations in class, for it was so well curated for "illustrating ... taught in the school": Ibid.

which now consisted of about two thousand specimens: Ella N. Wade, "A Curator's Story of the Mütter Museum and College Collections," *Transactions & Studies of the College of Physicians of Philadelphia,* Ser. 4, vol. 42, no. 2 (October 1974)

"to advance the science of medicine and to thereby lessen human misery": This mission statement is on the "College History" page of the "About Us" section at the College of Physicians of Philadelphia website; http://www.collegeofphysicians.org/about-us /college-history/

which always wanted to be seen as a place for medical professionals ... science and an art: Ibid.

"for the services of a curator, for an honorarium for a yearly lecturer and ... museum": Wade, "A Curator's Story"

condition: that the college provide a fireproof building for his collection ... four years: Ibid.

started a building fund in 1849—but despite their efforts ... let alone the fireproof one: Ibid.

"rapidly failing health": McCaw and Otis, *Virginia Medical Journal (1859)*

bequeath all his property of every description—"everything which I possess" ... exception: Robert E. Wright, State Reporter, *Pennsylvania State Reports,* Vol. XXX-VIII (Philadelphia: Kay & Brother, Law Booksellers, Publishers, and Importers, 1861)

"the arrangements entered into, but not completed, at the time of [his] departure for Europe": Ibid.

"It was better to relinquish quickly one's own terms": Slatten, "Thomas Dent Mütter"

"On our arrival we were not obliged to go to a hotel ... even dinner was awaiting us": Ibid.

where he could spend the winter in Nice: Pancoast, *A Discourse Commemorative*

the winter of 1856 was one of "unusual severity" in Europe: Ibid.

"His old malady renewed its attacks ... with its customary frequency": Ibid.

publish in the popular journal *Medical News*: Transcribed from the files of the Mütter Museum of the College of Physicians of Philadelphia

"the basis of a future contract between the College": Transcribed from the files of the Mütter Museum

"advantageous to both parties": Ibid.

"It will be seen from the foregoing that I have in every way attempted ... professional life": Ibid.

"Linen for Mary, Laudanum for me!": Alsop Family Papers, Yale University Library

"weary with the endless torture of disease": McCaw and Otis, *Virginia Medical Journal (1859)*

protracted residence abroad brought "no relief to the malad[ies]": Ibid.

"only remedy [to his condition] was to be its own last and fatal attack": Ibid.

those close to him sensed a growing impatience: Slatten, "Thomas Dent Mütter"

"feeble and dejected, with the graven lines of pain furrowed deeply on his brow": Levis, "Memoir of Thomas Dent Mütter"

"Conspicuous from his bright and manly bearing, which ... former associations": Pancoast, *A Discourse Commemorative*

had recently lost a child: Carter Papers

"My dear old friend ... "Ever since my arrival in this country I have ... to you at once": Ibid.

"It appears our heavenly father in his wisdom does by loss and . . . I love best in the world": Ibid.

"Now that I feel the approach of night . . . I know that soon I must lie down . . . sorrows": Ibid.

An Article of Agreement finalizing the organization's relationship . . . the Mütter Museum: *Article of Agreement between T. D. Mutter and the College of Physicians of Philadelphia with Extracts from Exemplification of Deed of Trust* (Philadelphia: Collins, Printer)

—CHAPTER TWENTY-SEVEN—

"This kind and Christian heart, this generous . . . there will be many to regret his loss": McCaw and Otis, *Virginia Medical Journal (1859)*

"The telegraph of the 17th heralded over the western world . . . the unknown ocean of Eternity": "In Memoriam," *The Medical and Surgical Reporter vol 2, no. 1.* April 2, 1859

"The subject of this memoir needs no eulogium . . . and to relieve the miseries of others": Levis, "Memoir of Thomas Dent Mütter"

"While I recount his manly form and noble bearing . . . my teacher, my friend, now no more": *The Medical and Surgical Report.*

"In every view of him, he was a 'good physician'" . . . His manner hopefully . . . to eternal rest": Levis, "Memoir of Thomas Dent Mütter"

"able hand" to write "the biography of this great . . . household word of American Surgery": *The Medical and Surgical Report.*

"Respect for his memory, and the gratitude . . . history of American Surgery": Levis, "Memoir of Thomas Dent Mütter"

"Yet again shall we meet him . . . where preceptor and . . . where sorrows are unknown!": Ibid.

"It is indeed impossible for me even now to revert . . . thorny paths of a surgical career": Pancoast, *A Discourse Commemorative*

"Dr. Mütter died early . . . too early . . . one of the noblest branches of the healing art": Ibid.

"Dr. Mütter raised his reputation to the highest pitch during his life. . . . records of science": Ibid.

"Often has he talked over such a project with me . . . our wishes and their fulfillment": Ibid.

hereditary gout and lung hemorrhages "greatly harassed, distressed, and weakened him": Ibid.

"forced upon him by slow degrees, and to the great regret of his colleagues" . . . leave Philadelphia: Ibid.

"The prospect of having to abandon his duties . . . *like the rending away of his right arm*": Ibid.

"For myself especially, who lived so long in his gentle . . . a similar sort of retrospection": Ibid.

"Such, gentlemen, was the surgeon whom the science . . . and name we shall ever cherish": Ibid.

fourth edition of his textbook . . . when news of Mütter's death broke: Meigs, *Memoir*

thirty-seven acres of land in Delaware County, eighteen miles from the city: Ibid.

a barn and a stable, a tenant house, a springhouse, an icehouse, and a workshop: Ibid.

"the Indian name of a small river in Connecticut [where] his forefathers had settled": Ibid.

"luxuriant growth of noble woods": Ibid.

"Men ought to retire from public appointments . . . judging of their own fitness for duty": Ibid.

Meigs agreed to give one more course of lectures . . . "though against his will or wishes: Ibid.

"I am now old and well stricken in years . . . and yet I labor in my calling! How long!": Ibid.

"This afternoon I delivered my last lecture at the Jefferson . . . simply glad to get out of it": Ibid.

"entirely weary of all medical responsibilities": Ibid.

"lost . . . taste for medical literature, and rarely looked into a medical book": Ibid.

If any battle of disastrous end should be known . . . "he should whistle twice as often": Ibid.

"favorite and pride among all his descendants . . . looked for at the hands of this grandson": Ibid.

"in one of the most luckless engagements of our war": Ibid.

"mind rose faithful still, and strong, above the dreadful sorrow": Ibid.

"The Angel of Death had not gone back to his abode . . . vulnerable state of my grandfather": Ibid.

"the keenness of [Meigs's] grief had begun to lose its edge": Ibid.

"She was not my grandfather's better half; she was his whole . . . would gladly have left it": Ibid.

"slowly pining away in grief both of soul and body": Ibid.

suffered "untold distresses with a bodily infirmity that took away his peace": Ibid.

"whose hot red bricks and monotonous lanes he had long ago learned to hate": Ibid.

"the distressed women and dying children that he had known as [the city's] inmates": Ibid.

"Cooped up in a second-story room, he pined for the peace . . . happiness in the fields alone": Ibid.

"a quiet night and an end of [my] toils": Ibid.

"There was only a little left of his mortal self . . . and he pined for dissolution": Ibid.

"All of him thought his life was now near its end . . . proud of its own strength": Ibid.

"full of misery and rent with shame": Ibid.

"repository for specimens, models, historical instruments" . . . all over the world: Bauer, *Doctors*

lumber, carpentry, bricklaying, painting, and plumbing: Wade, "A Curator's Story"

cases and jars needed to accommodate the more than two thousand specimens: Ibid.

"without charge or fee": *The Medical News* Vol. XV. No. 169 (Philadelphia: Blanchard and Lea; 1857)

chairman of the committee on the Mütter Museum: Gibson Lamb Cranmer, ed., *History of Wheeling City and Ohio County, West Virginia.* (Chicago, IL: Biographical Publishing Company, 1902)

In 1880, Brinton was asked to give a speech . . . memories of the famous Faculty of '41: Brinton, "Alumni Address: The Faculty of 1841"

the sharpshooting street urchins who hit Mütter's students with snowballs: Ibid.

"[a] stove-maker's room and [a] bottler's upper stories": Ibid.

"savory oyster" and "a steaming midnight cup of coffee . . . of the [exhausted] watcher": Ibid.

the story of Meigs and the etherized sheep that refused to die: Ibid.

"beloved, nay almost worshiped by his class": Ibid.

"his great charm lay in his enthusiasm and in his power . . . his own spirit to hearers": Ibid.

("powers and capabilities which shone so conspicuously"): Ibid.

"the anticipations and cherished hopes of its founder": Ibid.

"Time in his flight brings many changes . . . great professors . . . and we owe them much": Ibid.

"This world is no place of rest. . . . but for effort. Steady continuous undeviating effort": Mütter, *Introductory Lecture,* 1847

"Thus, in dying . . . has he left a precious heritage to the profession": Pancoast, *A Discourse Commemorative*

"While these bodies may be ugly . . . there is a terrifying beauty . . . endure these afflictions": Worden, *Mütter Museum*

"Place no dependence on your own genius . . . nothing is obtained without it": Mütter, *Introductory Lecture,* 1847

"This world is no place of rest. . . . Our work should never be done . . . nothing more to accomplish": Ibid.

IMAGE CREDITS

PROLOGUE

Bust of Thomas Dent Mütter **by Peter Charles Reniers.** Plaster bust of Thomas Dent Mütter by Peter Charles Reniers, circa 1850s. The College of Physicians of Philadelphia (ST 514). The image of this object is used by kind permission of The College of Physicians of Philadelphia. Photograph by Evi Numen. Copyright 2014 by The College of Physicians of Philadelphia. Used by permission.

CHAPTER ONE

Wax Model of Madame Dimanche. Wax model of a human horn (cornu cutaneum). Successfully removed after six years' growth from Madame Dimanche, a Parisian widow, in the early nineteenth century. From the original collection of Dr. Thomas Dent Mütter (1811–1859). Mütter Museum Collection (#6002). The image of this object is used by kind permission of The College of Physicians of Philadelphia. Photograph by Evi Numen. Copyright 2014 by The College of Physicians of Philadelphia. Used by permission.

"Woman with Ulcer of the Face" woodcut from *Lectures on the Operations of Surgery* by Robert Liston, with numerous additions by Thomas Dent Mütter. From the Author's personal collection.

"Man with Tumor of the Jaw" woodcut from *Lectures on the Operations of Surgery* by Robert Liston, with numerous additions by Thomas Dent Mütter. From the Author's personal collection.

"Woman with Severe Burns of the Face" woodcut from *Lectures on the Operations of Surgery* by Robert Liston, with numerous additions by Thomas Dent Mütter. From the Author's personal collection.

CHAPTER TWO

Title page of *An Account of the Bilious Remitting Yellow Fever* **by Benjamin Rush.** Courtesy of Thomas Jefferson University, Archives & Special Collections, Philadelphia.

Portrait of Lucinda Gillies Mutter, date and artist are unknown. Courtesy of Virginia Historical Society.

Portrait of John Mutter, date and artist are unknown. Courtesy of Virginia Historical Society.

CHAPTER THREE

Panorama Views of Philadelphia from the State House Steeple (**North, South, East and West**) by John Caspar Wild. Courtesy of The Library Company of Philadelphia.

Sabine Hall, date and artist are unknown. Courtesy of Virginia Historical Society.

Clothing Bill for a Young Thomas Mutter, courtesy of Carter Papers, Special Collections Research Center, Swem Library, College of William and Mary.

CHAPTER FOUR

The Medical School of the University of Pennsylvania, **circa early nineteenth century.** Artist unknown. Courtesy of Thomas Jefferson University, Archives & Special Collections, Philadelphia.

George McClellan. Daguerreotype by firm of John Plumbe, Jr. Courtesy of Thomas Jefferson University, Archives & Special Collections, Philadelphia.

CHAPTER FIVE

Jefferson Medical College at the Tivoli Theater, **1825–1829**. Lithograph by Frank J. Taylor. Courtesy of Thomas Jefferson University, Archives & Special Collections, Philadelphia.

"Surgery on Nathaniel Dickey" woodcut from *Lectures on the Operations of Surgery* by Robert Liston, with numerous additions by Thomas Dent Mütter (Philadelphia: Lea & Blanchard, 1846). From the Author's personal collection.

CHAPTER SIX

Woman posed in the Sims position for gynecological examination. James Wood Album, Historical Medical Photography Collection, Mütter Museum (HMP box 50). The image of this object is used by kind permission of The College of Physicians of Philadelphia. Copyright 2014 by The College of Physicians of Philadelphia. Used by permission.

Charles D. Meigs. Artist Unknown. Courtesy of Thomas Jefferson University, Archives & Special Collections, Philadelphia.

CHAPTER SEVEN

Muscle Man. Attributed to Gaspar Becerra from *Opera quae extant, omnia . . .* Johannes van der Linden, 1645. Courtesy of Thomas Jefferson University, Archives & Special Collections, Philadelphia.

Portrait of Benjamin Franklin. Painting by unknown artist, after Joseph Siffred Duplessis. Courtesy of Thomas Jefferson University, Archives & Special Collections, Philadelphia.

Portrait of Franklin Bache. Artist Unknown. Courtesy of Thomas Jefferson University, Archives & Special Collections, Philadelphia.

CHAPTER EIGHT

Portrait of an Unidentified Jefferson Medical College Student. Hand-colored ambrotype by unknown photographer. Courtesy of Thomas Jefferson University, Archives & Special Collections, Philadelphia.

CHAPTER NINE

The Clinic in the Amphitheater of Jefferson Medical College. Photographer unknown. Courtesy of Thomas Jefferson University, Archives & Special Collections, Philadelphia.

College Clinic Operating Table by unknown manufacturer. Photographer unknown. Courtesy of Thomas Jefferson University, Archives & Special Collections, Philadelphia.

Surgeon's Amputation Kit. Courtesy of Thomas Jefferson University Archives & Special Collections, Philadelphia.

Portrait of John K. Mitchell. Artist Unknown. Courtesy of Thomas Jefferson University, Archives & Special Collections, Philadelphia.

Joseph Pancoast, **1841.** Artist Unknown. Courtesy of Thomas Jefferson University, Archives & Special Collections, Philadelphia.

CHAPTER TEN

Portrait of Thomas Dent Mütter. Painting by Thomas Sully, circa 1842. Courtesy of Thomas Jefferson University, Archives & Special Collections, Philadelphia.

Title page of *On Recent Improvements in Surgery: An Introductory Lecture* **(1842) by Thomas Dent Mütter.** Courtesy of Thomas Jefferson University, Archives & Special Collections, Philadelphia.

CHAPTER ELEVEN

The Drunkard's Progress. From the Author's Personal Collection.

"Woman with Ulcer of the Cheek" woodcut from *Lectures on the Operations of Surgery* by Robert Liston, with numerous additions by Thomas Dent Mütter (Philadelphia: Lea & Blanchard, 1846). From the Author's personal collection.

CHAPTER TWELVE

The Life & Age of Woman: Stages of Woman's Life from the Cradle to the Grave. by N. Currier. Courtesy of The Library Company of Philadelphia.

CHAPTER THIRTEEN

"Woman with Severe Burns of the Face" woodcut from *Lectures on the Operations of Surgery* by Robert Liston, with numerous additions by Thomas Dent Mütter. From the Author's personal collection.

"Man with Nose Being Reconstructed from Forehead" woodcut from *Lectures on the Operations of Surgery* by Robert Liston, with numerous additions by Thomas Dent Mütter. From the Author's personal collection.

CHAPTER FOURTEEN

"Woman with Severe Burns of the Face, Before Mütter Flap Surgery" woodcut from *Lectures on the Operations of Surgery* by Robert Liston, with numerous additions by Thomas Dent Mütter. From the Author's personal collection.

"Woman with Severe Burns of the Face, During Mütter Flap Surgery" woodcut (2) from *Lectures on the Operations of Surgery* by Robert Liston, with numerous additions by Thomas Dent Mütter. From the Author's personal collection.

"Woman with Severe Burns of the Face, After Mütter Flap Surgery" woodcut from *Lectures on the Operations of Surgery* by Robert Liston, with numerous additions by Thomas Dent Mütter. From the Author's personal collection.

CHAPTER FIFTEEN

Jefferson Medical College Surgery Admission Ticket. Courtesy of Thomas Jefferson University, Archives & Special Collections, Philadelphia.

Advertisement for Jefferson Medical College, 1846–1847 Session. From the Author's personal collection.

Edward Robinson Squibb. Photographer Unknown. Courtesy of Thomas Jefferson University, Archives & Special Collections, Philadelphia.

Title page from *Lectures on the Operations of Surgery* by Robert Liston, with numerous additions by Thomas Dent Mütter. From the Author's personal collection.

CHAPTER SIXTEEN

William Thomas Green Morton Administering Ether. Engraving, etching, stipple by George R. Hall. Courtesy of Thomas Jefferson University, Archives & Special Collections, Philadelphia.

CHAPTER SEVENTEEN

Illustration of Thomas Dent Mütter Ether Surgery. By David Izenberg, from *JMC Clinic*, student yearbook, 1929. Courtesy of Thomas Jefferson University, Archives & Special Collections, Philadelphia.

CHAPTER EIGHTEEN

"Chloroform Anaesthesia." Image from *Bones Books & Bell Jars* by Andrea Baldeck (Philadelphia: College of Physicians of Philadelphia, 2012). Image provided by the Mütter Museum of the College of Physicians of Philadelphia. Photograph by Andrea Baldeck.

CHAPTER NINETEEN

Portrait of Thomas Dent Mütter. Lithograph by V. F. Harrison. Courtesy of Thomas Jefferson University, Archives & Special Collections, Philadelphia.

Ely Building Renovations. Engraving by Richard G. Harrison, ca 1846. Courtesy of Thomas Jefferson University, Archives & Special Collections, Philadelphia.

Woodcuts of various patients from *Lectures on the Operations of Surgery* by Robert Liston, with numerous additions by Thomas Dent Mütter. From the Author's personal collection.

CHAPTER TWENTY

Wet specimen of two hands with gout caused by lead poisoning. Mütter Museum Collection (#2201). The image of this object is used by kind permission of The College of Physicians of Philadelphia. Photograph by Evi Numen. Copyright 2014 by The College of Physicians of Philadelphia. Used by permission.

CHAPTER TWENTY-ONE

Portrait of Thomas Dent Mütter. Photographer Unknown. Courtesy of Thomas Jefferson University, Archives & Special Collections, Philadelphia.

CHAPTER TWENTY-TWO

The Famous Faculty of '41 Engraving by Robert Whitechurch. Courtesy of Thomas Jefferson University, Archives & Special Collections, Philadelphia.

CHAPTER TWENTY-THREE

Civil War American Flag. Manufactured by William G. Mintzer. Courtesy of Thomas Jefferson University, Archives & Special Collections, Philadelphia.

CHAPTER TWENTY-FOUR

Portrait of Charles D. Meigs. The College of Physicians of Philadelphia (Portrait Catalog PA 131). The image of this object is used by kind permission of The College of Physicians of Philadelphia. Photograph by Evi Numen. Copyright 2014 by The College of Physicians of Philadelphia. Used by permission.

Title page of *The History, Pathology, and Treatment of Puerperal Fever* by Charles D. Meigs. Courtesy of Thomas Jefferson University, Archives & Special Collections, Philadelphia.

CHAPTER TWENTY-FIVE

Ely Building Renovations. Photograph by unknown photographer, n.d. Courtesy of Thomas Jefferson University, Archives & Special Collections, Philadelphia.

Portrait of Carlos Finlay. Photographer Unknown. Courtesy of Thomas Jefferson University, Archives & Special Collections, Philadelphia.

President Lincoln on battlefield of Antietam, October, 1862. Courtesy of Library of Congress.

Photograph of John Hill Brinton as Soldier. Photographer Unknown. Courtesy of Thomas Jefferson University, Archives & Special Collections, Philadelphia.

John Hill Brinton's Certificate of Commission as a Brigade Surgeon of Volunteers. Engraving by John Peter Van Ness Throop and Orrameal Hinkley Throop, 1861. Courtesy of Thomas Jefferson University, Archives & Special Collections, Philadelphia.

Dr. William H. Pancoast's Anatomy Dissection Laboratory. By unknown photographer. Courtesy of Thomas Jefferson University, Archives & Special Collections, Philadelphia.

CHAPTER TWENTY-SIX

Encysted tumor from the shoulder. Original donation by Dr. Mütter. Mütter Museum Collection (6512). The image of this object is used by kind permission of The College of Physicians of Philadelphia. Photograph by Evi Numen. Copyright 2014 by The College of Physicians of Philadelphia. Used by permission.

Wet specimen of tumor extracted from the scalp. Original donation by Dr. Mütter. Mütter Museum Collection (6535.05). The image of this object is used by kind permission of The College of Physicians of Philadelphia. Photograph by Evi Numen. Copyright 2014 by The College of Physicians of Philadelphia. Used by permission.

Humerus, hypertrophic ostitis. Infectious right humerus. This specimen is a complete right humerus with a possible fracture at the distal epiphysis. The distal epiphysis, just above the trochlea shows signs of osteomyelitis and necrosis. There are also signs of periostitis. Donor: Dr. Mütter. Mütter Museum Collection (1269.32). The image of this object is used by kind permission of The College of Physicians of Philadelphia. Photograph by Evi Numen. Copyright 2014 by The College of Physicians of Philadelphia. Used by permission.

CHAPTER TWENTY-SEVEN

Portrait of Thomas Dent Mütter. Hand-tinted engraving by unknown artist. Mütter Museum Archives, The College of Physicians of Philadelphia (P998). The image of this object is used by kind permission of The College of Physicians of Philadelphia. Copyright 2014 by The College of Physicians of Philadelphia. Used by permission.

Portrait of Joseph Pancoast. Artist Unknown. Courtesy of Thomas Jefferson University, Archives & Special Collections, Philadelphia.

Photograph of the Mütter Museum from the turn of the century. Mütter Museum Archives, The College of Physicians of Philadelphia. The image of this object is used by kind permission of The College of Physicians of Philadelphia. Copyright 2014 by The College of Physicians of Philadelphia. Used by permission.

Early photograph of the Mütter Museum. Mütter Museum Archives, The College of Physicians of Philadelphia. The image of this object is used by kind permission of The College of Physicians of Philadelphia. Copyright 2014 by The College of Physicians of Philadelphia. Used by permission.

John Hill Brinton, M.D. (1832–1907). Photograph by Frederick Gutekunst, ca 1880–1890. Courtesy of Thomas Jefferson University, Archives & Special Collections, Philadelphia.

Current Photograph of the Mütter Museum, taken from lower level. This image is used by kind permission of The College of Physicians of Philadelphia. Photograph by Evi Numen. Copyright 2014 by The College of Physicians of Philadelphia. Used by permission.

Current Photograph of the Mütter Museum, taken from upper level. This image is used by kind permission of The College of Physicians of Philadelphia. Photograph by Evi Numen. Copyright 2014 by The College of Physicians of Philadelphia. Used by permission.

Portrait of Thomas Dent Mütter painted by Daniel Huntington, oil on canvas (donor and date of donation unknown) in situ at the Mütter Museum. The College of Physicians of Philadelphia (Portrait Catalog PA89). This image is used by kind permission of The College of Physicians of Philadelphia. Photograph by Evi Numen. Copyright 2014 by The College of Physicians of Philadelphia. Used by permission.

ENDPAPERS

Early photograph of the Mütter Museum. Mütter Museum Archives, The College of Physicians of Philadelphia. The image of this object is used by kind permission of The College of Physicians of Philadelphia. Copyright 2014 by The College of Physicians of Philadelphia. Used by permission.

INDEX

Note: Page numbers in *italics* refer to illustrations

–N–

–O–

–P–

ABOUT THE AUTHOR

CRISTIN O'KEEFE APTOWICZ was born and raised in Philadelphia and first visited the Mütter Museum during a class trip in the fourth grade. A decade and a half later, her feature-length biographical screenplay, *Mütter*, won screenwriting awards at the Hamptons International Film Festival and the Philadelphia Film Festival and earned her a fellowship from the Alfred P. Sloan Foundation, directly inspiring her to research and write this book. She is the author of six books of poetry, most recently *The Year of No Mistakes*, as well as the nonfiction book *Words in Your Face: A Guided Tour through Twenty Years of the New York City Poetry Slam*. Her recent awards include a National Endowment for the Arts Literature Fellowship, the ArtsEdge Writer-in-Residency at the University of Pennsylvania, and the Amy Clampitt Residency. She lives in Austin, Texas.

For more information, including forthcoming appearances, please visit:
www.aptowicz.com

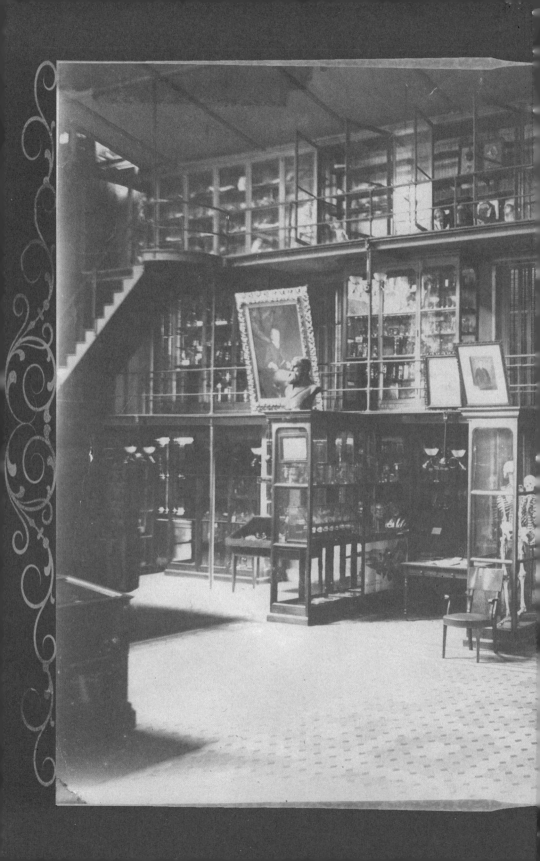